WOUNDS AND LACERATIONS

EMERGENCY CARE AND CLOSURE

WOUNDS AND LACERATIONS

EMERGENCY CARE AND CLOSURE

ALEXANDER T. TROTT, M.D.

Professor of Emergency Medicine
University of Cincinnati College of Medicine
Cincinnati, Ohio

SECOND EDITION

with **332** *illustrations*

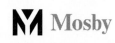 Mosby

An Affiliate of Elsevier Science

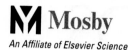
Mosby

An Affiliate of Elsevier Science

Vice President and Publisher: Anne Patterson
Senior Managing Editor: Kathryn H. Falk
Project Manager: Patricia Tannian
Production Editor: Melissa Mraz Lastarria
Book Design Manager: Gail Morey Hudson
Manufacturing Manager: Dave Graybill
Cover Design: Teresa Breckwoldt

SECOND EDITION

Printed in the United States of America

Mosby, Inc.
11830 Westline Industrial Drive
St. Louis, Missouri 63146

ISBN 0-8151-8853-6

03 04 05 06 / 9 8 7

Contributors

JAVIER A. GONZALES DEL REY, M.D.
Assistant Professor of Pediatrics
University of Cincinnati College of Medicine
Cincinnati, Ohio

GREGG A. DIGIULIO, M.D.
Assistant Professor of Pediatrics
University of Cincinnati College of Medicine
Cincinnati, Ohio

To my wonderful, bright, and beautiful children
Buffy, Hays, Alexandra, and **Jacqueline**
who are constant reminders of what is really important

and to my wife
Jennifer
the personification of love and strength of spirit.

Preface

. . . .

Since the publication of the first edition of *Wounds and Lacerations: Emergency Care and Closure,* clinical and scientific advancements have occurred to significantly improve the care of patients who require emergency wound care. Historically, improvements in wound care have relied on clinical experience that was then passed from clinician to clinician. In recent years, each step in modern care—from cleansing to wound dressings —has been subject to both laboratory and clinical investigations. Complementing the growth in the science has been a proliferation of wound care educational courses and seminars for physicians and allied healthcare professionals. It is reasonable to assume, therefore, that there has been an overall improvement in the delivery and the quality of care of wounds and lacerations.

The second edition not only reflects the growth in scientific knowledge but also has a more structured, guideline approach to wound care. Chapter 1 contains the *Clinical Policy for the Initial Approach to Patients Presenting a Penetrating Extremity Trauma* as published by the American College of Emergency Physicians. This guideline reflects the consensus of many experts who care for extremity wounds. Throughout the book are specific guidelines developed by the author that address a variety of wound care problems.

In addition to updating the text with the latest available information regarding the many aspects of wound and laceration care, two new chapters have been added. Because pediatric patients make up a large portion of wound care patients, a new chapter, *The Approach to the Pediatric Patient,* has been added to provide specific information targeted to their needs. Although not directly relevant to wound care, a chapter entitled *Cutaneous Abscesses* has been added because abscess drainage is a common companion procedure carried out in wound care areas. Abscess drainage has many instruments, anesthetics, and techniques in common with wound care.

One of the most important additions to the text is a section on the use of cyanoacry-late wound adhesives. Approval by the Food and Drug Administration is anticipated in the near future. These agents have the potential to significantly alter the management of uncomplicated lacerations under low tension. With advances such as tissue adhesives, the future of wound care holds great promise for continuing improvement in materials and techniques.

For the many and varied tasks necessary to produce this book I thank Kerri Myhand for her diligence and prompt attention to even the smallest detail. A special debt is owed to Gail McGarrahan who compiled and processed the bulk of the final manuscript. Her sharp eye for style and clarity of expression are much appreciated.

The artwork and special photographic processing were expertly produced by the Ob-servatory Group of Cincinnati led by Timothy Mullican, DVM. I also want to thank Wendell Day for the excellent photographs.

Finally, I am grateful to the many colleagues, residents, and medical students who have critiqued the first edition and made suggestions for the second.

Alexander T. Trott

Contents

1 *Patient Evaluation and Wound Assessment*

. . . .

Initial Steps
    Patient Comfort and Safety
    Initial Hemostasis
    Jewelry Removal
    Pain Relief

Wound Care Delay
    Children with Lacerations
Basic History
Screening Examination
Wound Assessment

Approximately 11.5 million patients with wounds are managed each year in emergency departments.[10] This group represents 12% of the 93 million emergency department visits in the United States in 1993.[6] Of 1000 patients whose clinical findings were entered into a wound registry, 74% of the patients were male with an average age of 23.[7] The average laceration was between 1 to 3 centimeters in length, and 13% were considered significantly contaminated. The majority of wounds occurred on the face and scalp (51%) followed by the upper (34%) and lower (13%) extremities. The remainder occurred on various sites of the truncal areas and proximal extremities. Approximately 3.5% to 6.3% of laceration wounds in adults treated in the emergency department become infected.[5, 9, 14, 15] Infection is more likely to occur with bite wounds, in lower extremity locations, and when foreign material is retained in the wound. The rate of infection in children, on the other hand, is only 1.2% for lacerations of all types.[3]

Before wound or laceration repair is initiated, a thorough evaluation of the patient must be carried out. It is important to keep in mind that all wounds, no matter how trivial, can be the result of a serious underlying disorder or the manifestation of a life- or limb-threatening injury. The combination of wound characteristics, anatomic sites, and underlying host conditions affects the management of every wound. Each patient is unique and requires individualized treatment. The basic history, general physical examination survey, and wound area examination will help define the repair strategy and will identify more serious injuries or problems that may necessitate more specialized or intensive care.

INITIAL STEPS
Patient Comfort and Safety

If there is the slightest question about a patient's ability to cope with his or her injury, the patient is placed in a supine position on a stretcher. Loss of blood, deformity, and pain are sufficient to provoke vasovagal syncope (fainting), which can cause further injury from an unexpected fall during evaluation or treatment. Fig. 1-1 demonstrates the recommended and not recommended patient positions for evaluation and treatment of emergency wound care problems. Also note the attire of the caregiver who is observing universal precautions. Because wound care can be strenuous, the caregiver should be comfortable and relaxed before proceeding. Note the seated position in Fig. 1-1, A.

Be aware that relatives or friends accompanying the patient can also respond in a similar manner. As a rule, relatives and friends are encouraged to sit in the waiting area, unless the physician or nurse determines that staying with the patient will be beneficial, for example, to comfort the injured child. Make sure to ask the parent or friend if he or she feels comfortable with that arrangement.

Initial Hemostasis

Any bleeding can be stopped with simple pressure and compression dressings. There is no need for dramatic clamping of bleeders. Clamping is reserved for the actual exploration and repair of the wound under controlled, well-lighted conditions. Blind application of hemostats in an actively bleeding wound can lead to the crushing of normal nerves, tendons, or other important structures.

Jewelry Removal

Rings and other jewelry must be removed as quickly as possible from injured hands or fingers. Swelling of the hand or finger can progress rapidly after wounding, causing rings to act as constricting bands. A finger can become ischemic and the outcome disastrous. Most items of jewelry can be removed with soap or lubricating jelly. Occasionally, ring cutters have to be used (Fig. 1-2). Never let the sentimental value of a wedding ring impede good medical judgment. A jeweler can always restore a ring that has been cut or damaged during removal. Another technique for ring removal that does not require cutting is described in Chapter 12.

Pain Relief

Pain relief begins with gentle, empathic, and professional handling of the patient. Occasionally it is necessary to give pain reducing or sedative medications to patients being treated in the emergency wound care setting. Sedation and specific pain relief measures are discussed more completely in Chapter 5.

Wound Care Delay

If there is going to be a delay from initial wound evaluation to repair, the wound is covered with a saline-moistened dressing to prevent drying. The dressing need not be

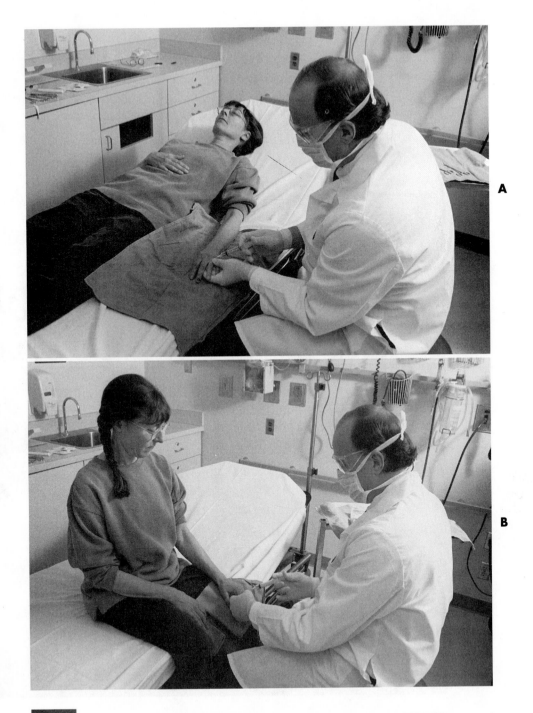

FIG. 1-1 **A,** Correct position for patient during assessment and treatment. Both patient and caregiver are in comfortable positions. **B,** Incorrect patient position. Any pain or apprehension can cause the patient to undergo a vasovagal response. From the sitting position, the patient can be injured during a fall.

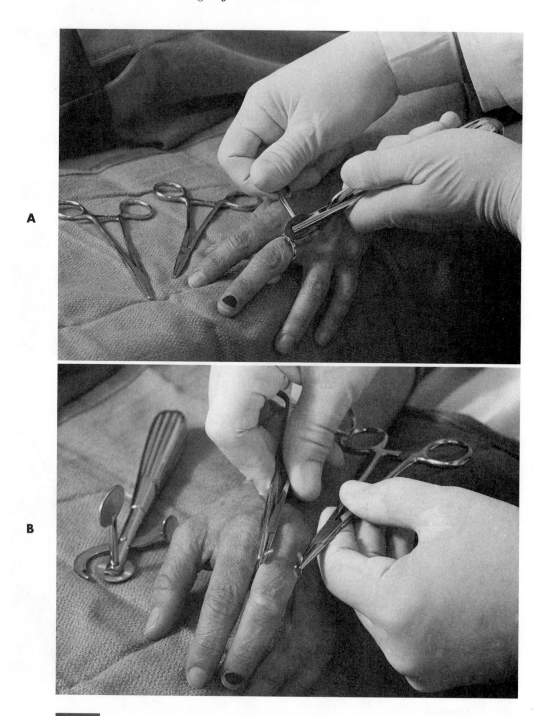

FIG. 1-2 For legend see opposite page.

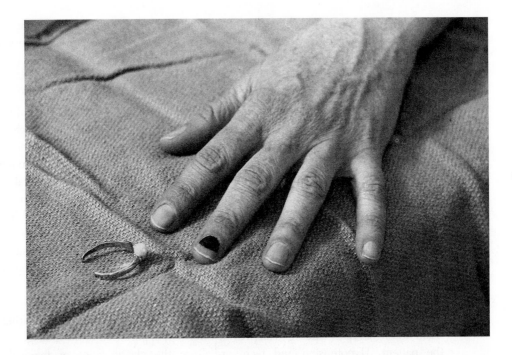

C

FIG. 1-2 **A,** Ring removal. Rings can be removed with a ring cutting device. A through and through cut is made in the thinnest portion of the ring. **B,** Large hemostats are clamped to each side of the cut portion. Taking care not to harm the finger, the ring is gently pried open. **C,** Once removed, the ring can be repaired by a jeweler and restored to its original shape.

soaked and dripping wet. Delays that extend beyond an hour or more require that the wound be thoroughly cleansed and irrigated before the saline dressing is applied.[13] If extended delays are inevitable, antibiotics are occasionally considered to suppress bacterial growth. If antibiotics are administered, they should be given early to provide the maximum protective benefit.[4, 11] Chapter 8 discusses further recommendations for the early administration of antibiotics.

Children with Lacerations

Particular care has to be taken with children who have wounds and lacerations. The pain and fear generated by the experience can be significantly reduced by a few simple measures. Allow the child to remain in the parent's lap for as long as possible before the actual wound repair. Most of the physical examination can be carried out at that time. If hemostasis is required and if the parent is willing to cooperate, allow him or her to tamponade small, bleeding wounds. Parents can also apply topical anesthetics. Careful judgment has to be used when handling children and their parents. It is not uncommon for some parents to be unable to tolerate the sight of their child in pain, and they often do better in the waiting room while care is being delivered. It is remarkable how some children stop crying once the parent has left the treatment area. A complete discussion of the pediatric considerations in wound care is contained in Chapter 4.

BASIC HISTORY

The historical items collected and recorded in the wound care patient's medical record need not be lengthy and excruciatingly detailed. However, key facts, such as mechanism, age of wound, allergies, and tetanus immunization status, are virtually always pertinent.

The patient's current and past medical history and present medications are frequently elements of the wound care assessment. Diseases such as diabetes and peripheral vascular disease can increase the risk of wound infection and cause delayed or poor wound healing.[2,8] It is well known that corticosteroids adversely affect the normal healing process.[12] Finally, a careful detailing of allergies is necessary to prevent an untoward reaction to local anesthetics or antibiotics that might be administered to the patient. Table 1-1 contains the basic history and physical elements of a wound care charting document.[1]

SCREENING EXAMINATION

The examination of every patient with a laceration or injury includes measuring the basic vital signs. Each vital sign can provide information pertinent to the management of the patient. Hypotension and tachycardia are the classic signs of hypovolemia. Innocuous-looking scalp wounds can bleed profusely, causing clinically significant blood loss with concomitant hypotension. Because alcohol is a cutaneous vasodilator, this complication is not uncommon in the intoxicated patient.

Wounds and lacerations are often the result of or the cause of systemic problems and illnesses. Patients who fall and sustain minor injuries may need to be questioned and examined for causes of syncope. That same scalp laceration, when caused by blunt trauma, has the possibility of being associated with a serious intracranial injury. In addition to the wound assessment, a trauma-oriented neurologic examination is often necessary.

A rapid general survey of the patient can reveal other injuries not reported. Because of the nature of a traumatic occurrence, patients often cannot accurately report all that has happened to them. A man who falls on an outstretched hand may only be aware of a bleeding hand laceration on arrival at the emergency department. Only when the caregiver examines the elbow and provokes pain might an underlying radial head fracture be revealed.

WOUND ASSESSMENT

When examining the wound, several features and findings must be noted and recorded in the medical record, as discussed in Table 1-1. Each wound characteristic and examination finding becomes a significant variable that influences repair decisions and all aspects of care, including wound preparation, anesthesia, closure strategy, and dressing choice.

Table 1-1   *Suggested History and Physical Examination of the Emergency Wound Care Patient with Penetrating Extremity Trauma*

Rule*	Guideline†
SOLICIT AND RECORD A HISTORY THAT INCLUDES:	**CONSIDER THESE ASPECTS OF THE HISTORY:**
Mechanism of injury	Potential contaminants and foreign bodies, associated crush injury, species of animal if bite or scratch, description of wounding agent, high-pressure injection injuries
	Circumstances (e.g., self-infliction, assault, domestic violence, or work-related)
Approximate age of wound Tetanus immunization status Allergies	
	Associated symptoms: pain, paresthesia, anesthesia, weakness, loss of function
	Treatment before arrival in the emergency department
	Social history: handedness, vocation/avocations
	Prior medical history: prior injury, prior disability, prior deficits, immunosuppression, diabetes mellitus, valvular heart disease, keloid formation, asplenia, peripheral vascular disease, bleeding disorders, internal prosthetic devices, current medications
CONDUCT AND RECORD A PHYSICAL EXAMINATION THAT INCLUDES:	**CONSIDER THESE ASPECTS OF THE PHYSICAL EXAMINATION:**
	Vital signs: blood pressure, pulse, respirations, temperature; weight of child
Inspection of the area of injury	Location, length, estimated depth and shape of the wound, nerve function, tendon function, vascular integrity, entrance, exit, hematoma, hemorrhage, evidence of foreign body or contamination, evidence of fracture, palpation, range of motion (active, passive, functional), exploration throughout range of motion when anatomically feasible

*An action reflecting principles of good practice in most situations. There may be circumstances when a rule need not or cannot be followed; in these situations, it is advisable that deviation from the rule be justified in writing. Inability to comply with rules should be incorporated in institutional policies.

†Guideline: An action that should be considered but may or may not be performed, depending on the patient, the circumstances, or other factors. Thus guidelines are not always followed, and there is no implication that failure to follow a guideline is improper.

Continued

Table 1-1 *Suggested History and Physical Examination of the Emergency Wound Care Patient with Penetrating Extremity Trauma—cont'd*

Implement ACTIONS based on the FINDINGS for the following VARIABLES:

Variable	Finding	Action	
HISTORY		**RULE**	**GUIDELINE**
Mechanism of injury	Potential for foreign body in wound	Explore when anatomically feasible	Imaging
	Potential for underlying injury	Explore when anatomically feasible	Imaging
	High potential for infection due to contamination	Attempt decontamination	Antibiotic administration
	Mammalian bite		Rabies risk assessment
			Antibiotic administration appropriate for biting species
	Human bite		Assess for joint penetration when proximate to joint
			Possible delayed closure
			Antibiotic administration
	Dog bite to asplenic or immunosuppressed patient		Antibiotic administration to prevent infection with *Capnocytophagia canimorsus* (DF-2)
			Consult
	High-pressure injection injury	Consult	
Age of wound	Delayed presentation		Possible delayed closure
			Antibiotic administration
Comorbidity	Valvular heart disease, immunosuppression, diabetes mellitus, internal prosthetic device		Antibiotic administration
	Keloid formation		Consult/referral
	Inadequate tetanus prophylaxis	Provide tetanus prophylaxis	Refer to ACEP information paper on tetanus immunization

Table 1-1 *Suggested History and Physical Examination of the Emergency Wound Care Patient with Penetrating Extremity Trauma—cont'd*

Implement ACTIONS based on the FINDINGS for the following VARIABLES:

Variable	Finding	Action	
PHYSICAL EXAMINATION		*RULE*	*GUIDELINE*
Location of wound	Over metacarpophalangeal joint or other joints	Assess potential for joint penetration	Assess potential for human bite Immobilization Consult
	Palmar puncture wound		Imaging Antibiotic administration Immobilization Consult
	Plantar puncture wound		Imaging Consult No weight bearing
Inspection, palpation, exploration, neurovascular examination, range of motion	Nerve injury		Immobilization Consult
	Suspicion of significant vascular injury	Control bleeding	IV access Immobilization Consult
	Tendon injury		Immobilization Repair or consult
	Deformity suggestive of underlying fracture	Image	Immobilization
	Open fracture	Image	Antibiotic administration Immobilization Consult
	Suspicion of joint violation		Imaging Wound exploration Antibiotic administration Immobilization Consult

Continued

Table 1-1 *Suggested History and Physical Examination of the Emergency Wound Care Patient with Penetrating Extremity Trauma—cont'd*

Implement ACTIONS for the following VARIABLES:

Variable	Finding	Action	
PHYSICAL EXAMINATION		**RULE**	**GUIDELINE**
	Joint violation	Joint irrigation or consult	Imaging
			Antibiotic administration
			Immobilization
	Visible wound contamination	Attempt decontamination	Wound irrigation and cleansing
			Debridement
			Antibiotic administration
			Consult
	Foreign body in wound		Imaging
			Removal of foreign body
	Significant avulsion injury		Grafting
			Consult

Implement ACTIONS based on the FINDINGS for the following VARIABLES:

Variable	Action	
DISPOSITION	**RULE**	**GUIDELINE**
Admission	Transfer care to accepting physician	
Transfer	Follow ACEP and other applicable transfer principles*	
Discharge	Provide referral for follow-up care	Advise patient about wound care, signs and symptoms of infection, signs and symptoms of compartment syndrome, the possibility of retained foreign body, methods for relieving pain, signs and symptoms suggestive of occult bone or tendon injury, follow-up, suture removal, care of the immobilized extremity/splint
	Provide instructions regarding treatment and circumstances that require return to ED	

*American College of Emergency Physicians: Appropriate interhospital patient transfer, *Ann Emerg Med* 22:766-767, 1993.

REFERENCES

1. American College of Emergency Physicians: Clinical policy for the initial approach to patients presenting with penetrating extremity trauma, *Ann Emerg Med* 23:1147-1156, 1994.
2. Altemeier W: Principles in the management of traumatic wounds and in infection control, *Bull NY Acad Med* 55:123-138, 1979.
3. Baker MD, Lanuti M: The management and outcome of lacerations in urban children, *Ann Emerg Med* 19:1001-1005, 1990.
4. Burke JF: The effective period of preventive antibiotic action in experimental incisions and dermal lesions, *Surgery* 50:161-168, 1961.
5. Gosnold JK: Infection rate of sutured wounds, *Practitioner* 218:584-591, 1977.
6. *Health Facts of Ohio*, Cleveland, 1995, Greater Cleveland Hospital Association.
7. Hollander JE, Singer AJ, Valentine S, Henry MC: Wound registry: development and validation, *Ann Emerg Med* 25:675-685, 1995.
8. Hunt T: Disorders of wound healing, *World J Surg* 4:271-277, 1980.
9. Hutton PA, Jones BM, Law DJ: Depot penicillin as prophylaxis in accidental wounds, *Br J Surg* 65:549-550, 1978.
10. McCraig LF: *National hospital ambulatory medical survey: 1992 emergency department survey*. Advance draft from Vital Health Statistics, #245. Hyattsville, Md, 1994, National Center for Health Statistics.
11. Morgan WJ, Hutchinson D, Johnson HM: The delayed treatment of wounds of the hand and forearm under antibiotic cover, *Br J Surg* 67:140-141, 1980.
12. Pollack S: Systemic medications and wound healing, *Int J Dermatol* 21:489-496, 1982.
13. Robson MC, Duke WF, Krizek TJ: Rapid bacterial screening in the treatment of civilian wounds, *J Surg Res* 14:426-430, 1973.
14. Rutherford WH, Spence R: Infection in wounds sutured in the accident and emergency department, *Ann Emerg Med* 9:350-352, 1980.
15. Thirlby RC, Blair AJ, Thal ER: The value of prophylactic antibiotics for simple lacerations, *Surg Gynecol Obstet* 156:212-216, 1983.

2 Anatomy of Wound Repair

· ·

The primary anatomic focus in surface wound care is the skin. Underlying the skin are two equally important structures, the superficial (subcutaneous) fascia and the deep fascia. The skin is a complex organ that provides basic protection against mechanical trauma, heat injury, and bacterial invasion. The skin serves to regulate heat loss and gain through its rich vascular network and sweat glands. It contains the sensory organs that register stimuli from the environment. The fascias act not only as a supportive base to the skin, but also carry nerves and vessels that eventually branch into it.

All the layers of the skin and fascia are present in every body site, but they vary considerably in thickness. Most skin is 1 to 2 mm thick, but can increase to 4 mm over the back. This variability often dictates the choice of suture needles. Larger, stronger needles are required to penetrate the skin on the palms of the hand and soles of the feet. Very small and delicate needles should be used on the thin skin of the eyelids. Knowledge of these and other properties of the skin, which are discussed in the following section, helps in the choice of the correct wound care materials and appropriate closure techniques.

ANATOMY OF THE SKIN AND FASCIA

Although the skin and fascia consists of a complex system of organs and anatomic features, it is the layer arrangement that is most important for wound closure (Fig. 2-1). These layers include the epidermis, dermis, superficial fascia (commonly referred to as the subcutaneous or subcuticular layer), and deep fascia. These layers should be thought of as planes that need to be carefully and accurately reapproximated when disrupted by trauma. Each one has its own set of characteristics that are important to proper wound closure and healing.

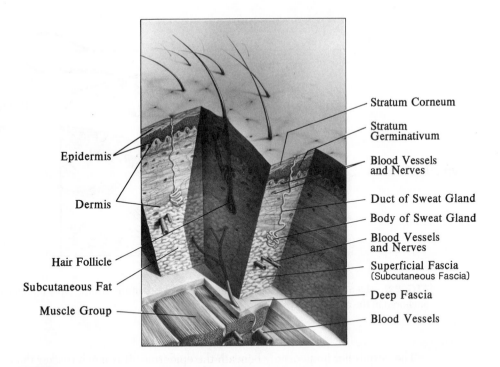

Epidermis

Dermis

Hair Follicle

Subcutaneous Fat

Muscle Group

Stratum Corneum

Stratum
Germinativum

Blood Vessels
and Nerves

Duct of Sweat Gland

Body of Sweat Gland

Blood Vessels
and Nerves

Superficial Fascia
(Subcutaneous Fascia)

Deep Fascia

Blood Vessels

FIG. 2-1 Anatomy of the skin illustrating structures pertinent to wound repair.

Epidermis and Dermis (Skin or Cutaneous Layer)

The epidermis is the outermost layer of the skin or cutaneous layer. It is also called the cutaneous layer. The epidermis consists totally of squamous epithelial cells and contains no organs, nerve endings, or vessels. Its primary function is to provide protection against the ingress of bacteria and toxic chemicals and the inappropriate egress of water and electrolytes.

There are four microscopic layers of the epidermis, of which two are important in surface wound care. The stratum germinativum, or basal layer, is the parent layer for new cells. This layer provides the cells for new epidermis formation during wound healing after injury. The stratum corneum is the keratinized or horny layer that is derived from migrating and maturing basal cells. This is the outermost, visible layer and gives skin its final cosmetic appearance.

Although the epidermis is an anatomically separate layer, it is only a few cell layers thick. During wound repair, it cannot be seen by the naked eye as being separate from the dermis. Therefore correct approximation of the epidermis will naturally result from careful apposition of the lacerated edges of the dermis.

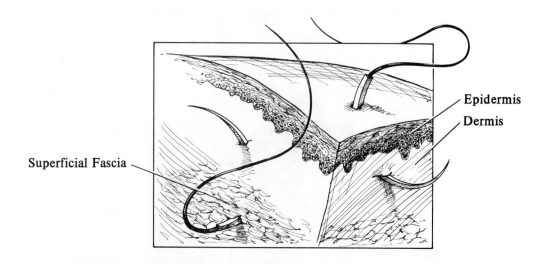

FIG. 2-2   Demonstration of either percutaneous or deep suture closure. Note that the needle is anchored in the dermis for each suture placement.

The dermis lies immediately beneath the epidermis. It is much thicker than the epidermis and is primarily composed of connective tissue. The main cell type in the dermis is the fibroblast, which elaborates collagen, the basic structural component of skin. Other cells found in the dermis are macrophages, mast cells, and lymphocytes. Along with fibroblasts, these components are active during wound healing.

The dermis is composed of two layers, the papillary dermis and the reticular dermis. The richly vascular papillary dermis interdigitates with the epidermis and provides nutrients to that layer. The deeper reticular dermis contains the bulk of adnexal structures of the skin. These include the hair follicles and vascular plexus. Nerve fibers branch and differentiate into specialized nerve endings that invest both layers of the dermis.

The dermis is the key layer for achieving proper wound repair. It is easily identifiable and provides the anchoring site for both percutaneous and deep sutures (Fig. 2-2). Every effort is made to cleanse, remove debris, and accurately approximate the dermal edges to allow for optimal wound healing with minimal scar formation. Whenever dermis is devitalized or severely damaged, sharp debridement is often necessary to remove it. It is important to remember, however, that tissue excision and trimming must only include that which is truly unsalvageable. Because dermal defects are replaced by scar tissue, any unnecessary dermis removal increases the size and prominence of that scar.

Superficial Fascia (Subcutaneous Layer)

Deep to the dermis is a layer of loose connective tissue that encloses a varying amount of fat. Fat makes the superficial fascia easily recognizable in a laceration. Superficial fascia provides insulation against heat loss, as well as some measure of protection against trauma.

There are several consequences of injury to this layer. Devitalized fat can promote bacterial growth and infection.[4] Unlike dermis, it can be liberally debrided so that any devitalized portion can be completely excised. Injuries to the superficial fascia also have the potential for creating "dead" space. Failure to evacuate this space of contaminants and clots can lead to an increased risk of infection.

The sensory nerve branches to the skin travel in the superficial fascia just deep to the dermis. When injecting a local anesthetic, the needle is directed along the plane between the dermis and superficial fascia (see Fig. 5-1). Anesthetic spreads easily along the "floor" of the dermal layer and quickly abolishes sensation from the skin.

Deep Fascia

Deep fascia is a relatively thick, dense, and discrete fibrous tissue layer. It acts as a base for the superficial fascia and as an enclosure for muscle groups. This layer is recognized as an off-white sheath for the underlying muscles. The main function of the deep fascia is to support and protect muscles and other soft tissue structures. It also provides a barrier against the spread of infection from the skin and superficial fascia into muscle compartments. Lacerations of the deep fascia are easily recognized and require closure to reestablish the protective and supportive functions of this layer.

SKIN TENSION LINES

There are two types of skin tension—static and dynamic—that have an important impact on the final scar structure of healed lacerations. Because *all* wounds scar, knowledge of skin tension is required when considering repair strategy or educating the patient about eventual healing outcome.

As it tautly clings to the body framework, skin is under constant static tension.[7] Static tension lines are commonly known as Langer's lines. The arrangement, orientation, and distensibility of collagen fibers cause most wounds to retract open. The degree to which wound edge retraction, or "gaping," takes place is an indicator of how wide the resulting scar might be. Gaping of 5 mm or greater is indicative of significant tension and increased risk for wide scar formation.[2] Lacerations of the lower extremity, particularly over the anterior tibia, tend to retract under great tension and scar conspicuously. A horizontal laceration of the skin of the eyelid, on the other hand, is under little tension with little gaping. These lacerations become virtually unnoticeable with time.

Static skin tension plays an important role in wound edge debridement and revision. It is tempting to want to excise jagged wound edges to convert an irregular laceration into a straight one. If the wound is already gaping because of static tension, then debridement of tissue might increase the force necessary to pull the new straight edges together. Scar width will be increased and the purpose of the edge excision will be defeated. An irregular laceration under little tension will often heal with a less notice-

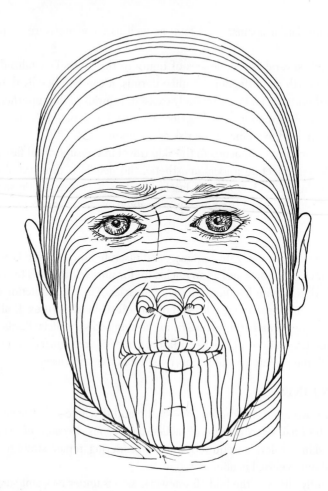

FIG. 2-3   Skin tension lines of the face. Incisions or lacerations parallel to these lines are less likely to create widened scars than those that are perpendicular to these lines. (Adapted from Simon R, Brenner B: *Procedures and techniques in emergency medicine*, Baltimore, 1982, Williams & Wilkins.)

able scar than a straight wound under greater tension. As a rule, a ragged wound with viable tissue edges is repaired best by putting the "puzzle pieces" back together to preserve as much tissue as possible. If the wound needs later revision, the "extra" tissue will be welcomed by the plastic surgeon.

Different from static forces but equally important are dynamic forces on the skin, illustrated by Kraissl's lines in Figs. 2-3 and 2-4.[6] These forces are created by the underlying pull of muscles in any given body area and correspond to wrinkles created by compression of the skin during muscle contraction.[1] These forces are most dramatically

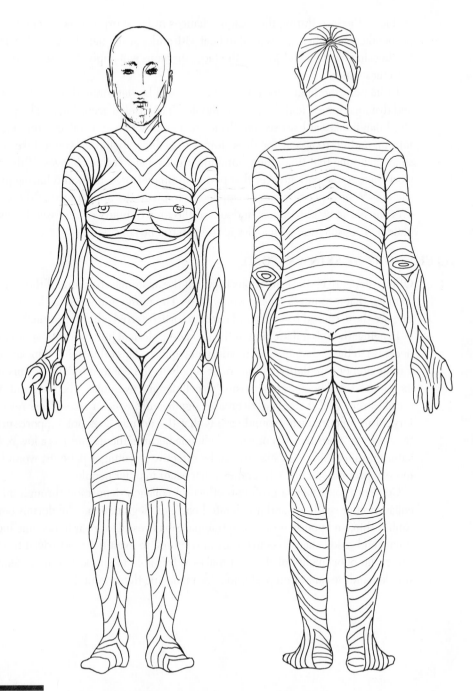

FIG. 2-4   Skin tension lines of the body surface. (Adapted from Simon R, Brenner B: *Procedures and techniques in emergency medicine*, Baltimore, 1982, Williams & Wilkins.)

visible in the face during the various changes in facial expression. Lacerations that are perpendicular to these lines tend to heal with wider scars than do those that are parallel. In choosing elective incisions of the face, surgeons will apply the scalpel to correspond with these lines.

Ultimately, the final appearance of a scar will be determined, in part, by both static and dynamic forces, and the patient should be counseled accordingly. The patient is advised that it takes at least six months for scar contraction and collagen remodeling to diminish, and up to a year for these forces to stabilize before a wound takes on its final shape.[5] During that time, the wound undergoes many visible changes. If the scar is still worrisome to the patient after that period of time elapses, tension relieving procedures, such as W- or Z-plasties, can be applied to improve the appearance of the scar. Whenever the cosmetic outcome is in doubt at the time of injury or the issue is raised by the patient, a consultation with a plastic surgeon can be considered.

ALTERATIONS OF SKIN ANATOMY

Often, there are clinical situations in which the anatomic structure of the skin is altered so much that it requires special wound care. The most common skin changes in this setting are those caused by aging and chronic corticosteroid administration.[3,8]

In aging, there is a flattening of the dermo-epidermal junction with an accompanying decrease in the prominence of the dermal papillae. This effacement appears to result in a reduction of vascularity and nutrient supply to the epidermis. The dermis itself loses its thickness and becomes increasingly acellular and avascular. The net result is that the tensile strength of the dermis decreases significantly, which makes it less resistant to injury. More important to wound care is that the dermis does not support sutures well: they tend to "tear" the skin or cause ischemia because the dermis has a low resistance to suture tension. Although sutures can be effective in younger patients, wound tapes are more appropriate in many lacerations that occur in older people.

Corticosteroids have a profound effect on collagen deposition through inhibition of collagen fiber synthesis and accelerated collagen degradation. The dermis becomes atrophic, thin, and poorly resistant to trauma. Small vessels appear to become increasingly fragile and readily cause ecchymoses in response to even the most trivial trauma. As in aging, the poor quality of the skin makes it less able to support sutures. Skin tapes or simple bandages are often preferable for managing these wounds.

REFERENCES

1. Borges A, Alexander J: Relaxed skin tension lines, Z-plasties on scars and fusiform excision of lesions, *Br J Plast Surg* 15:242-254, 1962.
2. Edlich RF, Rodeheaver GT, Morgan RF, Berman DE, Thacker JG: Principles of emergency wound management, *Ann Emerg Med* 17:1284-1302, 1988.
3. Gilchrest B: Age-related changes in skin. In Cape R, Coe R, Rossman I, editors: *Fundamentals of geriatric medicine*, New York, 1983, Raven Press.
4. Haury B, Rodeheaver G, Vensko J, et al: Debridement: an essential component of traumatic wound care, *Am J Surg* 135:238-242, 1978.
5. Hollander JE, Blaski B, Singer AJ, et al: Poor correlation of short- and long-term cosmetic appearance of repaired lacerations, *Acad Emerg Med* 2:983-987, 1995.
6. Kraissl C: The selection of lines for elective surgical incisions, *Plast Reconstr Surg* 8:1-28, 1951.
7. Thacker IG, Iachetta FA, Allaire PE, et al: Biomechanical properties: their influence on planning surgical excisions. In Krizek TI, Hoopes PE, editors: *Symposium on basic science in plastic surgery*, St Louis, 1975, Mosby.
8. Warrenfeltz A, Graham W: Avulsion injuries in patients receiving corticosteroids, *Am Fam Prac* 11:74-81, 1975.

3 *Surface Injury and Wound Healing*

One of the realities of wound care is that many of the elements of scar formation are beyond the control of the operator repairing a traumatic wound. Unlike surgical incisions, wounds and lacerations are not planned with regard to location, length, depth, or cosmetic concerns. Wounds caused at random present a variety of biologic and technical problems that need to be solved to produce the best repair result. It is incumbent on the operator to have a thorough understanding of the mechanisms of injury and the process of wound healing to increase the chances of achieving a cosmetically acceptable scar. Age, race, body region, skin tension lines, associated conditions and diseases, drugs, type of wound, and technical considerations all affect scar formation. The choice of repair strategy depends on these and other factors. Finally, knowledge of the spectrum of wound healing will ensure that patients with traumatically induced wounds receive the proper advice and counseling.

MECHANISM OF INJURY

The mechanism of injury is important because it is a significant determinant in the choice of management technique, as well as in estimating the probability of wound infection. The injury mechanism also plays a role in scar formation and in the eventual cosmetic outcome. The mechanism of injury can be described as three forces that are applied to the skin under injury conditions: shearing, tension, and compression forces.[10, 32] The various causes of emergency department wounds and their frequency are listed in Table 3-1.

Table 3-1   *Etiology of Traumatic Wounds**

Cause of Wound	Number of Cases*
Blunt object	417 (42%)
Sharp (non glass)	338 (34%)
Glass	133 (13%)
Wood	35 (4%)
Bites	
Human	5 (1%)
Dog	29 (3%)
Other	15 (2%)
Totals	972 (99%)

From Hollander JE, Singer AJ, Valentine S, Henry MC: Wound registry: development and validation, *Ann Emerg Med* 25: 675-685, 1995.
*Taken from a study of 1000 wounds. The etiology of the wound was not described in 28 cases.

Shearing

Shearing injuries, which result in a simple dividing of tissues, are those caused by sharp objects such as knives or glass (Fig. 3-1). This mechanism accounts for the majority of lacerations that present to the emergency department.[9] The skin is divided traumatically, but little energy is imparted to the tissues and minimal cell destruction occurs. Such lacerations can be repaired primarily (primary intention), and they have a low incidence of wound infection. The resulting scar is usually thin and cosmetically acceptable.

Tension

Tension injuries occur as a result of a blunt or semiblunt object striking the skin at a glancing angle (Fig. 3-2). Under these conditions a triangular flap, a partial avulsion, of skin is often created. Because the blood supply is interrupted on two sides of the flap, ischemia can occur, leading to devitalization and necrosis. The remaining blood vessels entering the flap from the base have to be preserved by careful handling and special suturing techniques, which are described in Chapter 10. If the flap base is distally based, that is, the flap tip points back against the regional arterial flow, the compromise is even greater. The energy necessary to create this type of wound is greater than that caused by shearing forces. The combination of potential ischemia and greater cell destruction, therefore, can increase the risk of wound infection. These wounds also tend to lead to greater scar formation.

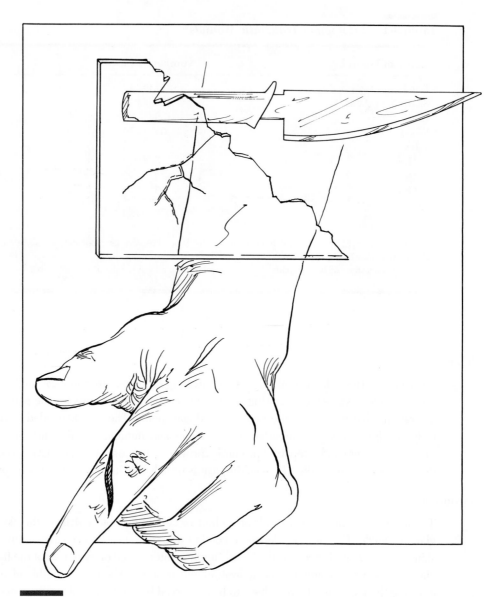

FIG. 3-1   Examples of injuring objects and a resulting laceration caused by shearing forces.

Compression

Crushing or compression injuries occur when a blunt object strikes the skin at right angles (Fig. 3-3). These lacerations often have ragged or shredded edges and are accompanied by significant devitalization of skin and superficial fascia (subcutaneous tissue).

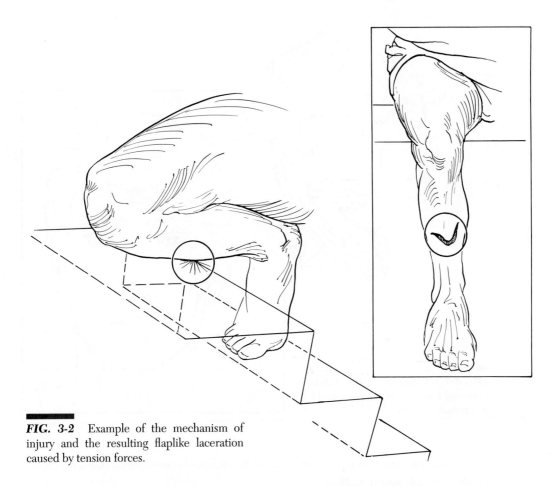

FIG. 3-2 Example of the mechanism of injury and the resulting flaplike laceration caused by tension forces.

Under these conditions, there is increased susceptibility to infection.[2] Such wounds require extensive cleansing, irrigation, and debridement. In spite of a meticulous primary repair, the resulting scars can be cosmetically poor in appearance.

NORMAL WOUND HEALING

Once injury has occurred, by whatever mechanism, normal wound healing is a process that proceeds unimpeded unless there is undue interference from infection, tissue devitalization, poor repair technique, or underlying conditions such as diabetes and healing-inhibiting drugs. In recent years, there has been an explosion in research on and knowledge of the biochemical aspects of wound healing, specifically of growth factors.[16] Virtually all healing events—inflammation, angiogenesis, epithelialization, fibroblast growth, scar remodeling—are under the control of specific mediators derived from a variety of sources: platelets, macrophages, lymphocytes, etc. These mediators, particularly growth factors, are already being applied therapeutically in the chronic wounds.[31] The

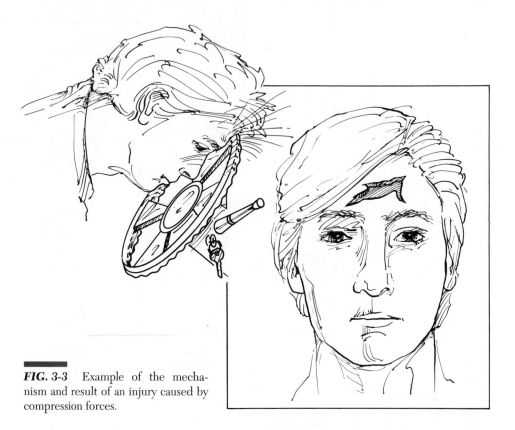

FIG. 3-3   Example of the mechanism and result of an injury caused by compression forces.

future of acute wound care promises to bring biochemical interventions that will considerably enhance wound healing.

Although wound healing is commonly described as discrete events, it is actually a continuum of overlapping phases. For the sake of clarity, these phases are described separately, and their interrelationships are graphically depicted in Fig. 3-4.

Immediate Response to Injury: Hemostasis

At the moment of injury, several events take place that culminate in rapid hemostasis. The traumatic insult causes changes in skin architecture that result in wound edge retraction and tissue contraction, which lead to compression of small venules and arterioles. Vessels also undergo intense reflex vasoconstriction for up to 10 minutes. Platelets begin to aggregate in the lumens of the severed vessels, as well as on the exposed wound surfaces. The clotting cascade is activated by tissue clotting factors, and within minutes, the wound begins to fill with a hemostatic coagulum. As hemostasis is secured, vasoactive amines are released into the wound region, leading to the dilatation of uninjured capillaries and the initiation of wound exudation.

ACTIVITY OF WOUND HEALING COMPONENTS

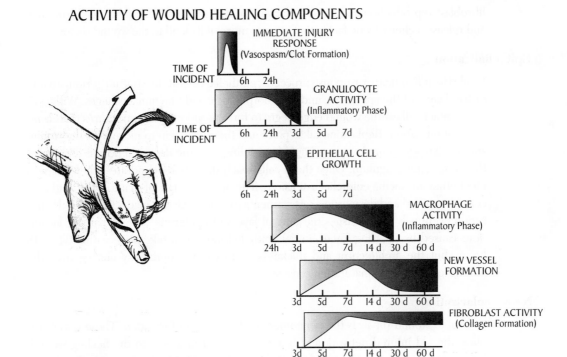

FIG. 3-4   Graphic illustration of the various components of wound healing and their time frames.

Inflammatory Phase

Once hemostasis has been achieved and exudation begins, the inflammatory response rapidly follows. The complement system is activated, and chemotactic factors, which attract granulocytes to the wound area, are released. These cells are followed shortly by lymphocytes. Peak granulocyte numbers can be found between 12 and 24 hours after the injury has been sustained. The chief function of granulocytes and lymphocytes appears to be the control of bacterial growth and therefore the suppression of infection. These cells are aided by immunoglobulins that are included in the wound exudate. In most simple wounds granulocyte counts markedly diminish after 3 days.

After 24 to 48 hours, macrophages can be detected in large numbers, and by day 5, they are the predominant inflammatory cells in the wound area. These cells play a major role in the inflammatory responses and in the early fibroblast and collagen formation. Their first responsibility appears to be phagocytosis and ingestion of wound debris. As part of this process, these cells return usable substrates (amino acids and simple sugars) back to the wound exudate. Macrophages also appear to be important in stimulating fibroblast reproduction and neovascularization. Finally, these remarkable cells produce and release a chemotactic factor that attracts more of its kind to the wound region.

Epithelialization

While the inflammatory response proceeds, epithelial cells at the stratum germinativum, or basal layer of the epidermis, undergo morphologic and functional changes. Within 12 hours intact cells at the wound edge begin to form pseudopod-like structures that facilitate cell migration. Replication takes place and the cells begin to move over the wound surface. An advancing layer can be seen traveling over the damaged dermis and under the hemostatic coagulum. Once these cells reach the inner wound area, they begin to meet other advancing epithelial extensions. The original cuboidal shape of the epithelial cells is regained and desmosomal attachments to other cells are made. Continued replication eventually reestablishes the normal layers of epidermis. After repair for lacerations caused by shearing forces, initial epithelialization can take place within 24 to 48 hours, but the architecture and thickness of this layer continually change over the months of the wound maturation process.

Neovascularization

Crucial to wound repair is the phenomenon of new vessel formation. These vessels replace the old injured network and bring oxygen and nutrients to the healing wound. Neovascularization is evident by day 3 and is most active by day 7. The marked erythematous appearance of the wound at the time of suture removal can thus be explained. Vascularity decreases rapidly by day 21, with continued regression as the wound matures. New vessels form loops of capillaries that are surrounded by actively growing fibroblasts. These two components on the wound surface give it the classic appearance referred to as granulation. Granulation tissue is most often seen in open wounds that are allowed to heal by secondary intention.

Collagen Synthesis

With the establishment of a vascular supply and stimulation by macrophages, fibroblasts rapidly undergo mitosis. They begin to produce new collagen fibrils by the second day. Peak synthesis occurs between days 5 and 7, and the wound has its greatest collagen mass by 3 weeks. By then, the wound is devoid of inflammatory infiltrate and edema.

New collagen is laid down in a random, amorphous pattern. It is a gel with little tensile strength. Over the months, however, this gel continually remodels itself, creating an organized basket-weave pattern that is achieved by the cross-linking of collagen fibers. In order for this process to proceed without excess collagen formation, collagen lysis takes place. Hydrolysis and collagenase activity break down old and damaged collagen, permitting ingestion by macrophages. New collagen takes its place. The balance between synthesis and lysis creates a vulnerable period approximately 7 to 10 days after injury, when the wound is most prone to unwanted opening or dehiscence. The wound

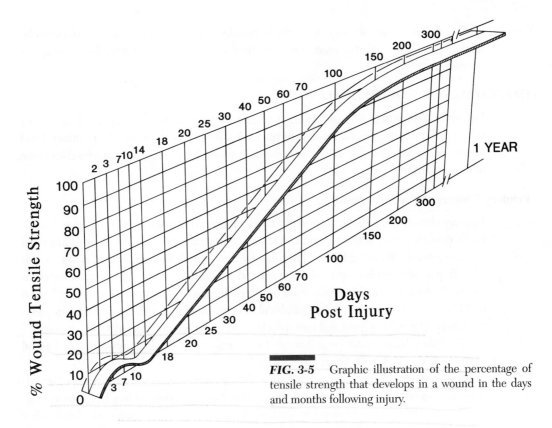

FIG. 3-5 Graphic illustration of the percentage of tensile strength that develops in a wound in the days and months following injury.

will have only 5% of its original tensile strength at 2 weeks and 35% at 1 month (Fig. 3-5). Final tensile strength is not achieved for several months.

Wound Contraction and Remodeling

Every wound undergoes scar remodeling over a period of several months. With this remodeling comes some degree of wound contraction. It is most pronounced in full-thickness skin losses. The scar that forms gradually contracts centripetally over the wound defect through the action of specialized fibroblasts called myofibroblasts. Contraction pulls normal surrounding skin over the defect. Practically speaking, a properly everted suture line will contract to a flat, cosmetically acceptable scar, whereas a wound closed with the edges already inverted will form an unsightly depression in the epidermis that will stand out because of shadow formation from incident light (see Chapter 9 for further details).

As scars remodel, they change appearance as well. In an important study of scar appearance at suture removal versus appearance 6 to 9 months later, there was little correlation.[15] Biologic determinants such as skin tension, wound remodeling, and body location ultimately determine final scar appearance. Patients need to be advised that the final appearance may not be evident for 6 months to 1 year. Only then can a decision be made on whether plastic reconstruction might be necessary if cosmesis remains a concern.

CATEGORIES OF WOUND HEALING

For clinical purposes, wound healing is often categorized into three types of closure or intentions: primary, secondary, and tertiary (Fig. 3-6). Based on time from injury, level of contamination, and degree of tissue devitalization, this classification guides the choice of closure strategy.

Primary Closure (Primary Intention)

Primary closure can only be carried out on lacerations that are relatively clean and minimally contaminated, with minimal tissue loss or devitalization. These wounds are most often created by shearing forces. They can be closed with sutures, wound tapes, or staples. Repair of wounds is optimal when carried out within 6 to 8 hours, often referred to as the "Golden Period," from the time of injury. In practice, this period can vary from 6 to 24 hours according to body region, level of contamination, and degree of tissue devitalization. The risk for hand and foot infection increases significantly after 4 to 6 hours.[22] On the other hand, some practitioners feel comfortable closing uncomplicated facial lacerations up to 24 to 36 hours after injury.[3, 28]

Because there are no hard and fast rules that govern every possible situation, the following recommendation is made: any injury that can be converted to a fresh-appearing, slightly bleeding, nondevitalized wound, with no visible contamination or debris after aggressive cleansing, irrigation, and debridement, is a candidate for primary closure.

Secondary Closure (Secondary Intention)

Skin infarctions, ulcerations, abscess cavities, punctures, small cosmetically unimportant animal bites, and partial-thickness (dermal base preserved) abrasions are often better left to heal by secondary intention. They are not closed with sutures and are allowed to gradually heal by granulation and eventual reepithelialization. After an appropriate program of wound care, they can become candidates for later skin coverage, if necessary, by grafting. These wounds have a pronounced inflammatory response and are prone to significant wound contraction over time.

Tertiary Closure (Delayed Primary Closure)

Certain wounds are candidates for closure after being cleansed, debrided, and observed for 4 to 5 days.[1, 7, 18] These are wounds that are too contaminated to close primarily, but have not suffered significant tissue loss or devitalization. Wounds that fall into this category are often older; excessively contaminated with soil, feces, saliva, or vaginal secretions; caused by human or animal bites (see Chapter 14 for a detailed discussion of bite wounds); or the result of high-velocity missiles, such as bullets. Wounds created after

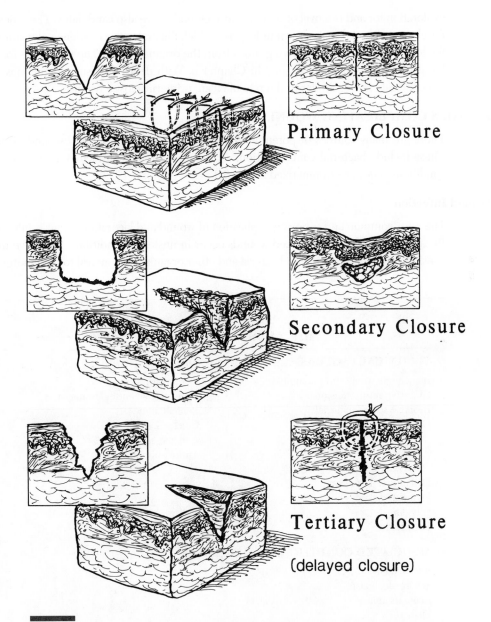

Primary Closure

Secondary Closure

Tertiary Closure

(delayed closure)

FIG. 3-6 Primary closure is accomplished by closing the wound with sutures at the time of presentation to the emergency department. Secondary closure occurs as a result of natural healing without intervention other than cleansing and debridement. Tertiary closure (delayed primary closure) is carried out approximately 4 to 5 days after the injury.

exploration for and removal of noninert foreign bodies are also candidates. The rationale for closure after 4 days is shown in Fig. 8-1, which illustrates the incidence of wound infection following injury at varying times from the original injury. The technique for delayed wound closure is described in Chapter 8. With delayed closure techniques, the infection rate is 4%, similar to the rate of clean, primarily closed wounds.[33]

FACTORS COMPLICATING WOUND HEALING

There are many sources of potential interference with uncomplicated wound healing. These include bacterial contamination, anatomic and technical factors, and associated conditions. They are summarized in Box 3-1.

Wound Infection

The most common and serious complication of wound and laceration repair is infection. Because all accidentally induced wounds occur in unsterile conditions, they have to be considered contaminated with bacteria and other organisms on arrival to the emergency

---

BOX 3-1

Alterations of Wound Healing

TECHNICAL FACTORS

Inadequate wound preparation
Excessive suture tension
Reactive suture materials
Local anesthetics

ANATOMIC FACTORS

Static skin tension
Dynamic skin tension
Pigmented skin
Oily skin
Body region

ASSOCIATED CONDITIONS AND DISEASES

Advanced age
Severe alcoholism
Acute uremia
Diabetes
Ehlers-Danlos syndrome
Hypoxia
Severe anemia
Peripheral vascular disease
Malnutrition

DRUGS

Corticosteroids
Nonsteroidal antiinflammatories
Penicillamine
Colchicine
Anticoagulants
Antineoplastic agents

department. The stratum corneum of the epidermis normally acts as an effective barrier against the penetration of bacteria into the deeper layers of the skin and superficial fascia. Any violation of the epidermis provides a pathway for bacterial invasion. Not only do environmental microorganisms find their way into wounds, but the skin, which is populated with a variety of indigenous microflora, can also harbor a potentially infective inoculum of pathogenic bacteria.[21] Areas of the body with high concentrations of bacteria include scalp, perineum, axillas, mouth, feet, and nail folds. The trunk and proximal extremities are sparsely populated.

A critical factor in determining whether contaminating bacteria go on to cause an established wound infection is the time elapsed from injury to cleansing and repair. It has been established that 100,000 (10^5) bacteria per gram of tissue constitute an infective inoculum.[9] Wounds with counts below that number heal without event. If bacterial counts are above that number, the risk of infection increases manyfold.[19] In a series of patients studied in an emergency department setting, it was observed that wounds less than 2.2 hours old contained 100 (10^2) bacteria per gram of tissue.[26] Wounds that were 3 hours old harbored between 10^2 and 10^6 bacteria per gram of tissue. Wounds more than 5 hours old consistently grew more than 10^6 bacteria per gram of tissue. In spite of experimental support for bacterial growth and invasion early after injury, the true clinical significance has not been established. It remains prudent, however, to cleanse and irrigate wounds in a timely manner. If antibiotics are considered necessary, early administration is appropriate.

Technical Factors

Soil, in particular clay, can impair healing in two ways.[27] The threshold infective inoculum is reduced to 10^2 bacteria, even in the presence of a small amount of dirt.[13] Second, soil and grit of any kind can lead to permanent tattooing if not aggressively removed. Consultation with a plastic surgery specialist may be indicated if wound cleansing and debridement cannot eliminate grit that is visibly embedded in the epidermis and superficial dermis.

Excessive tension created by improper suture technique can cause unnecessary wound ischemia.[25] Ischemia promotes cellular necrosis with greater inflammatory and scarring responses. Deep sutures, undermining, and increasing the number of sutures per laceration are methods that can reduce the danger of excessive tension.

Because tissue reactivity and inflammation vary with different suture materials, these materials can have differing effects on the healing process.[30] Although silk has excellent mechanical properties, it has a propensity for causing marked tissue reactivity. Nylon and polypropylene, however, are the least reactive of the nonabsorbable materials. Absorbable sutures act as foreign material, and excessive numbers can increase the risk of infection and may provoke a greater scarring response.[8, 20] Wound tapes and staples are the least reactive of wound closure alternatives and are associated with low infection rates even in contaminated wounds.

Experiments have shown that local anesthetics can cause retardation of wound healing.[23] This negative effect is enhanced by increasing concentrations of local anesthetics, as well as the use of adrenaline in anesthetic solutions.[13] There is no question, however, that local anesthetics need to be used in wound care. Judicious amounts at the lowest concentrations possible are recommended.

Anatomic Factors

Body region and skin tension lines have a significant effect on wound healing, specifically on final scar morphology (see Chapter 2). Wounds over the anterior thorax or the extremities heal with the most evident scars, whereas wounds of the eyelid heal with the least obvious scars. Pigmented and oily skin also tends to heal with greater scar formation than fairer, less oily skin.

Associated Conditions and Diseases

Several conditions and diseases cause an alteration in wound healing. Advanced age has been implicated in slower healing of wounds.[12] However, if the patient is basically healthy, normal healing and scar formation ultimately take place.[11] Wound healing can be retarded in the patient with chronic alcoholism who has advanced liver disease and impaired protein synthesis. Acute uremia has long been thought to impede healing.[5] In patients with uremia, there is an inhibition of fibroblast growth and a decrease in tensile strength during wound healing. Patients with diabetes also have numerous problems with wound healing.[17] Not only do they have an increased chance of wound infection, but there is also retardation of neovascularization and collagen synthesis. A rare disease that causes problems with collagen formation and wound healing is Ehlers-Danlos syndrome.[4]

Any condition that leads to failure of oxygen and nutrient delivery to the wound profoundly affects wound healing.[14] Shock, severe anemia, peripheral vascular disease, and malnutrition all fall into this category. Patients with severe underlying diseases such as advanced cancer, hepatic failure, and severe cardiovascular disease exhibit one or more of these clinical states and are subject to poor wound healing. Victims of major trauma, particularly those who have undergone prolonged shock and complicated resuscitations, are also at risk for poor wound healing.

Drugs

Numerous drugs and pharmacologic preparations alter wound healing.[24] Drugs that appear to have negative effects include corticosteroids, nonsteroidal antiinflammatory agents (aspirin, phenylbutazone), penicillamine, colchicine, anticoagulants, and antineoplastic agents. Of these drugs, corticosteroids have the most profound effect on healing and interfere with the process at many points. They adversely alter the inflammatory response, fibroblast activity, neovascularization, and epithelialization. Nonsteroidal antiinflammatory compounds depress the normal inflammatory response and can decrease overall wound tensile strength. Anticoagulants and aspirin increase the possibility of wound hematoma formation with subsequent delays in healing time. Although in theory antineoplastic agents have a good reason to inhibit wound healing, in actual practice it is not clear that they do so in a clinically significant manner.

Vitamins C and A, zinc sulfate, and anabolic steroids have a generally positive effect on wound repair.[24] Vitamin C deficiency profoundly impairs collagen formation, but normal synthesis can be restored with administration of ascorbic acid. Vitamin A and anabolic steroids are able to reverse corticosteroid-induced suppression of the inflammatory response. Zinc deficiency appears to play a role in slowing the healing process. Correction of the deficiency reverses that effect. Use of zinc ointments in nonzinc-deficient patients can cause a cross-linking failure during collagen maturation.[24] Experimental evidence that zinc sulfate can retard wound contraction is supportive of this observation.[29]

SUTURE MARKS

Skin suture marks can be an unsightly and unnecessary complication of laceration repair. There are several causes of suture marks, some within and some out of the control of the operator.[6] These causes are:

Skin type: Some areas of the skin are more prone to retaining suture marks than others. These include the skin of the back, chest, upper arms, and lower extremities. On the face, skin of the lower third of the nose and cheeks adjacent to the nasal alae are also vulnerable. On the other hand, suture marks are unusual on the eyelids, palms of the hands, and soles of the feet.

Keloid tendency: Keloid formers have a higher risk of suture mark formation.

Suture tension: Excessive suture tension during knot tying can cause tissue constriction, which increases the risk for larger and more obvious suture marks.

Stitch abscess: Occasionally a small abscess forms adjacent to the suture itself. Because suture material is a foreign body, the risk of abscess formation, although small, is inherent. Silk and braided sutures are more likely to provoke an inflammatory response at the suture site than monofilament nylon or metallic staples.[30]

Duration sutures left in place: Sutures remaining in place for 14 days or longer uniformly leave behind suture marks.[6] By 14 days epithelialization of the suture track occurs and a permanent epithelial "plug" is left behind. Conversely, no suture marks remain if sutures are removed before 7 days. The period between 7 and 14 days is less predictable with regard to retention and permanency of suture marks. It should be noted that these findings are independent of needle type or suture size.

KELOID AND HYPERTROPHIC SCAR FORMATION

A keloid is an inappropriate accumulation of scar tissue that originates from a wound and extends beyond its original boundaries (Fig. 3-7). Keloids are more common in blacks, but can occur in darkly pigmented skin areas of people of different races. These

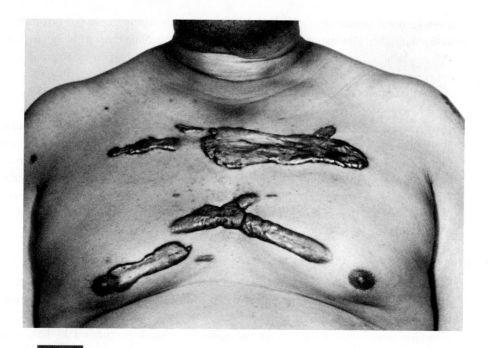

FIG. 3-7   An example of a keloid scar. Note that the scar extends beyond the margins of the original wound.

scars tend to be more commonly located on the ears, upper extremities, lower abdomen, and sternum. Treatments for keloids have included corticosteroid injection, compressive dressings, and surgical excision followed by radiation therapy. Eventual outcome and treatment depend on early recognition of keloid formation and prompt therapy.

Hypertrophic scars also have excessive bulk, but unlike keloids, they are confined to the original borders of the wound (Fig. 3-8). They tend to occur in areas of tissue stress, such as flexion creases across joints. The cause of this excessive scar response is not known. Physical therapy and splinting can be used during healing in patients who have a history of hypertrophic scarring. Corticosteroids and radiation therapy are other therapeutic alternatives.

SUMMARY OF WOUND HEALING: THE SUCCESSFULLY CLOSED WOUND

Although there are many factors that cannot be controlled regarding the final cosmetic outcome of a scar, the following is a summary of steps, which, if properly observed and taken, will yield the best results possible:

- Hemostases: All bleeding from the wound, except very minor oozing, should be controlled, usually with gentle, continuous pressure, before wound closure.

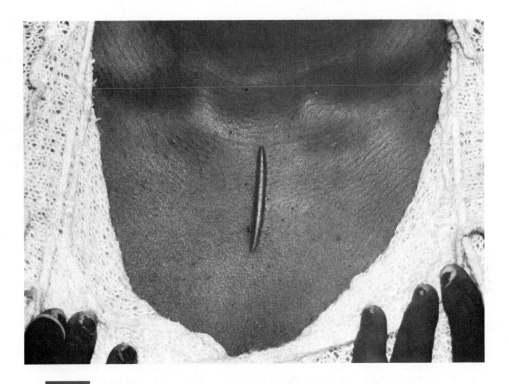

FIG. 3-8   An example of a hypertrophic scar. Note that the scar remains confined to the original borders of the wound.

- Anesthesia: Effective local anesthesia before wound cleansing allows the caregiver to thoroughly clean the wound without fear of causing unnecessary pain.
- Wound irrigation: This is the single most important step in reducing bacterial contamination and therefore the potential for wound infection.
- Removal of devitalized and contaminated tissue: Visibly devitalized and contaminated tissue that could not be removed through wound cleansing and irrigation needs to be completely but judiciously debrided.
- Tissue preservation: At the time of emergency department or primary closure, tissue excision should be resisted. It is best to tack down what remains of viable tissue, especially in complicated wounds. Because of the natural contraction of wounds, any cosmetic revisions done later can be successfully accomplished if sufficient tissue remains. Unnecessary tissue excision can lead to a permanent, uncorrectable, and unsightly scar.
- Closure tension: When wound edges are being brought together, they should just barely "touch." Excessive wound constriction when knot tying strangulates the tissue,

leading to a poor outcome. If necessary, tension reducing techniques such as the placement of deep sutures and undermining can be applied.

- Deep sutures: Because all sutures act as foreign bodies, as few as possible deep sutures are to be placed in any wound.
- Tissue handling: Rough handling of tissues, particularly when using forceps, can cause tissue necrosis and increase the chance of wound infection and scarring.
- Wound infection: Antibiotics are no substitute for wound preparation and irrigation. However, if the decision is made to treat the patient with antibiotics, the initial dose is most effective when administered intravenously as soon as possible after wounding.
- Dressings: Wounds heal best in a moist environment provided by a properly applied wound dressing.
- Follow-up: Well-understood verbal and written wound care instructions and timely return for either a short follow-up inspection or suture removal at the proper interval are essential to complete care.

REFERENCES

1. Brown SE, Allen HH, Robins RN: The use of delayed primary wound closure in preventing wound infections, *Am J Obstet Gynecol* 127:713-717, 1977.
2. Cardany R, Rodeheaver GT, Thacker TG, et al: The crush injury: a high risk wound, *J Am Coll Emerg Phys* 5:965-970, 1976.
3. Chisholm CD: Wound evaluation and cleansing, *Emerg Med Clinics North Am* 10:665-672, 1992.
4. Cohen I, McCoy B, Biegelmann, R: An update on wound healing, *Ann Plast Surg* 3:264-272, 1979.
5. Colin J, Elliot P, Ellis H: The effect of uraemia upon wound healing: an experimental study, *Br J Surg* 60:793-797, 1979.
6. Crikelair GF: Skin suture marks, *Am J Surg* 66:631-639, 1958.
7. Dimick AR: Delayed wound closure: indications and techniques, *Ann Emerg Med* 17:1303-1304, 1988.
8. Edlich RF, Rodeheaver G, Kuphal J, et al: Technique of closure: contaminated wound, *J Am Coll Emerg Phys* 3:375-381, 1974.
9. Edlich RF, Rodeheaver GT, Morgan RF, et al: Principles of emergency wound management, *Ann Emerg Med* 17:1284-1302, 1988.
10. Edlich R, Rodeheaver G, Thacker J: Technical factors in the prevention of disease. In Simmons RL, Howard RJ, Henriksen AI, editors: *Surgical infectious diseases*, New York, 1982, Appleton-Century-Crofts.
11. Goodson W Hunt T: Wound healing and aging, *J Invest Dermatol* 73:88-91, 1979.
12. Grove G: Age-related differences in healing of superficial skin wounds in humans, *Arch Dermatol Res* 272:381-385, 1982.
13. Haury BB, Rodeheaver GT, Pettry D, et al: Inhibition on nonspecific defenses by soil infection-potentiating factors, *Surg Gynecol Obstet* 144:19-24, 1977.
14. Hotter A: Physiologic aspects and clinical implications of wound healing, *Heart Lung* 11:522-530, 1982.
15. Hollander JE, Blasko B, Singer AJ, et al: Poor correlation of short- and long-term cosmetic appearance of repaired lacerations, *Acad Emerg Med* 2:983-987, 1995.
16. Howell JM: Current and future trends in wound healing, *Emerg Med Clinics North Am* 10:655-663, 1992.
17. Hunt T: Disorders of wound healing, *World J Surg* 4:271-277, 1980.

18. Johnson BW, Scott PG, Brunton JL, Petrik PK, Williams HT: Primary and secondary healing in infected wounds. An experimental study, *Arch Surg* 117:1189-1193, 1982.

19. Krizek TJ, Robson MC, Kho E: Bacterial growth and skin graft survival, *Surg Forum* 18:518-520, 1967.

20. Losken HW, Auchincloss JA: Human bites of the lip, *Clin Plast Surg* 11:773-775, 1984.

21. Marples M: Life on the human skin, *Sci Am* 220:108-115, 1969.

22. Morgan WJ, Hutchinson D, Johnson HM: The delayed treatment of wounds of the hand and forearm under antibiotic cover, *Br J Surg* 67:140-141, 1980.

23. Morris T, Appleby R: Retardation of wound healing by procaine, *Br J Surg* 67:391-392, 1980.

24. Pollack S: Systemic medications and wound healing, *Int J Dermatol* 21:491-496, 1982.

25. Price P: Stress, strain, and sutures, *Ann Surg* 128:408-421, 1948.

26. Robson MC, Duke WF, Krizek TJ: Rapid bacterial screening in the treatment of civilian wounds, *J Surg Res* 16:299-306, 1974.

27. Rodeheaver GT, Pettry D, Turnbull V: Identification of the wound infection-potentiating factors in soil, *Am J Surg* 128:8-14, 1974.

28. Rodgers KG: The rational use of antimicrobial agents in simple wounds, *Emerg Med Clin North Am* 10:753-766, 1992.

29. Soderberg T, Hallmans G: Wound contractions and zinc absorption during treatment with zinc tape, *Scand J Reconstr Surg* 16:255-259, 1982.

30. Swanson N, Tromovitch T: Suture materials: properties, uses and abuses, *Int J Dermatol* 21:373-378, 1982.

31. Trott AT: Chronic skin ulcers, *Emerg Med Clinics North Am* 10:823-845, 1992.

32. Trott AT: Mechanisms of surface soft tissue trauma, *Ann Emerg Med* 17:1279-1283, 1988.

33. Weiss Y: Delayed closure in the management of the contaminated wound, *Int Surg* 67(4 Suppl):403-404, 1982.

4 Wound Care and the Pediatric Patient

Javier A. Gonzalez del Rey and Gregg A. DiGiulio

- -

General Approach and Calming Techniques
    Assessing the Child
    Handling Parents
Restraint for Wound Care
Pediatric Patient Sedation

Local Anesthetic Techniques
Choice of Closure Materials in Children
Special Considerations for Different Anatomic
    Sites in the Pediatric Patient
Wound Aftercare

Children with lacerations are commonly seen in emergency departments, and lacerations represent approximately 30% to 40% of all injuries that present to a pediatric emergency department.[11, 24] Estimates of the annual rate of lacerations are 50 to 60 per 1000 children.[29, 31]

Lacerations commonly involve younger children who lack the experience, common sense, and motor coordination of older children. Males are involved twice as often as females. Lacerations frequently result from falls from stairways, bicycles, and furniture.[6] In children, 60% of the time the lacerations occur on the head followed by upper and lower extremities.[6] Overall, lacerations are one of the most common types of pediatric injury requiring both functional and cosmetic evaluation by a physician.

GENERAL APPROACH AND CALMING TECHNIQUES
Assessing the Child

The child with a laceration represents not only a technical challenge but also an emotional challenge for the caregiver, the child, and the parent. Realizing this, it is important to take time to explain the procedure, your approach, and possible discomforts to the child, as well as the parents. Time spent preparing the child will be time gained in the end.

Assuming that there are no life- or limb-threatening injuries, you should first obtain the history and at the same time gain the child's confidence. Do not immediately undress or examine the wound. Establish a rapport by talking directly to the child using age appropriate terms. Involve toddlers by asking them how they got their "boo-boo," but don't expect an adequate history; the specifics are better obtained from the parent. The child who is 4 or 5 years of age and older can frequently give the history, and additionally, this gives him or her a sense of control.

Distraction or imagery can be effective at any age. Ask about toys, friends, siblings, favorite colors, again at an age appropriate level. A general understanding of the developmental milestones is invaluable in allowing the physician to interact appropriately with a child. Table 4-1 summarizes the developmental abilities for various aged children.[13]

The history should focus on the events of the injury, as well as the potential for injury to other areas of the body. Consider physical abuse when the history is not consistent with the injury or when the event cannot be explained by the developmental age of the patient (e.g., a six month old *climbing* onto and falling from a counter). There are also some specific injury patterns that should raise the specter of abuse: immersion pattern,

Table 4-1 *Childhood Developmental Abilities by Age*

Age (Yr)	Development Issues	Fears	Techniques
Infancy 0 - 1	Minimal language Feel like an extension of parents Sensitive to physical environment	Stranger anxiety	Keep parents in sight Address possible hunger Use warm hands Keep room warm
Toddler 1 - 3	Receptive language more advanced than expressive See themselves as individuals Assertive will	Brief separation Pain	Maintain verbal communication Examine in parent's lap Allow some choices (if possible)
Preschool 3 - 5	Excellent expressive skills Rich fantasy life Magical thinking	Long separation Pain Disfigurement	Allow expression Encourage fantasy and play Encourage participation in care
School age 5 - 10	Fully developed language Understanding of body structure and function Able to reason and compromise Experience with self-control	Disfigurement Loss of function Death	Explain procedures Explain pathophysiology and treatment Project positive outcome Stress child's ability to master situation Respect physical modesty
Adolescence 10 - 19	Self-determination Decision making Realistic view of death	Loss of autonomy Loss of peer acceptance Death	Allow choices and control Stress acceptance by peers Respect autonomy

Based on data from Stein MT: Interviewing in a pediatric setting. In Dixon SD, Stein MT, editors: *Encounters with children*, ed 2, St Louis, 1992, Mosby.

linear marks or lacerations consistent with a belt or hanger, or an unusual location not usually prone to injury. A social services referral is necessary for any case where abuse is suspected.

Pay special attention to the immunization status. Simply asking the parent if the child's shots are up-to-date most often elicits a positive response whether or not this is actually true. It is better to inquire about the number of "shots" and the age when the last one was given.

Next, the wound is assessed. Allowing the child to remain with the parent for as long as possible facilitates the examination. Confidence can be gained by telling the child that initially you are just going to "look." Continue to involve the parent in the evaluation process, so that the child knows that the physician is there to help. Generally, kindness and patience should be accompanied by a thorough and directed approach. The examination should begin away from the injury especially in the toddler or younger child. If the injury is on the hand or face, start by playing gently with a foot so that the child realizes that you are not going to hurt him or her and slowly advance to the site of the injury. Direct probing of the wound is painful and should not be done until after anesthesia is achieved. In cases where hemostasis is necessary, pressure should be applied and can often be done safely by the parent.

Once the wound is evaluated, take time to explain the procedure to the child and the parent. Use words that the child can understand ("numbing medicine," "I'm going to make this spot go to sleep," "magic string [suture material]—it's magic because it doesn't hurt"). Tell the child which part of the procedure may be uncomfortable and for how long. Allow the parents to participate as much as their level of comfort allows. A parent can be of great help in calming and distracting the child, and if the parent wants to be at the bedside, encourage him or her to stay. However, give parents the option of going to the waiting area if close by. Some parents cannot tolerate invasive treatment of their child, but this lack of tolerance should not be perceived as a lack of caring.

Children often cry during a procedure, and although this is disturbing, it does not always imply pain. A cry can also be a sign of fear or a display of frustration with immobilization. The frightened cry often increases as the examiner approaches the patient. The painful cry occurs consistently when the wound is manipulated.

Handling Parents

Parents may be upset because their child has been injured and may appear to be angry. Fear of the outcome or guilt because the child was injured when they were supposed to be their child's protector often underlies the parents' behavior. Allay their fears by explaining the procedure, involving them in the process, and informing them of the expected outcome. Regardless of the circumstances, any exhibition of judgmental behavior by the caregiver is unwarranted.

Often parents bring in their child for seemingly minor cuts and wounds. Although this can be frustrating when faced with a busy office or emergency department, keep in mind that the parent may be seeking your professional opinion as to whether the wound requires a formal repair. Sometimes local care and a bandage is the most appropriate care. Most parents can accept the care decision, no matter how minor, when clearly explained.

Explain to the parent and child your proposed management of the wound and that you will do everything that you can to alleviate pain by using an anesthetic. A parent can be one of your greatest allies when faced with a frightened child, so allow the parent to participate if he or she so desires. However, question them about their tolerance for the procedure. If there is any risk for parental vasovagal syncope, have them leave the care area. Warn parents that the child may cry with touching or the sensation of pressure and this does not necessarily mean pain. If the child appears to feel pain, strongly consider reanesthetizing the area. This will greatly enhance parental satisfaction.

Explain what to expect from the laceration repair. Overall satisfaction is greatly improved if the parent understands the healing process and the truth that the laceration repair decreases but not completely eliminates scarring. The discussion should include the changing appearance of the scar over time and the fact that all wounds scar and their final appearance may not be known for several months.

Verbal and written follow-up instructions are as important as the procedure itself. Printed discharge instructions detailing wound care, the signs and symptoms of infection, and the timing of suture removal are recommended. During the time of the visit, the parents are frequently anxious and may not recall the myriad of verbal instructions given to them.

RESTRAINT FOR WOUND CARE

Most children are frightened and anxious about being in a doctor's office or an emergency department. A conscientious physician spends time with the patient and parents to minimize this anxiety. If the previously described calming techniques do not allay the fears of the uncooperative child, restraints may be necessary. The decision of whether or not to use restraints can often be determined by the initial observation of child's behavior, as well as parental report of the child's overall ability to cooperate. There are several methods of restraint available: physical, chemical, and "imagery."

Physical restraints should be considered in the preverbal child because imagery and verbal calming techniques are ineffective. Their limited language and ability to comprehend their situation makes it difficult for them to cooperate with caregiver. Papoose boards are usually well tolerated, and it is our experience that once in place, the infant or toddler frequently becomes less agitated after infiltration is performed.

Regardless of the method used, always take the time to explain the need for restraints to the parents. Restraints protect the child and caregiver during the procedure and also ensure the best result. Their use however is not without complication. Restraints limit the child's protective reflexes should he or she vomit. Excessive crying increases gastric pressure and together with a full stomach the possibility of emesis increases. Suction should be readily available, and the child should be turned to a lateral decubitus position while in the papoose if emesis occurs.

Even when restraints are used, the assistance of a nurse or technician is still necessary to maintain immobilization of the head for facial lacerations or of an extremity for hand, arm, foot, or leg lacerations. These personnel need formal training in restraining techniques. For example, when immobilizing the face of a child, the holder needs to use his or her palms rather than fingertips to prevent bruising and to achieve better head control (Fig. 4-1). Care is always taken to maintain an unobstructed airway and a thorax free to provide adequate ventilation.

Mental imagery can be used with children who are 4 or 5 years of age and older. The outcome frequently relates to the verbal abilities of the individual child. Imagery includes distraction or fantasy. Ask the child to tell you about his or her friends, favorite toys, or what activities he or she likes. Or have the child describe what makes him or her feel good. Keeping up-to-date on the latest toys can be invaluable. Often a parent can be your ally and help distract the child if he or she is permitted and wants to be at the bed-

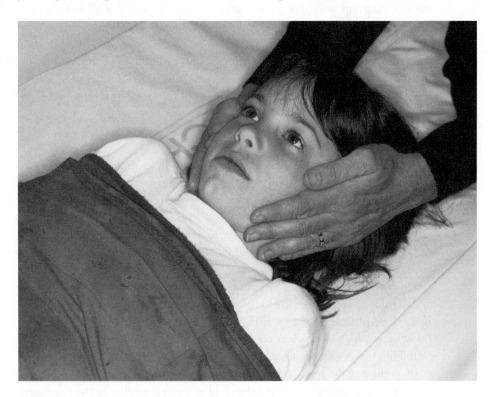

FIG. 4-1   When restraining a pediatric patient for a facial repair, the head is held with the palms of the hands. The airway remains unobstructed and undue pressure with fingertips is avoided.

side. An assistant can also play an important role in encouraging imagery and distracting the child.

PEDIATRIC PATIENT SEDATION

Despite caregivers' best efforts, there is the occasional child who does not cooperate. When the child's inability to cooperate interferes with your ability to perform an adequate repair or poses a danger to the caregivers or to the child themself, consider the use of pharmacologic sedation. The type, location, and complexity of the laceration, as well as the emotional state of the child, determines the type of sedative to use. In small, simple lacerations, the risk of sedation may outweigh the benefits. In our experience and by using the previously described techniques, we are able to repair the vast majority of lacerations including facial lacerations without the use of sedatives.

For the repair of a laceration, the physician usually wants to induce conscious or light sedation. In this state, the child maintains protective reflexes, maintains his or her own airway, and is able to respond to a directed command. All sedation techniques can evolve into deep sedation, which is a more depressed state of consciousness where the child is not easily aroused and cannot maintain protective reflexes or an open airway. Titrating the sedative dose to the desired level of sedation may help prevent the evolution of conscious to deep sedation. In the office setting or emergency department, conscious sedation should be limited to children with ASA classifications I and II (class I is a normally healthy patient; class II is a patient with mild systemic disease).[2]

Choosing the appropriate method of sedation should take into consideration the following questions: is the procedure painful?, does the child need to be motionless?, what is the duration of the procedure?, what safety resources are available for the procedure?, and when was the patient's last meal? In general, a recent meal is not a contraindication to sedation for urgent procedures.

The suite where sedation is performed must have equipment available for airway and cardiovascular interventions for children of all ages and sizes. The physician must have the ability to handle a sudden change in the child's status. Whenever sedatives are used, there should be one practitioner present whose sole job is to monitor the patient and assist in any resuscitative measures that become necessary. Continuous monitoring of pulse oximetry and pulse and intermittent documentation of respiratory rate and blood pressure is necessary in all of these patients. We recommend that each institution develop a policy appropriate to its setting using the American Academy of Pediatrics Guidelines for Sedation or the American College of Emergency Physicians Guidelines for Pediatric Sedation.[2, 4] Monitoring of any child who has received a sedative continues until discharge criteria are met. Discharge criteria include an ability to converse at an age appropriate level, to maintain his or her airway, to have stable cardiovascular function, and to sit unaided. Regardless of the agent used, parents should be informed of type of sedative to be used and potential side effects. Consent should be documented in accordance with hospital, local, and state requirements.

Table 4-2 *Selected Drugs for Sedation*

Medication	Recommended Dose	Route of Administration	Additional Instructions
Fentanyl (Sublimaze)	1-3 mcg/kg	IV	Titrate slowly (1mcg/kg/min); effect within mins; max dose 5 mcg/kg over 1 hr
Morphine	0.1-0.15 mg/kg	IV	Effect within mins; max dose 10 mg over 1 hr for opioid-naive pts; up to 20 mg over 1-2 hr for pts who get opioids often
Midazolam (Versed)	0.1-0.15 mg/kg	IV	Titrate over 3 min to desired effect; effect within 3-5 min; max initial dose 5 mg
	0.3-0.5 mg/kg	PO	Add to juice; effect delayed 20-30 min; max initial dose 10 mg; may repeat in 30 min if pt; not sedated well
	0.2-0.3 mg/kg	IN	Slowly drip into nostrils; effect delayed 5-10 min; max dose 10 mg
	0.2 mg/kg	IM	Effect delayed 10-15 min; max dose 8 mg
Diazepam (Valium)	0.1-0.2 mg/kg	IV	Titrate over 3 min; to desired effect; max initial dose 10 mg
	0.2 mg/kg	IM	Effect delayed 10-15 min; max dose 10 mg
Chloral hydrate	50-75 mg/kg	PO, PR	Effect delayed 30-60 min; may repeat an additional 25-50 mg/kg in 30 min if pt; not sedated well; max dose 100 mg/kg; consider use for noninvasive procedures such as CT, ultrasound, and Echo
REVERSAL AGENTS			
Naloxone (Narcan)	1. mg/kg, MAX 2. 0.4 mg, MAX	IV, IM	For opiate reversal (fentanyl, morphine); repeat in 5 min if no effect
Flumazenil (Romazicon)	0.01 mg/kg or 0.2 mg	IV	For benzodiazepine reversal (midazolam, diazepam); repeat 0.2 mg/min up to 1 mg if no effect

Sedative agents can be administered orally, intranasally, parenterally, rectally, or through inhalation. Table 4-2 lists some commonly used agents and gives dosing recommendations. For each agent that he or she uses, the physician should become familiar with the dose, administration, and side effects. The most common, significant side effect is respiratory depression, although cardiovascular changes can also occur.

Fentanyl is a synthetic opioid agonist 100 times more potent than morphine. It is commonly used as a sedative when analgesia is also needed during conscious sedation.[7] The benefits of this agent are rapid onset, short duration, and predictability. It is often combined with a short-acting benzodiazepine (i.e., midazolam) for painful procedures. It must be used with caution, especially when combined with another sedative agent because of an increased risk of respiratory depression. It should be titrated in 1 mcg/kg increments with a maximum dose of 5 mcg/kg over 1 hour. Higher doses administered rapidly can induce chest wall rigidity with impaired ventilation. Morphine and Demerol are also commonly used for analgesia but, because of their longer half-life and their requirement for prolonged monitoring before discharge, these agents are not the first choice for short procedures.

Midazolam is a short-acting benzodiazepine frequently used in children.[17] The main attributes of this drug are the provision of effective anxiety reduction and anterograde amnesia, combined with a favorable overall safety profile.[12, 22, 26] It can be administered intravenously, orally, or intranasally. The intranasal route is commonly used in toddlers and young children with lacerations and obviates the need for an intravenous catheter. The IV solution is drawn up into a tuberculin syringe, the needle is removed and then with the child supine, the dose is administered in aliquots of two drops per nostril over 2 to 5 minutes. The solution can be irritating to the mucosa, and it is prudent to warn the child and parent of a stinging sensation. Sedation usually occurs within 5 to 10 minutes. Because of a significant and variable first pass effect, there is considerable variation in the dose required to induce sedation. When effective, the child often becomes mildly sedated and the caregiver and parents can talk with him or her through the procedure. Rarely, a paradoxic reaction occurs, and the child can become more agitated and anxious.

Chloral hydrate is a mild sedative with an excellent safety record. Its major drawbacks are the relatively long time to onset and long duration of action.[3] It probably does not require monitoring beyond the observation of the child's mental status.

Nitrous oxide in concentrations less than 50% has been commonly used in pediatric dentistry. It has anxiolytic, sedative, and mild analgesic properties. It has been used as an adjunct to local infiltration or nerve block in wound repair.[21] The delivery and scavenging systems are expensive, making this technique difficult to use outside of a surgical or dental suite. It also has been reported to carry some risk to caregivers.[32]

Ketamine (4 mg/kg IM) is a dissociative agent that provides effective sedation without loss of airway reflexes. Its effectiveness and safety have been demonstrated in children in a variety of painful emergency department procedures. Some disadvantages include increased secretions and the possibility of hallucinations (emergent reactions).

Some drug combinations, such as Meperidine, Promethazine, and Chlorpromazine (DPT), have been used for sedation with very good results in children.[35] Because this combination is difficult to titrate and because of the recent development of other faster and safer agents, many caregivers no longer recommend this combination.

Remember that no matter which agent or combination is used, sedation does not imply analgesia, and a local anesthetic must still be used.

LOCAL ANESTHETIC TECHNIQUES

Always anesthetize the area before cleansing and irrigation. Wound cleansing is painful, and often the adequacy of anesthesia can be assessed during irrigation. Cleansing and irrigation techniques are the same for children and adults and are fully described in Chapter 6.

Recently, topical anesthetics (TAC [tetracaine 0.5%, adrenaline 0.5%, and cocaine 11.8%] or LET [lidocaine 4%, epinephrine 0.1%, and tetracaine 0.5%] solution or gel) are being used more frequently and are equally effective.[34, 36] Preparations of TAC containing half-strength (5.9%) cocaine have also been used with good results.[36] These combinations are very effective in lacerations of the face and scalp. Some authors have found that TAC provides inconsistent anesthesia for wounds located on extremities, often necessitating the use of supplemental infiltration with lidocaine.[8] All of the combinations provide anesthesia without causing the discomfort associated with an injection and do not distort the local anatomy. Another potential advantage that we have noted is that we need to use physical restraints less often when we use these agents. TAC should not be used in, or directly adjacent to, the nasal mucosa, oral mucosa, or the conjunctiva because the cocaine component can be absorbed from these areas in sufficient quantities to cause systemic toxicity. Care must also be taken not to allow the solution to drip into any of these areas. This solution should not be used in areas of end artery flow, such as fingers, toes, and ears.

These topical anesthetics should be used before wound cleansing and repair. Saturate a small pledget of cotton or piece of gauze that is of similar size to the wound with the solution. The maximum dose is 0.1 ml/kg. It has been clearly demonstrated that less than 3 ml of TAC is sufficient to anesthetize the majority of lacerations encountered in children.[8, 9, 33] Remove any blood coagulum from the wound. The pledget is then placed directly into the wound and can be held in place by a Band-Aid, Tegaderm, tape, or held directly by the parent using gloves to prevent absorption through the fingers. It is left in place for 10 to 15 minutes. Effective application usually blanches the skin around the wound. Further discussion of topical and local anesthetic techniques is contained in Chapter 5.

Regional blocks are another useful method of anesthesia for children. They do not distort the anatomy at the site of the injury and may be less traumatic as they often require one or at most two injections as opposed to the multiple injections required for local anesthesia. Digital, infraorbital, mental, and supraorbital blocks are probably the most commonly used, although all of the blocks described in Chapter 5 may be used in children.

CHOICE OF CLOSURE MATERIALS IN CHILDREN

A wide array of suture material and size is available to the practitioner. Personal preferences often determine which material is used. In general, the choice of material to use is the same as described for adults. In children, there are particular situations that may be more amenable to other means of closure. Because suture removal is often fraught with the same anxiety and difficulties as suture application, the use of absorbable suture is sometimes the best option. For nail bed and scalp lacerations we often use chromic gut. If the sutures still remain at 7 days, we ask the parent to facilitate removal by gently rubbing the material with gauze. This should be done parallel to the wound to minimize the potential for wound dehiscence. Skin staples are a fast, effective method of closing scalp lacerations especially in the uncooperative child. They have the same cosmetic outcome as standard sutures.

Skin tapes are an alternative method of repair for simple lacerations. The advantage is that they are easy to apply, they leave no marks, and follow-up is not necessary. However, the tapes are not reliable for infants and young children who may remove them. Tissue adhesive, although used in Europe and Canada, is not presently available for routine use in the United States. In anticipation of approval of tissue adhesives, closure techniques using these agents are discussed in Chapter 13.

SPECIAL CONSIDERATIONS FOR DIFFERENT ANATOMIC SITES IN THE PEDIATRIC PATIENT
Scalp

Careful examination and palpation of the wound is necessary to ensure that there is no skull fracture. If the mechanism of injury is unlikely to cause a fracture or if an adequate examination can be performed, then radiographs are not necessary. Further exploration of the wound can be performed once the laceration is anesthetized. Direct observation of the periosteum and skull is frequently possible. Use cotton tipped swabs to assist in probing, especially in smaller lacerations.

Simple, small scalp lacerations that are not grossly contaminated, are not actively bleeding, and have not interrupted the galea may be closed using the hair-tie technique. An adequate length of hair from opposite sides of the wound is necessary. Twist the hair strands on both sides of the suture line (the number of knots should be equal to the number of stitches that would normally have been used in the care of this wound), pull them across the wound and then knot them. Postclosure wound care is similar to that of a routine scalp closure. The knot is allowed to grow away from the wound edge and can be cut free in 1 to 2 weeks.

As previously noted, chromic gut can be used to close scalp wounds to eliminate the return visit for suture removal.

Face

An assistant is invaluable and necessary when closing facial wounds in children. The assistant is needed to maintain immobilization, and this is best accomplished if he or she uses firm, consistent pressure, being careful to use the flat surfaces of his or her hands or forearms (see Fig. 4-1) to immobilize the head. Avoid using fingertips that cause localized pressure and pain. When closing chin lacerations firm, consistent pressure can be applied to keep the jaw closed and minimize "quivering" of the chin.

Bandages are difficult to maintain on a toddler's face or scalp, and the frequent application of an antibiotic ointment is recommended to keep the wound moist and promote healing.

Hand

Difficulties arise primarily during the evaluation of pediatric hand lacerations. Cooperation for formal nerve and tendon function is difficult to obtain. Young children are unable to follow commands and verbalize the concepts of numbness and paresthesias. Often the practitioner must rely on observation rather than formal testing. Observe the resting position of the extremity. Is there a consistency to the amount of resting flexion between digits? An extended finger while the others are flexed raises the suspicion of a tendon injury and should prompt further investigation. Watch for spontaneous movement of the injured part. Does the child withdraw from touch or noxious stimuli? Once anesthesia is obtained, does the depth of the wound suggest tendon or nerve involvement?

In children less than 5 years of age, the classic sensory examination is modified. Two methods are available to determine the sensory innervation in the area distal to the wound. The first method is based on the principle that denervated fingers do not sweat. If you run the body of a clean plastic pen along an area with normal innervation, the sweat will create a slight drag. In the denervated area, the pen will move swiftly. Another popular method is the submersion test. Normal skin becomes wrinkled after 20 minutes of being under water. Denervated skin usually remains smooth.

Frequently, the final answer cannot be determined at the initial encounter. Under such circumstances, only the skin should be closed, and serial examinations over the following few days help clarify if there is any nerve or tendon involvement. Consultation with a hand specialist is indicated at this time. Most hand surgeons reevaluate the initial injury within 3 to 5 days. Tendon or neuronal repair can be done within the first 3 weeks following the injury with good results. Fingertip avulsions are common pediatric injuries. These injuries occur in toddlers when windows and doors close on their fingers. Older children are more prone to injuries from sharp objects.

In cases of complete fingertip amputation, several studies have shown superior results when the fingertip is allowed to regenerate on its own.* The granulation tissue that develops contains neural buds and provides superior sensation when compared with a graft. In cases of partial amputation or a flap laceration of the fingertip, the flap may be reattached once blood clots are removed. In most cases, obtain an x-ray to exclude the presence of a fracture. For a distal tuft fracture, copious irrigation should be followed by the use of prophylactic antibiotics. More proximal, open fractures should be managed in consultation with a hand specialist. In cases where the laceration involves the nail bed use the same principles described in Chapter 12. Formal splinting of the injury after repair protects the repair and the injury. The prognosis of these injuries depends on how much of the tip is involved. These injuries may take weeks for complete healing. It is advisable to arrange follow-up with a plastic or an orthopedic surgeon.

Foot

Foot injuries present the problems and challenges of the injury itself and also the difficulties that the injury causes in ambulation. Unless the child is older than 6 to 8 years old, crutches are not be recommended because of insufficient motor coordination. Younger children may need to be carried or encouraged to crawl. Be prepared to commiserate with the stress that this can impose on the family.

Puncture wounds present their own unique controversies. There have been no prospective studies that address this common entity. Although some authors recommend routine coring for puncture wounds, we discourage this because coring is uncomfortable, increases local pain, makes ambulation difficult, and does not have proven efficacy.[19] However, every puncture wound has the potential to harbor foreign material that increases the risk of infection. Most foreign bodies are not radiodense and are difficult to find on probing. Removal of any organic material or identifiable foreign body is recommended and opening the wound with a small incision may be necessary in these instances. Chapter 15 contains further discussion of plantar puncture wounds.

Serious complications can occur for puncture wounds through tennis shoes. Pseudomonas osteomyelitis has been reported in 4% of these cases.[18] Most authors agree, and it is our opinion that antibiotics are not routinely required following puncture wounds to the feet. If cellulitis develops within the first few days of the injury, then antibiotic coverage is needed and is directed toward staphylococcus and streptococcus sp. The quinolones that are frequently used in the adult population are relatively contraindicated in preadolescents because of a concern for inhibition of cartilage growth and development. Pseudomonas osteomyelitis should be considered in cases of persistent inflammation despite adequate antistaphylococcal coverage or increasing bony tenderness over time.

*References 1, 5, 14, 16, 20, 23, 25, 28.

Perineum/Straddle Injuries

Careful and complete examination is necessary when evaluating these injuries. Blunt straddle injuries occur when the perineum strikes a fixed object such as the crossbar of a bicycle. This mechanism is associated with trauma to the labia and posterior fourchette.[10] However if there is a penetrating injury as occurs with falling onto a fence post, then vaginal injury is more likely.[15] If there is any concern of vaginal lacerations, unexplained bleeding, or lacerations involving the rectum, then a complete examination is required.[30] Often, the use of general anesthesia and a referral to a subspecialist is necessary. Straddle injuries can be accompanied by trauma to the urethra and concomitant urinary retention.[27] Foley catheterization is sometimes necessary if watchful waiting is unsuccessful. Small superficial labial lacerations can be sutured in the emergency department. Because children are very afraid of a stranger manipulating their genitalia, sedation is usually recommended even in small lacerations. Chromic gut or any other appropriate absorbable material is recommended to avoid the stress and anxiety of suture removal.

WOUND AFTERCARE

Wound care after a laceration repair is the same as previously described. Bandages and dressings should be applied but need to be adequately secured because of the child's curiosity. Materials such as Coban may be used, but be careful to avoid creating a tourniquet effect. Sutures in general can be removed earlier than is done for the adult. Give both oral and written discharge instructions. They must be clear and concise, indicating possible complications, follow-up care, and timing of suture removal. Written instructions are invaluable since parents often may not recall the details of the instructions once the children are discharged.

Other important issues are related to the psychologic well-being of the child. Remember to always give a reward such as a sticker or a sucker. Encourage the parents to minimize the stress of the accident by making the event a positive experience and not a punishment. Throughout the encounter try to engage the child, gain his or her confidence and possibly become a friend. In the end you will be rewarded with a satisfying experience for the child, the parents, and yourself.

REFERENCES

1. Allen MJ: Conservative management of finger tip injuries in adults, *Hand* 12:257, 1980.
2. American Academy of Pediatrics: Guidelines for monitoring and management of pediatric patients during and after sedation for diagnostic and therapeutic procedures, *Pediatrics* 89:257-262, 1992.
3. American Academy of Pediatrics: Use of chloral hydrate for sedation in children, *Pediatrics* 92:471-473, 1992.
4. American College of Emergency Physicians: The use of pediatric sedation and analgesia, *Ann Emerg Med* 22:626-627, 1993.

5. Ashbell TS, Kleinert HE, Putcha SM, et al: The deformed finger nail, a frequent result of failure to repair nail bed injuries, *J Trauma* 7:177, 1967.

6. Baker MD, Selbst SM, Lanuti M: Lacerations in urban children, *AJDC* 144:87-92, 1990.

7. Billmire DA, Neale HW, Gregory RO: Use of IV fentanyl in the outpatient treatment of pediatric facial trauma, *J Trauma* 25:1079-1080, 1985.

8. Bonadio WA, Wagner V: Efficacy of TAC topical anesthetic for pediatric laceration repair, *Am J Dis Child* 142:203-205, 1988.

9. Bonadio WA, Wagner V: Half-strength TAC for selected dermal lacerations in children, *Clin Pediatr* 27:495-498, 1988.

10. Bond GR, Dowd MD, Landsman I: Unintentional perineal injury in prepubescent girls: a multicenter, prospective report of 56 girls, *Pediatrics* 95:628-631, 1995.

11. Chenoweth A: Health problems of infants and children. In: Wallace HM, Gold EM, Liss EF, editors: *Maternal and child health practices*, Springfield, Ill, 1973, Charles C. Thomas Publisher.

12. Diament MJ, Stanley P: The use of midazolam for sedation of infants and children, *Am J Roentgenol* 150:377-378, 1988.

13. Dixon SD, Stein MT: *Encounters with children: pediatric behavior and development,* St Louis, 1992, Mosby.

14. Douglas BS: Conservative management of guillotine amputation of the finger in children, *Aust Pediatr J* 8:86, 1972.

15. Dowd MD, Fitzmaurice L, Knapp JF, Mooney D: The interpretation of urogenital findings in children with straddle injuries, *J Pediatr Surg* 29:7-10, 1994.

16. Farrell RG, Disher WA, Nesland RS, et al: Conservative management of fingertip amputations, *JACEP* 6:273, 1977.

17. Feld LH, Negus JB, White PF: Oral midazolam preanesthetic medication in pediatric outpatients, *Anesthesiology* 73:831-834, 1990.

18. Fischer MC, Goldsmith JF, Gilligan PH: Sneakers as a source of Pseudomonas aeruginosa in children with osteomyelitis following puncture wounds, *J Pediatr* 106:607-614, 1985.

19. Fitzgerald R, Cowan J: Puncture wounds of the foot, *Orthop Clin North Am* 6:965-972, 1975.

20. Fox JW, Golden GT, Rodeheaver G, et al: Nonoperative management of fingertip pulp amputation by occlusive dressings, *Am J Surg* 133:255, 1977.

21. Gamis AS, Knapp JF, Glenski JA: Nitrous oxide analgesia in a pediatric emergency department, *Ann Emerg Med* 18:177-181, 1989.

22. Hennes HM, Wagner V, Bonadio WA, et al: Effect of oral midazolam on anxiety of preschool children during laceration repair, *Ann Emerg Med* 19:1006-1009, 1990.

23. Holm A, Zachariae L: Fingertip lesions: an evaluation of conservative treatment versus free skin grafting, *Acta Orthop Scand* 45:382, 1974.

24. Izant RJ, Hubay CA: Annual injury of 15,000,000 children: a limited study of childhood accidental injury and death, *J Trauma* 6:65-74,1966.

25. Lamon RP, Cicedro JJ, Frascone RJ, et al: Open treatment of fingertip amputations, *Ann Emerg Med* 12:358, 1983.

26. Levine MF, Spahr-Schopfer IA, Hartley E, et al: Oral midazolam premedication in children: the minimum time interval for separation from parents, *Can J Anaesth* 40:726-729, 1993.

27. Levne PM, Gonzalez ET: Genitourinary trauma in children, *Urol Clin North Am* 12(1):53, 1985.

28. Louis DS, Palmer AK, Burney RE: Open treatment of digital tip injuries, *JAMA* 244:697, 1980.

29. Manheimer DI, Dewey J, Mellinger GD, Corsa L: Fifty thousand child-years of accidental injuries, *Public Health Rep* 81:519-533, 1966.

30. Muram D: Genital tract injuries in the prepubertal child, *Pediatr Ann* 15:616, 1986.

31. Rivara FP, Bergman AB, LoGerfo JF, Weiss, NS: Epidemiology of childhood injuries, II: sex differences in injury rates, *AJDC* 136:502-506, 1982.

32. Rowland AS, Baird DD, Weinberg CR, et al: Reduced fertility among women employed as dental assistants exposed to high levels of nitrous oxide, *N Engl J Med* 327:993-997, 1992.

33. Schaffer D: Clinical comparison of TAC anesthetic solutions with and without cocaine, *Ann Emerg Med* 14:1077-1080, 1985.

34. Schilling CG, Bank DE, Borchert BA, et al: Tetracaine, epinephrine and cocaine versus lidocaine, epinephrine and tetracaine for anesthesia of lacerations in children, *Ann Emerg Med* 25:203-208, 1995.

35. Terndrup TE, Cantor RM, Madden CM: Intramuscular meperidine, promethazine, and chlorpromazine; analysis of use and complications in 487 pediatric emergency department patients, *Ann Emerg Med* 18:528-533, 1989.

36. Terndrup TE: Pain control, analgesia and sedation. In Barkin RM, editor: *Pediatric emergency medicine: concepts and clinical practice*, St Louis, 1992, Mosby.

5 *Infiltration and Nerve Block Anesthesia*

Effective anesthesia is essential for a successful patient intervention and wound repair. As with any procedure, success depends on a thorough understanding of the properties of anesthetic solutions and injection techniques. The choice of anesthetics and techniques must be individualized for every patient. The type, location, extent of the wound, and estimated length of time for repair are variables that make each patient unique. Besides technical considerations, patients have differing emotional characteristics and responses. They often fear that injections and needles will cause excessive pain. Therefore a clear explanation of the procedure and gentle handling will gain the confidence of the patient and ease any apprehension.

PHARMACOLOGY OF LOCAL ANESTHETICS

Although the knowledge and science of local anesthetics are extensive, there are characteristics and behaviors of these solutions specific to the wound care setting. These characteristics are described in the following sections: mechanism of blockade, onset of action, duration of anesthesia, differential blockade, and addition of epinephrine.

Mechanism of blockade: On injection, local anesthetics infiltrate tissues and diffuse across neural sheaths and membranes. They act by interfering with neural depolarization and transmission of impulses along axons. Prevention of sodium influx across

53

nerve membranes is considered the physiologic basis for impulse conduction blockade. As sodium influx decreases, there is a decrease in the rate of rise in amplitude of the polarization. As a result there is inadequate formation of action potential and, with no action potential, there is no nerve impulse. Without nerve impulses, anesthesia is achieved.

Onset of action: Although onset of action is just one of many physiologic actions of local anesthetics, it is important to a busy emergency physician because the saving of even a few minutes can contribute to the overall effectiveness of that physician in a hectic emergency department. Onset of action is influenced by technique of injection, concentration of the solution, nerve fiber diameter, total dose, the addition of epinephrine, pH manipulations, and physiochemical determinants such as pKa, lipid solubility, and protein binding. Local infiltration of a laceration brings on rapid anesthesia. If the anesthetic is delivered at the interface of the superficial fascia and dermis, nerve fibers are very vulnerable to immediate blockade. Wound cleansing and suturing can begin almost immediately. A slightly shorter onset of action is yielded by 2% solutions than 1% solutions, but clinically speaking, this effect is negligible.[19] The addition of epinephrine and the buffering of local anesthetics also can shorten the onset of action and is discussed later in this chapter.

When blocking larger nerve trunks such as digital nerves, onset of action is significantly slower. Technique of delivery is very important, and knowledge of anatomy can mean the difference between a successful and an unsuccessful blockade. A bolus of local anesthetic delivered immediately adjacent to a digital nerve can lead to complete digital anesthesia within 1 to 2 minutes. Poor technique and delivery of that bolus even 2 or 3 ml from the nerve trunk can delay onset of action or lead to inadequate blockade and the need for repeat injection.

The two most commonly used wound care anesthetics, lidocaine and mepivacaine, have similar physiochemical profiles with similar onsets of action. Bupivacaine, on the other hand, has physiochemical properties that delay onset of action but in return provides for much greater duration of action than lidocaine or mepivacaine.

Duration of anesthesia: Protein binding of local anesthetic solutions is the primary determinant of duration of action. Bupivacaine, which is 95% protein bound, remains in the sodium channel longer than lidocaine (64% bound) and mepivacaine (78% bound). Duration of action is significantly affected by vasoactivity of the anesthetic, blood supply of the region anesthetized, and the addition of epinephrine to anesthetic solutions. Of the commonly used anesthetics, lidocaine produces the most vasodilation. The duration of action can be significantly shortened in areas such as the face. Additionally, vasodilation can cause excessive bleeding in a wound during repair. The addition of epinephrine to lidocaine eliminates unwanted bleeding and extends the action of lidocaine by 1 hour on facial lacerations and up to 5 hours for extremity injuries.[30] Bupivacaine, without epinephrine, also extends the duration of action 2 to 4 hours when compared with lidocaine alone.

Differential blockade: Myelin sheath coverings of nerve fibers within axons vary in diameter and thickness. Fibers that carry stimuli from pain receptors in the skin have no myelin sheath and have the smallest diameter. The sensations of pressure and touch, as well as motor impulses, are transmitted by larger, myelinated fibers. The thin pain fibers are more rapidly and easily blocked by local anesthetic solutions. This fact is significant in wound care because a solution of 1% lidocaine might only block pain stimuli but not the sensation of touch and pressure. Therefore an overly anxious patient may react to touch and pressure as if it were pain. A higher concentration of lidocaine or mepivacaine, for example, 2%, abolishes all awareness of stimuli and allows for unimpeded repair. Adding epinephrine to these solutions also achieves the same effect.

Addition of epinephrine: Adding epinephrine to local anesthetic solutions increases the duration of action and the amount of drug that can be used. The extended action ranges from 1.3 times to 10 times longer than lidocaine alone.[30] The extension of time is shorter on the face than other body locales. The most useful property of epinephrine is to decrease the amount of bleeding in a wound during laceration repair. There are potential but infrequent complications to its use. The most serious side effect, ischemia, can occur if epinephrine containing anesthetics are improperly injected into fingers, toes, tip of the nose, pinna of the ear, or penis. In susceptible patients, it can cause palpitations and tremors. Because the concentrations used are low (1:100,000 or 1:200,000) and the amounts small, risk is limited. Aspiration before injection is particularly important when using anesthetic solutions with epinephrine to avoid the potential serious consequences of direct intravascular bolusing. Known coronary artery disease and hypertension are relative contraindications to the use of these solutions.

TOXICITY OF LOCAL ANESTHETICS

The injection of local anesthetics can cause three toxic reactions. These are cardiovascular reactions, excitatory central nervous system effects, and vasovagal syncope secondary to pain and anxiety. Cardiovascular reactions include hypotension and bradycardia and are caused by a myocardial inhibitory effect of the anesthetic.[11] Local anesthetic solutions can cause excitatory phenomena in the central nervous system that ultimately can culminate in seizure activity. Both the cardiovascular and nervous system effects are commonly caused by an inadvertent injection of a solution directly into a vessel, causing a bolus effect on the heart or brain. Therefore a key principle in the use of local anesthetics is always to aspirate the syringe before injection to check for blood return. If blood is aspirated, the needle has to be moved to avoid injecting the solution into a vein or artery.

The most common reaction to local anesthetics is vasovagal syncope (fainting). The anxiety and pain of injection can cause dizziness, pallor, bradycardia, and hypotension. This reaction can largely be avoided with gentle handling of the patient; proper counseling; and slow, careful injection technique. No anesthetic infiltration is ever carried out on a patient who is not in the supine position. Preferably, the patient should also be placed so that he or she cannot see the injection being administered.

Local complications to anesthetic infiltration are unusual but can include infection; hematoma formation; and, potentially, permanent nerve damage to peripheral nerves anesthetized during block procedures.

Management of the Toxic Reaction

Treatment of toxic reactions is largely supportive. The airway is appropriately protected and ventilations are maintained. Hypotension and bradycardia are usually self-limited and can be reversed by placing the patient in the Trendelenburg position. An intravenous line is started with normal saline, and a bolus of 250 to 500 ml is infused to counteract hypotension in any patient who does not respond to that maneuver. Cardiac monitoring with frequent vital signs is instituted. Seizures are also self-limited but may need to be controlled by intravenous diazepam (Valium).

ALLERGY TO LOCAL ANESTHETICS

Allergic reactions are uncommon with the newer amide local anesthetics, such as lidocaine, mepivacaine, and bupivacaine. Reactions were more frequent with the older ester solutions, procaine and tetracaine.[22] Multiple-dose vials still contain the preservative methylparaben, which has been implicated as a possible mediator of allergic responses.[19] Allergic reactions are characterized by either delayed appearances of skin rashes or the acute onset of localized or general urticaria. Rarely, outright anaphylactic shock can occur. True allergic responses occur in less than 1% of patients receiving local anesthetics.[22] This observation has been confirmed in a study of 59 patients who reported prior reactions to local anesthetic agents. None responded adversely to skin testing and provocative drug challenge.[9]

Management of Allergic Responses

Allergic responses are managed in the standard manner with airway control; establishment of intravenous access; and by administering epinephrine, diphenhydramine, and steroids as needed.

Alternatives for the Allergic Patient

Because patients cannot always accurately describe a prior adverse reaction to a local anesthetic and it is usually impossible to perform skin testing in an emergency department setting, the clinician may be faced with a patient who is truly allergic to local anesthetics. The following strategies are suggested:

- Use no anesthetic at all for calm patients who have very small lacerations. Often the pain of injection exceeds the pain of placing two or three sutures.
- Ice placed directly over the wound can provide a short period of decreased pain sensation.

- Because the preservative methylparaben has been implicated in allergic reactions, use local anesthetic preparations prepared for spinal, epidural, and intravenous anesthesia. They are preservative free. They can be obtained from the operating suite of the hospital.
- If the allergy-causing drug can be identified as an ester (tetracaine, benzocaine, chloroprocaine, cocaine, procaine), then it can be substituted with an amide (lidocaine, mepivacaine, bupivacaine, Benadryl).
- Diphenhydramine (Benadryl) has similar properties to standard local anesthetics.[24] When compared with lidocaine, it provides adequate anesthesia for laceration repair for at least 30 minutes.[12] When compared with lidocaine, it is not as effective for procedures longer than 30 minutes. A 50 mg (1 ml) vial is diluted in a syringe with 4 ml of normal saline to produce a 1% solution. Local infiltration is carried out in the usual manner. Diphenhydramine is more painful to inject than lidocaine, and this pain is not reduced by buffering.[13, 28]

PATIENT SEDATION

Patient sedation for emergency procedures has become a common strategy in the emergency department. Wound care can cause significant anxiety and discomfort, and patients can benefit by the administration of anxiolytics or pain relievers that supplement local anesthesia. Opiates, such as fentanyl and Demerol, and the benzodiazepines—midazolam and diazepam—can be delivered orally or parenterally for this purpose. They can also be given in combination for good effect. Other sedative agents that have been studied in this setting include nitrous oxide; ketamine; and the combination "cocktail" of Demerol, promethazine, and chlorpromazine. Commonly used sedative agents are summarized in Table 5-1.

Midazolam is an effective anxiolytic that comes in oral, intranasal, parenteral, and rectal forms.[16, 27, 32] Intravenously it achieves sedation in 3 to 5 minutes and has an elimination half-life of 1 hour. Alone, or in combination with fentanyl, it has become a commonly used emergency department sedative. When administered intranasally, orally, or rectally, its onset of action is slower and elimination half-life longer. Because of midazolam's bitter taste, it becomes more acceptable when mixed with fruit juice. Intranasally it can cause a burning sensation. Hypoxia and oversedation are its most significant, but uncommon, side effects. Therefore administration needs to be in a controlled setting with readily available airway and resuscitation equipment. The reversal agent, flumazenil, is effective if needed to reverse the actions of this benzodiazepine.

Fentanyl is a synthetic opioid with properties that make it an excellent agent for immediate pain relief and support invasive procedures.[5] Peak effect after intravenous administration is 2 minutes with a duration of action of 30 to 90 minutes. Unlike other opioids, fentanyl does not commonly cause nausea and vomiting (less than 1% of patients). Its most serious side effect is respiratory depression that can be readily reversed with naloxone.

Table 5-1   *Agents for Sedation in Wound Care Procedures*

Agent(s)	Initial Dose[†]	Route
Midazolam	0.03–0.05 mg/kg	IV
	0.2–0.3 mg/kg	Intranasal*
	0.3–0.5 mg/kg	Oral
Diazepam	0.05–0.10 mg/kg	IV
Fentanyl	0.5–1.0 µg/kg	IV
	20–25 µg/kg	Oral transmucosal*
Meperidine	1.0–2.0 mg/kg	IV, IM
DPT (Demerol/Phenergan/ Thorazine)	2:1:1 mg/kg (maximum 50:25:25 mg in children)	IM*

From Yealy DM, Dunmire SM, Paris PM: Pharmacologic adjuncts to painful procedures. In Roberts TR, Hedges TR, editors: *Clinical procedures in emergency medicine,* Philadelphia, 1991, Saunders.
*Suggested for pediatric sedation and analgesia.
[†]Often two doses are needed to obtain adequate sedation in many patients. The use of additional doses should be based on individual responses. In the elderly, smaller doses should be used in an incremental fashion. IV, intravenously; IM, intramuscularly.

A well-studied, and commonly used since the 1950s, sedation method is the combination of meperidine (Demerol), promethazine (Phenergan), and chlorpromazine (Thorazine).[29] Onset of action after intramuscular administration is approximately 30 minutes with a duration of action of 1½ to 2 hours. Serious complications, such as hypoxia, are uncommon, but vomiting can occur in as many as 10% to 15% of patients. Full recovery, that is, back to normal activity, averages almost 20 hours.[29] The newer, shorter acting agents have effectively replaced this drug combination.

Although ketamine has been in use for years to sedate pediatric patients for invasive procedures, there is less experience in its use in the emergency department.[5] Most experience with ketamine use is in the intravenous or intramuscular form. This drug can cause a dissociative reaction in the patient during administration, as well as an emergence reaction in which there is misperception by the patient of visual and auditory stimuli. Only recently has ketamine been studied in its oral form in patients requiring laceration repair.[26] Significant anxiety reduction and sedation were noted without the occurrence of major side effects. Minor side effects, however, occur in up to 26% of patients. Parenteral ketamine requires significant experience and operator comfort with its sedation profile. Further studies of its oral use in wound care are needed to fully delineate its appropriate use in that setting.

Nitrous oxide is both a sedative and an analgesic substance that can provide effective

BOX 5-1

Procedure for Conscious Sedation in Painful Wound Care and Abscess Drainage Interventions

1. Establish an intravenous infusion of normal saline (18-gauge catheter preferred in adults) in the supine patient with the bed rails in the up position.
2. Pulse, respiratory rate, blood pressure, and level of consciousness should be recorded intially, *after every dose of each agent, and every 5 to 10 minutes throughout the procedure.*
3. Continuous monitoring of oxygen saturation with a pulse oximeter probe (to maintain at >95% or no less than 3% to 5% less than the initial value) must be performed. Supplemental oxygen via nasal prongs can be administered based on need. ECG monitoring is optional but suggested in the elderly or those with a cardiac history.
4. A resuscitation cart with a bag-valve mask, oral and nasal airways, endotracheal tubes, and a functioning laryngoscope must be nearby. Suction equipment and naloxone should be at the bedside.
5. Administer 1 mg midazolam over 30 to 60 seconds; if after 3 to 5 minutes there is no evidence of mild sedation (subjective relaxation by the patient with mild drowsiness and normal or minimally altered speech), additional 1-mg doses can be administered in a similar fashion, up to a maximum of 0.1 mg/kg.* The goal is *mild sedation and anxiolysis,* achievable in most patients with 1 to 2 mg of midazolam.
6. Reassess clinical status (see 2).
7. Administer fentanyl[†] 100 µg (2 ml) over 60 seconds; this may be repeated in 0.5 to 1.0 µg/kg (50 to 100 µg) increments every 3 to 5 minutes until adequate analgesia and sedation have been obtained (slurred speech, ptosis, drowsy but responsive to painful and verbal stimuli, and good analgesia with initial stages of procedure). The maximal total dose recommended is 5 to 6 µg/kg.*
8. Administer local anesthesia if indicated (this often serves to help gauge effectiveness of systemic analgesia).
9. Perform the procedure. Additional doses of fentanyl may be required based on the response and length of the procedure.
10. If hypoxemia, deep sedation, or slowed respirations unresponsive to external stimuli are seen during or after procedure, ventilation should be assisted with a bag-valve mask and naloxone (0.4- to 0.8-mg increments) should be administered. Naloxone should not be given routinely at the termination of procedures, since it will abruptly reverse all analgesia.
11. Continue close observation until the patient is awake and alert, and discharge the patient only after a minimum 1 hour of further observation. Instruct the patient not to drive or operate dangerous machinery for at least 6 hours.

From Yealy DM, Dunmire SM, Paris TML: Pharmacologic adjuncts to painful procedures. In Roberts TR, Hedges TR, editors: *Clinical procedures in emergency medicine,* Philadelphia, 1991, Saunders.
*For children, fentanyl alone is suggested in 0.5 µg/kg increments up to a maximum total dose of 2 to 3 µg/kg.
[†]Sublimaze 50 µg/ml.

procedure sedation. Equipment requirements and operator experience make this a method of sedation with limited usefulness in laceration repair and wound care.

The "best" sedative for anxious and frightened patients, particularly children, is an empathic, calm, and sensitive approach resulting from experience. Most patients, if handled appropriately, can overcome their anxiety and cooperate with laceration repair and minor wound care. Active sedation has its place for complex and painful procedures, but the style and demeanor of the physician or nurse cannot be overemphasized.

Techniques for Sedation

Techniques, agents, and doses for sedation of children are covered in Chapter 4. Conscious sedation for adults is described in detail in Box 5-1.

ANESTHETIC SOLUTIONS

There are three anesthetic solutions commonly in use for local infiltration and simple nerve block (Table 5-2). These are lidocaine (Xylocaine 1% and 2%, with and without epinephrine), mepivacaine (Carbocaine 1% and 2%), and bupivacaine (Marcaine 0.25% and 0.5%). The amide derivatives have largely replaced the older ester compounds like procaine (Novocain).

Lidocaine (Xylocaine)

Lidocaine is the most commonly used anesthetic solution. The drug has a rapid onset of action that is almost immediate in local infiltration. Lidocaine's tissue-spreading proper-

Table 5-2 *Local Anesthetic for Wound Care*

Agent	Concentration	Onset of Action Infiltration	Block	Duration of Action for Blocks	Maximum Allowable Single Dose
Lidocaine (Xylocaine)	1%, 2%	Immediate	4-10 Min	30-120 Min	4.5 mg/kg of 1% (30 ml per average adult)
Lidocaine with epinephrine	1%	Immediate	4-10 Min	60-240 Min	7 mg/kg of 1% (50 ml per average adult)
Mepivacaine (Carbocaine)	1%, 2%	Immediate	6-10 Min	90-180 Min	5 mg/kg of 1% (40 ml per average adult)
Bupivacaine (Marcaine, Sensorcaine)	0.25% 0.5%	Slower	8-12 Min	240-480 Min	3 mg/kg of 0.25% (70 ml per average adult) 30cc
Topical anesthesia	See text	5-15 Min	—	20-30 Min	2-5 ml of mixture

ties are good, and it readily penetrates nerve sheaths. Duration of action for nerve blocks is approximately 75 minutes with a range of 60 to 120 minutes. Although there is no clear information in the literature concerning the duration of action for direct wound infiltration, the anesthetic effect appears to wear off much sooner, in approximately 20 to 30 minutes. A small group of patients appear to metabolize lidocaine very rapidly and require repeated local injections. With the addition of epinephrine, the duration of action is increased, and local hemostasis is better achieved. The maximum allowable doses of lidocaine and the other local anesthetics are summarized in Table 5-2.

Mepivacaine (Carbocaine)

Mepivacaine is widely used as an emergency wound anesthetic but has some properties that are different from lidocaine. The drug has a slightly slower onset of action: 6 to 10 minutes for a simple block. The duration of action is 30 to 60 minutes, somewhat longer than lidocaine. Mepivacaine has less of a vasodilatory effect than lidocaine and usually does not require the use of epinephrine for local wound area hemostasis.

Bupivacaine (Marcaine)

Bupivacaine is a newer amide that is becoming more widely used in emergency wound care. Although it is a very effective anesthetic, its chief drawback is that it has slow onset of action, approximately 8 to 12 minutes for simple blocks of small nerves. The main advantage of bupivacaine is its duration of action, which is considerably longer than lidocaine and mepivacaine. In a study comparing lidocaine with bupivacaine, no significant difference was noted in the pain of local infiltration, onset of action, and level of satisfactory anesthesia.[15] Because the anesthetic effects of bupivacaine lasted four times longer than lidocaine and significantly extended the period of pain relief, bupivacaine was recommended by the authors to be considered for anesthesia of lacerations sutured in the emergency department.

REDUCING THE "PAIN" OF ANESTHESIA
Anesthetic Buffering

Local anesthetic solutions are maintained at an acidic pH to ensure stability of the preparation and solubility. The low pH decreases the concentration of nonionized anesthetic, which is contrary to its mechanism of action. As a consequence, injection of unbuffered local anesthetic causes significant discomfort to the patient, and it has to undergo a pH change in the tissues to affect blockade.

It makes physiologic sense, and there are ample studies to support the addition of bicarbonate to local anesthetic solutions to reduce the pain of injection.[3, 20, 23] Additionally, buffering reduces the time to onset of anesthesia and increases the intensity of the blockade. However, buffering does reduce the shelf life of local anesthetics, and the excessive addition of bicarbonate can cause visible precipitation within the anesthetic vials. It appears that lidocaine alone when buffered with bicarbonate has a shelf life of at least 7 days.[4] Buffering has also been shown to degrade epinephrine, up to 20% of the total, within 24 hours in open containers exposed to light.[21] On the other hand, buffered solutions containing epinephrine do not show any significant epinephrine degradation in a 72-hour period if kept in a closed container that is stored in the dark. Shelf life studies of buffered mepivacaine and bupivacaine have not been carried out.

The following techniques are recommended for the buffering of local anesthetics:

- Lidocaine (Xylocaine): 1 ml of bicarbonate per 9 ml of 1% lidocaine; buffering of 2% solutions may cause precipitates; shelf life 7 days
- Mepivacaine (Carbocaine): 0.5 to 1 ml of bicarbonate per 9 ml of mepivacaine; shelf life unknown after 24 hours
- Bupivacaine (Marcaine): 0.1 ml of bicarbonate per 20 ml of bupivacaine; shelf life unknown after 24 hours

When mixing a 20 ml lidocaine or mepivacaine vial, remove 2 ml of anesthetic and replace it with 2 ml of the bicarbonate. This technique not only ensures the correct buffering mixture but also maintains the original volume of solution in the vial. Because shelf life is shortened, the vial should be marked or labeled with the date of preparation.

Bicarbonate is available in solutions of 8.4% sodium bicarbonate stored as 50 milliequivalents per 50 ml (1 mEq/ml). Multidose vials of this preparation are available. An easily available supply of bicarbonate, although an expensive and inefficient use of this preparation, is the standard 50 ml 8.4% sodium bicarbonate Abboject syringe used during major patient resuscitations.

Anesthetic Warming

The warming of local anesthetics has not been conclusively shown to reduce the pain of anesthetic injection. While some investigators have reported a benefit, others have not.[1, 18] The added effort of warming either vials or syringes of anesthetic to 37° to 40° C and rapidly injecting the solution before cooling might not add real value to the care of the patient.

Choice of Needles

Experienced operators doing wound care often limit themselves to 27- or 30-gauge needles. Not only is a small gauge likely to reduce the pain of needle insertion but it reduces the rate of injection. Rapid injection and tissue expansion is significantly more painful than slow injection.[1]

On the other hand, considerable experience is necessary in handling small diameter needles. They bend easily, and it can be difficult to judge the amount of anesthetic injected without observing plunger movement past the syringe hatch marks. It is recommended that inexperienced operators become familiar with the properties of a 25-gauge needle before proceeding to smaller gauge 27- and 30-gauge needles. The 25-gauge 1½-inch needle can be used for most local infiltration procedures, as well as facial and digital blocks.

ANESTHESIA TECHNIQUES

Most minor lacerations and wounds can be managed by administering a local anesthetic directly into or around (parallel to) the wound area. Other wounds are best served by the application of a nerve block. The following are descriptions of the techniques for administering local anesthetics most useful in emergency wound and laceration repair.

Topical Anesthesia

Topical anesthesia is an established method to anesthetize uncomplicated lacerations.[22] Pediatric patients are ideal candidates for this technique. It requires no injection and can be administered by the parent. Because of the profuse vascularity of those areas, lacerations of the face and scalp are more effectively anesthetized than the trunk or proximal extremities. Because of tissue absorption of topical agents, this technique is best limited to lacerations of 5 cm or less. Contraindicated sites include the finger, toe, nose, pinna of the ear, and penis. Care is taken to avoid mucous membranes. The death of a 7½-month-old infant whose nasal mucous membranes and lips were inadvertently exposed to 10 ml of the solution underscores the need to be cautious.[10]

Experimentally TAC has been associated with a higher potential for wound infection.[2] However, in a study of 158 primarily pediatric patients this potential for increased infection was not observed when TAC was compared with local needle infiltration.[25]

Numerous topical anesthetic mixtures have a comparable efficacy. They can be divided into those solutions that do or do not contain cocaine. This ingredient increases the cost and raises issues of storage and handling. Because cocaine was one of the original components of TAC and this preparation has proven efficacy, it remains in use. On the other hand, preparations without cocaine are comparable in their effectiveness and are gaining favor with practitioners. Topical anesthetics are commonly prepared as liquids but can be mixed in gels.[7] Gels can decrease the risk of mucosal exposure and possibly reduce the total dose delivered. The following is a range of topical anesthetic alternatives:

- TAC: The original preparation contains tetracaine (0.5%), epinephrine (1:2000 concentration), and cocaine (11.8%)
- TAC, ½ strength: Tetracaine (1%), epinephrine (1:2000), and cocaine (4%)[31]
- TAC, ½ strength: Tetracaine (0.25%), epinephrine (1:4000), and cocaine (5.9%)[8]
- LAT: Tetracaine (1%), epinephrine (1:2000), and lidocaine (4%)[14]
- TLE: Lidocaine (5%) and epinephrine (1:2000)[6]

These figures represent the final concentrations and dilutions when calculated amounts of each ingredient are combined and brought to a predetermined volume with saline. Preparation of a topical anesthetic solution should be carried out by or under the supervision of a pharmacist.

Technique for Topical Anesthesia

A 2 × 2 inch sponge is saturated, but should not be dripping with solution. The sponge is placed in and around the laceration and left for at least 20 minutes. Shorter application

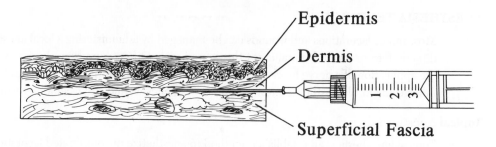

FIG. 5-1   The plane of anesthesia for local skin infiltration is just below the dermis at the junction of the superficial fascia (subcutaneous tissue).

times are associated with higher failure rates. Once the sponge is fashioned to conform with the wound, it can be secured with tape. Additionally, the caregiver or parent should apply gentle manual pressure over the taped sponge. Gloves are recommended to prevent absorption by the caregiver. Common errors include failure to place a sponge fold into the wound, "dabbing" the wound, or releasing the manual pressure prematurely. For small lacerations cotton swabs soaked with the solution can be used.

Complete anesthesia is reached when a zone of blanching is observed around the wound. The maximum dose of the solution is 2 to 5 ml. The average wound requires 2 to 3 ml. In approximately 5% of wounds supplemental infiltration is required to achieve complete anesthesia.[8]

Direct Wound Infiltration
Indications

Direct infiltration through the wound is indicated for most minimally contaminated lacerations in anatomically uncomplicated areas. Injecting directly into the wound is technically easy to do and, because intact skin is not pierced, needlestick pain is less. Some patients may express concern, or even alarm, at this prospect. Explaining the advantage of less pain will allay those fears.

Anatomy

The proper plane of injection is immediately beneath the dermis at the junction of the superficial fascia (Fig. 5-1). Tissue resistance is less in this plane, and sensory nerves are easily reached by the spreading solution. Trying to inject directly into the dermis meets with great resistance. Injecting deep down into the fatty fascia unnecessarily delays onset.

Technique for Direct Infiltration

Direct infiltration can be carried out with 25-, 27-, or 30-gauge needles of varying lengths (½ inch to 1¼ inches). Insert the needle through the open wound into the su-

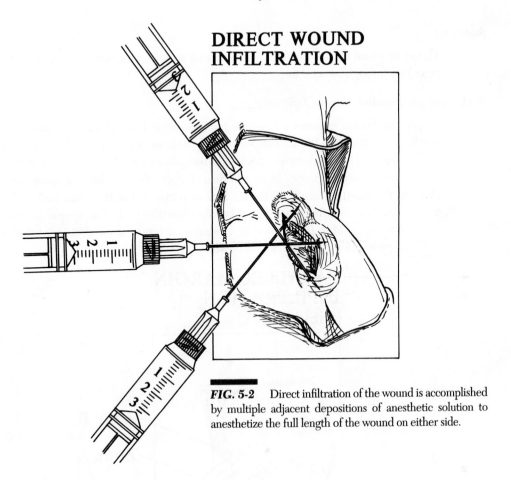

DIRECT WOUND INFILTRATION

FIG. 5-2   Direct infiltration of the wound is accomplished by multiple adjacent depositions of anesthetic solution to anesthetize the full length of the wound on either side.

perficial fascia (subcutaneous fat) parallel to and just deep to the dermis (Fig. 5-2). Inject a small bolus of anesthetic solution. Remove the needle and inject another bolus at an adjacent site, but just inside the margin of anesthesia of the previous injection. This ensures greater patient comfort. Repeat this process until all edges and corners of the wound are anesthetized. A simple laceration approximately 3 to 4 cm in length requires 3 to 5 ml of an anesthetic solution.

Parallel Margin Infiltration (Field Block)
Indications

This technique is an alternative to direct wound infiltration and has the advantage of requiring fewer needlesticks. It is preferred in wounds that are grossly contaminated so that the needle does not inadvertently carry debris or bacteria into uncontaminated tissues, although this potential complication has not been clearly documented.

Anatomy

The same plane as described earlier for direct wound infiltration is used, but it is approached through intact skin.

Technique for Parallel Margin Infiltration

Parallel infiltration requires a 1¼- to 2-inch needle at least 25 gauge in diameter. The needle is inserted into the skin at one end of the laceration. The needle is advanced to the hub parallel to the dermis-superficial fascia plane (Fig. 5-3). Aspiration is followed by slow injection of a "track" of anesthetic as the needle is withdrawn down the tissue plane to the insertion site. The needle is then reinserted at the distal end of the first track where the skin is beginning to become anesthetized. The second insertion (if needed) is less painful. Reinsertion and injection is repeated on all sides of the wound until complete infiltration has been achieved.

PARALLEL MARGIN INFILTRATION
(Field Block)

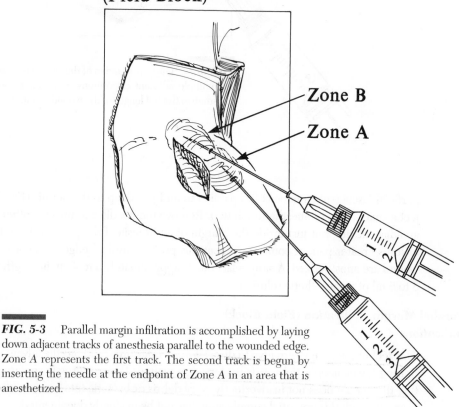

Zone B

Zone A

FIG. 5-3 Parallel margin infiltration is accomplished by laying down adjacent tracks of anesthesia parallel to the wounded edge. Zone A represents the first track. The second track is begun by inserting the needle at the endpoint of Zone A in an area that is anesthetized.

Supraorbital and Supratrochlear Nerve Blocks (Forehead Block)
Indications

Used for extensive lacerations and wounds of the forehead and anterior scalp.

Anatomy

The supraorbital and supratrochlear nerves supply sensation to the forehead and anterior scalp and exit from foramina located along the supraorbital ridge (Fig. 5-4).

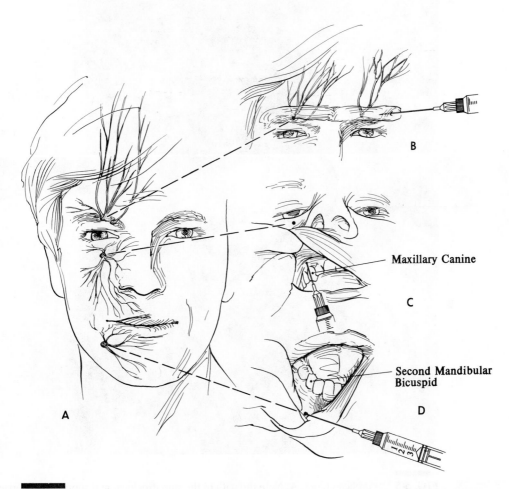

Maxillary Canine

Second Mandibular Bicuspid

FIG. 5-4   **A,** Position and course of the supraorbital, supratrochlear, infraorbital, and mental nerves. **B,** Technique for deposition of anesthesia to accomplish a supratrochlear and supraorbital (forehead) nerve block. **C,** Intraoral technique to anesthetize the infraorbital nerve. **D,** Intraoral technique to anesthetize the mental nerve.

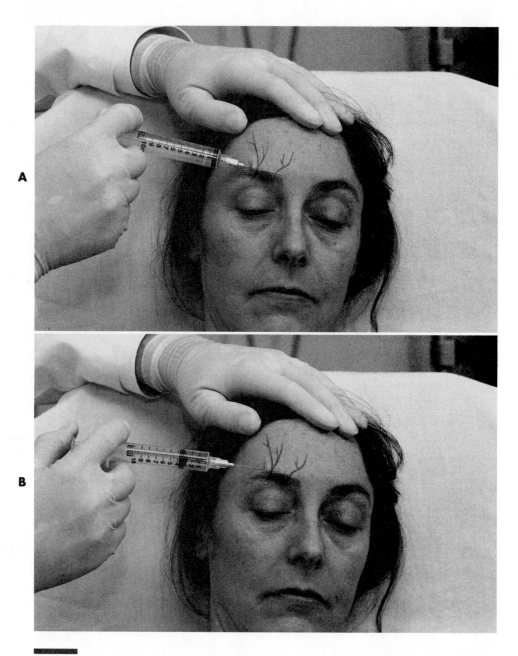

FIG. 5-5   Forehead block. **A,** Note the path of the supratrochlear and supraorbital nerves that originate from the superior orbital rim. The needle is inserted to its hub at the plane adjacent to the bone itself. **B,** Anesthetic is laid down in a continuous track as the needle is slowly withdrawn across the path of the nerves.

Technique for Forehead Block

The easiest manner to block the nerves, as well as their many branches, is to lay a continuous subcutaneous track at brow level as shown in Fig. 5-5. The actual injection technique is similar to that discussed earlier in the section on parallel margin infiltration. The plane of injection is just superficial to the bony plane. The needle is inserted to bone and then advanced until the hub is reached. The track laid down floods the nerves as they exit the foramina in the supraorbital rim.

Infraorbital Nerve Block
Indications

Lacerations of the upper lip are very common. Local anesthetic infiltration can cause anatomic distortion leading to difficulty with exact wound edge approximation and repair. An infraorbital nerve block can circumvent this problem. This block can also be used to repair lacerations of the lateral-inferior portion of the nose and lower eyelid.

Anatomy

The location and distribution of the infraorbital nerve is illustrated in Fig. 5-4, *A*. The infraorbital foramen is located approximately 1.5 cm below the inferior rim of the orbit and 2 cm from the lateral edge of the nose. This foramen can often be palpated. (Fig. 5-6, *A*).

Technique for Infraorbital Nerve Block

The infraorbital nerve can be approached both intraorally and extraorally, although the intraoral route has been shown to be significantly less painful. By the intraoral route the upper lip is retracted, revealing the maxillary canine tooth. Before actual injection, the site of needle entry into the buccal mucosa can be pretreated with a topical anesthetic like viscous lidocaine (Xylocaine viscous). A cotton-tipped applicator soaked in this solution is applied to the gingival-buccal margin for 1 to 2 minutes before the insertion of the needle (Fig. 5-6, *B*). The needle is introduced at the gingival-buccal margin at the anterior margin of the maxillary canine (Fig. 5-6, *C*). It is advanced parallel and just superficial to the maxillary bone until the infraorbital foramen is reached. If paresthesia results, pull the needle back slightly before injection to avoid injecting into the foramen and causing unwanted pressure on the nerve. Deposit 1 to 3 ml of anesthetic and anesthesia results within 4 to 6 minutes. If there is uncertainty about the precise location of the nerve, injection is carried out by depositing multiple small boluses in a "fan" configuration.

Mental Nerve Block
Indications

Used to repair lower lip lacerations without distorting the anatomy by local infiltration.

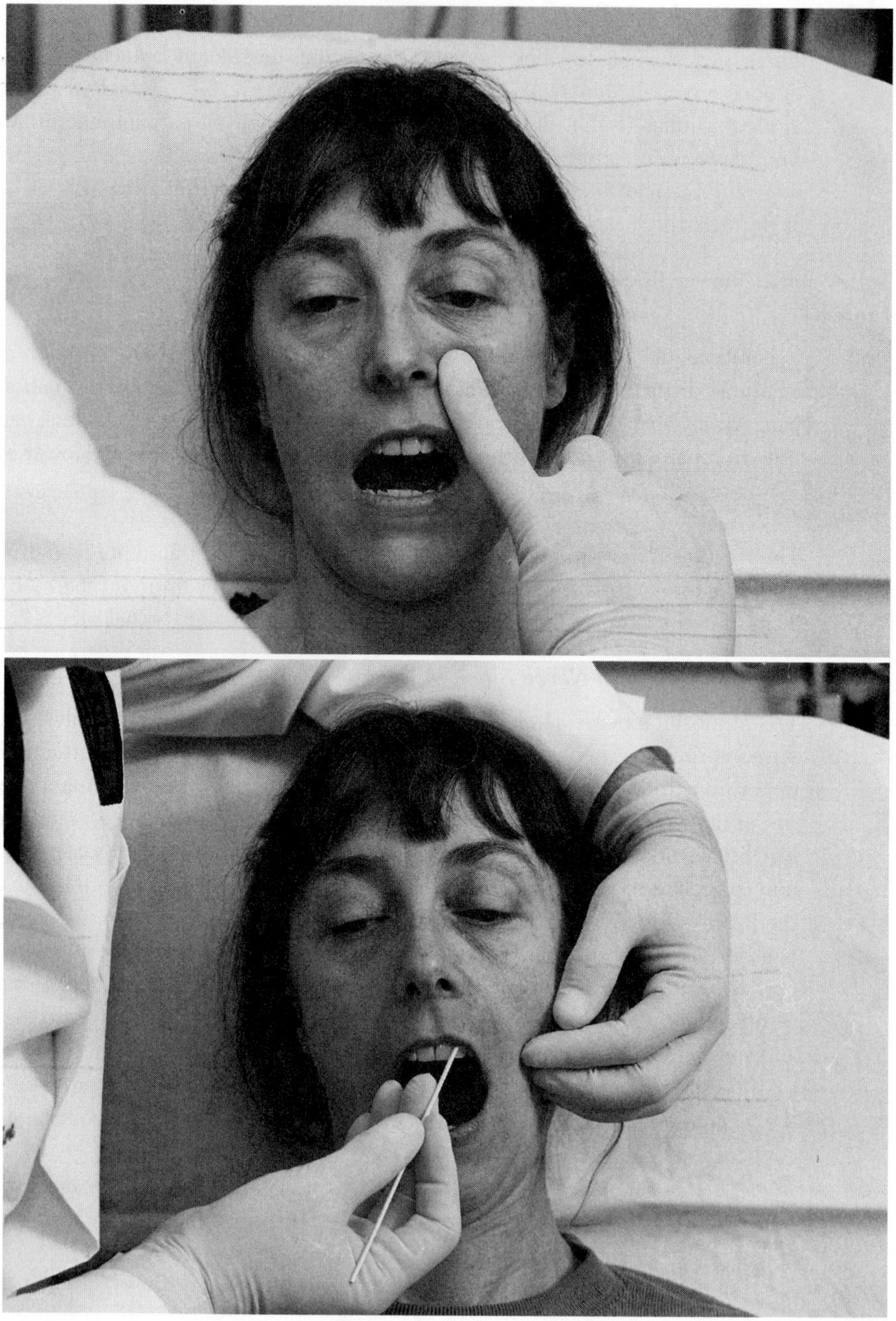

FIG. 5-6   For legend see opposite page.

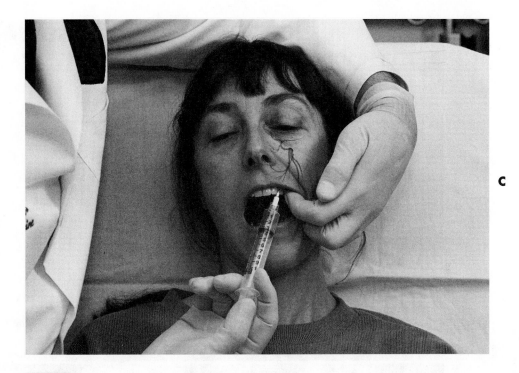

C

FIG. 5-6, cont'd   Infraorbital nerve block. **A,** The infraorbital foramen can be palpated before injection. **B,** A cotton-tip applicator soaked in a topical anesthetic, lidocaine gel, is applied to the mucosal site where the needle will be inserted. **C,** With gentle retraction of the lip, using the maxillary canine as the landmark, the needle is advanced, and anesthetic deposited at the infraorbital foramen. Note the path of the nerve as it exits the foramen.

Anatomy

The mental nerve foramen lies just inferior to the second mandibular bicuspid, midway between the upper and lower edges of the mandible, and 2.5 cm from the midline of the jaw. This nerve provides sensation to the lower half of the lip but only a portion of the chin. The mental foramen can be palpated as shown in Fig. 5-7, *A.*

Technique for Mental Nerve Block

As in the infraorbital technique, the mucosal injection site can be pretreated with viscous lidocaine as described earlier for the infraorbital nerve block (Fig. 5-7, *B*). The lower lip is retracted and the needle is introduced at the gingival-buccal margin inferior to the second bicuspid (Fig. 5-7, *C*). Once the foramen is approximated, 1 to 2 ml of anesthetic is injected after careful aspiration. Full anesthesia is achieved within 4 to 6 minutes. The fanning technique can be applied here as well.

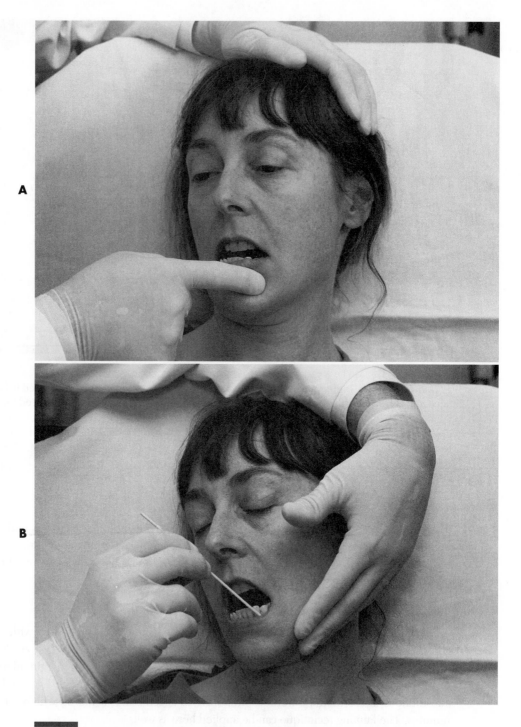

FIG 5-7   For legend see opposite page.

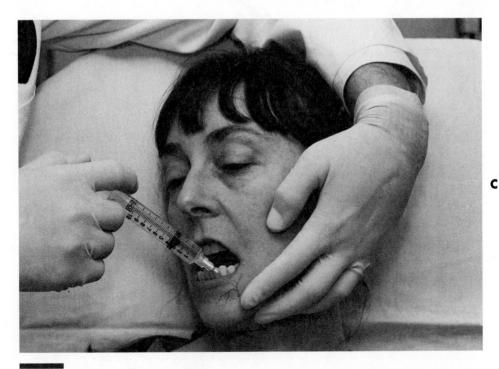

C

FIG 5-7, *cont'd*   Mental nerve block. **A,** The mental nerve foramen can be palpated before injection. **B,** Lidocaine gel is applied to the mucosal injection site. **C,** Using the second bicuspid as the landmark, the needle is advanced and the anesthetic is deposited at the foramen. Note the path of the nerve as it exits the foramen.

Auricular Block
Indications

Lacerations of the auricle of the ear are not uncommon. The skin is tightly adherent to the cartilaginous skeleton and the deposition of an anesthetic for large or complicated wounds can be difficult or may excessively distort the local tissue relationships. The auricular block is indicated for extensive repairs of the ear.

Anatomy

Sensory innervation of the auricle arises from branches of the auriculotemporal, greater auricular, and lesser occipital nerves. Sensory supply to the meatus derives additionally from the branch of the vagus. For this reason, an auricular block does not always completely block the meatal opening.

Technique for Auricular Block

The technical goal of the auricular block is to achieve circumferential anesthesia around the ear. Beginning just below the lobule, fully insert a 1½- to 2-inch 25-gauge needle attached to a preloaded syringe with 10 ml of anesthetic (without adrenalin) into the sul-

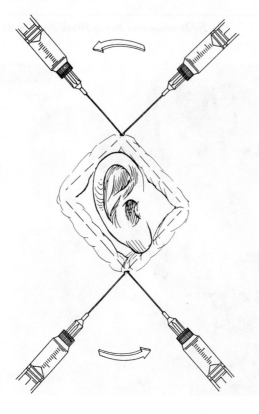

FIG. 5-8 Technique to achieve field anesthesia of the ear.

cus behind the ear, parallel and just superficial to the bone (Fig. 5-8). Leave approximately 2 to 3 ml of anesthetic in a track back to the insertion site. Without leaving the insertion site, redirect the needle anterior to the lobule and tragus. Leave a similar track in that area. Reload the syringe if necessary. Starting at a point just behind the superior portion of the helix, leave a similar track behind the superior portion of the ear. Again, without leaving the injection site, deposit a bolus of anesthetic backward from the tragus. Anesthesia should be complete in 10 to 15 minutes.

Digital Nerve Blocks (Finger and Toe Blocks)
Indications

The most common nerve block in minor wound care is the digital block. The block is the anesthetic method recommended for lacerations distal to the level of the midproximal phalanx of the finger or toe. It is the procedure preferred for nail removal, paronychia drainage, as well as repair of lacerations of the digits. A recent study has shown that digital block, as described here, is more effective and less painful than the metacarpal block to achieve finger anesthesia.[17]

Anatomy

There are four digital nerves for each finger or toe, including the thumb and great toe (Fig. 5-9). The palmar digital nerves have the most extensive sensory distribution and

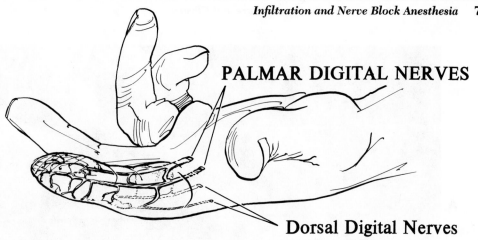

PALMAR DIGITAL NERVES

Dorsal Digital Nerves

FIG. 5-9 Illustration of the four digital nerves of the digit. Note that the two palmar digital nerves are dominant and provide sensation to the volar surface of the finger, as well as the entirety of the volar pad and nail bed area.

FIG. 5-10 Digital nerve block. To effectively block a digit, all four nerves, dorsal and volar, are approached as illustrated. The needle is introduced dorsally to first anesthetize the dorsal nerve. Without reinserting the needle, it is redirected towards the volar nerve and anesthetic deposited. The same procedure is carried out on the opposite side of the same digit to complete the block.

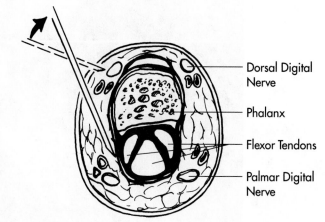

Dorsal Digital Nerve

Phalanx

Flexor Tendons

Palmar Digital Nerve

are responsible for distal finger and fingertip sensation, including the nail bed. Although the dorsal nerves have a lesser distribution, there is sufficient overlap with the palmar nerves that all four branches on each finger must be blocked to achieve complete digit anesthesia. The digital nerves are immediately adjacent to the phalanges and these structures act as landmarks for locating the nerves.

Techniques
Technique for Digital Block

Needle size can vary from 25- to 30-gauge. Small gauge needles, 27- and 30-gauge, require experience and technical comfort of the operator. The technique requires 2 needlesticks and 4 small injections of anesthetic. Fig. 5-10 illustrates the approach to the
Text continues on p. 80

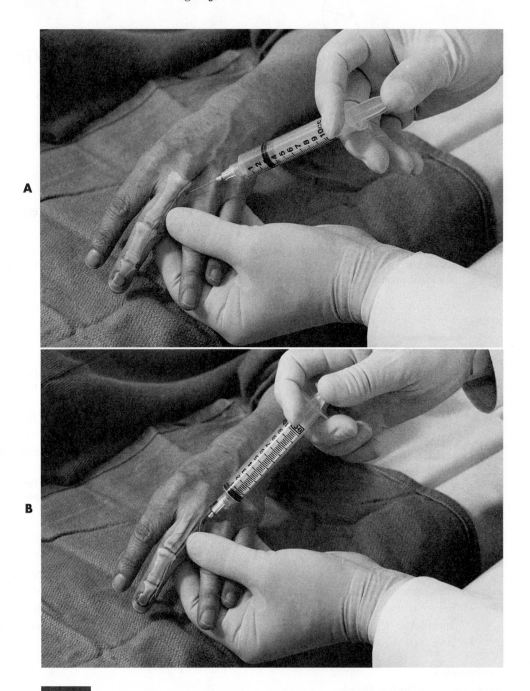

FIG. 5-11 Digital nerve block. Note the course of the volar and digital nerves. **A,** Within the web space, the needle is introduced and advanced towards the dorsal digital nerve. **B,** After deposition of the anesthetic, the needle is redirected, without withdrawing it from the skin, towards the volar nerve and anesthetic deposited.

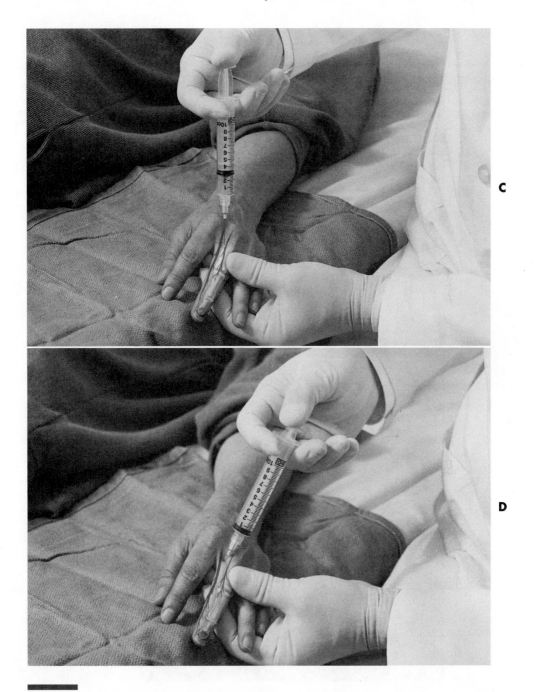

C

D

FIG. 5-11, *cont'd* **C** and **D,** Repeat the same steps on the opposite side of the same digit.

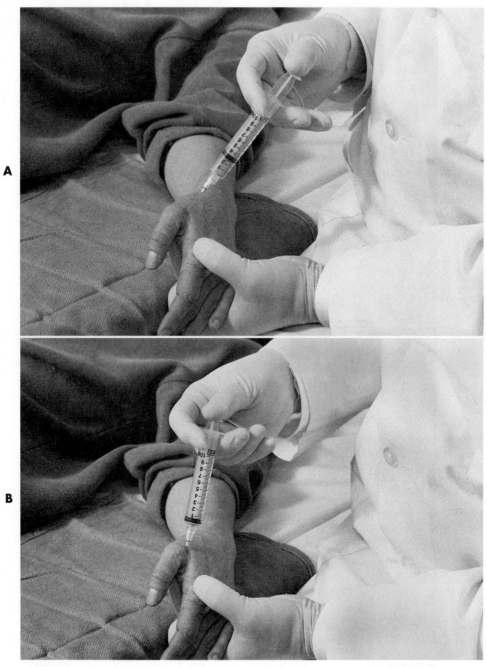

FIG. 5-12 Thumb block. The basic procedure for digital block can be carried out for the thumb. Note the nerve pathways as illustrated. **A,** Within the web space, the ulnar dorsal digital nerve to the thumb is blocked. **B,** Through the same injection site, the ulnar volar nerve is blocked after redirection of the needle.

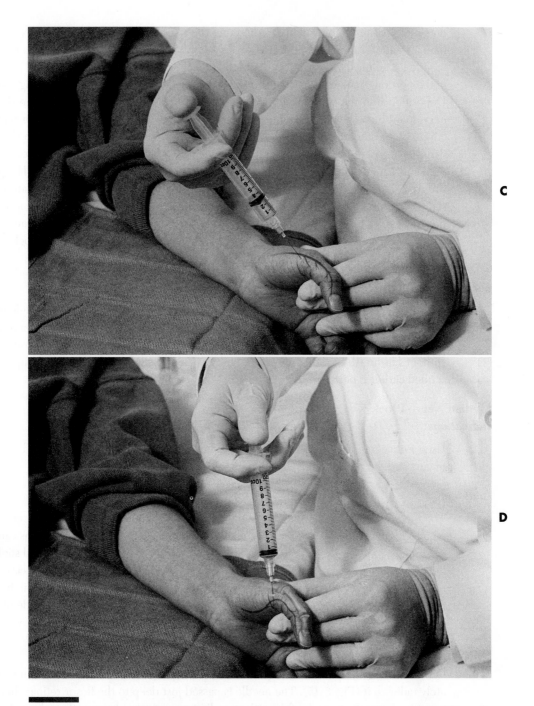

FIG. 5-12, *cont'd*   **C,** The radial dorsal digital nerve is approached as illustrated. **D,** After redirection, the radial volar nerve is blocked.

dorsal digital nerve followed by redirecting the needle to the palmar nerve. No more than a total of 4 ml of 1% lidocaine without epinephrine or 1% mepivacaine is recommended. The needle is introduced into the dorsal-lateral aspect of the proximal phalanx in the portion of the web space just distal to the metacarpal-phalangeal joint (Fig. 5-11). Deposition into the web space prevents build up of excessive pressure on the digital nerves and blood vessels. The needle is advanced until it touches bone. Approximately 0.5 ml of anesthetic is delivered to the dorsal digital nerve. The needle is then slightly withdrawn and redirected adjacent to the bone of the phalanx to the volar surface of the digit and 1 ml of solution is deposited at the site of the volar or palmar nerve. The procedure is repeated on the opposite side of the digit to achieve full finger or toe anesthesia. A complete block is usually achieved within 4 to 5 minutes. Maintaining close proximity of the nerve to the bone at all times will ensure good blockade because the course of the nerve is adjacent to bone. Fig. 5-12 illustrates the digital nerve block technique for the thumb.

Toe Block Technique

Because the second to fifth toes are relatively thin at the proximal phalanx, a single midline dorsal needlestick can be used to anesthetize both sides of the toe. After depositing the anesthetic on one side, the needle is withdrawn and passed down the opposite side without leaving the original puncture site (Fig. 5-13). Standard digital technique described earlier is best for the great toe.

Median Nerve Block
Indications

Used for lacerations and wounds of the palmar aspect of the thumb, index, and middle fingers and the radial half of the palm.

Anatomy

The median nerve can be found at the proximal flexor crease of the wrist between the palmaris longus and the flexor carpi radialis tendon (Fig. 5-14). The two tendons can be identified by having the patient voluntarily close his or her fingers into a fist and slightly flex the wrist. Some patients do not have a palmaris longus tendon, in which case the nerve is just radial to the flexor sublimis tendons of the fingers, which usually lie below the palmaris longus tendon. The nerve can also be located 1 cm to the ulnar side of the flexor carpi radialis.

Technique for Median Nerve Block

On identifying the palmaris longus tendon, a 25-gauge needle is introduced immediately radial to it (Fig. 5-15). The needle is passed just deep to the flexor retinaculum. A "popping" sensation can be felt as the needle traverses the dense retinaculum. An attempt is made to elicit paresthesias by passing the needle slowly deeper into the wrist. If

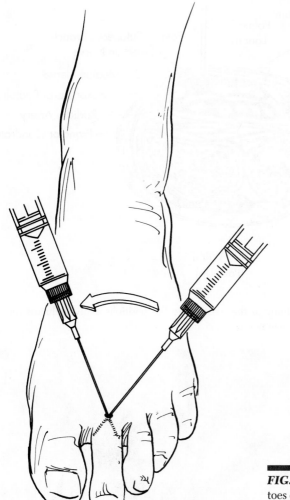

FIG. 5-13 Technique to provide anesthetic to toes other than the great toe (see text).

paresthesias are elicited, 2 ml of solution is deposited adjacent to but not into the nerve. If none are elicited, 3 to 5 ml of solution is injected, from deep to superficial as a track. Anesthesia might not be complete for at least 20 minutes.

Ulnar Nerve Block
Indications

Used for repair of wounds to the ulnar dorsal and palmar aspects of the hand, fifth finger, and ulnar side of the fourth finger.

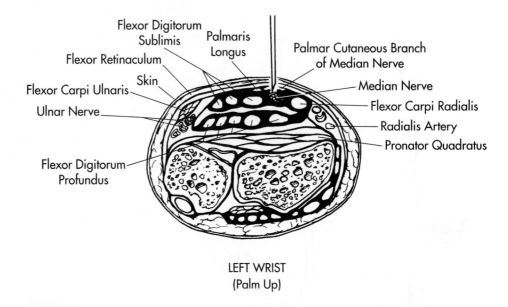

Flexor Digitorum Sublimis
Palmaris Longus
Palmar Cutaneous Branch of Median Nerve
Flexor Retinaculum
Skin
Flexor Carpi Ulnaris
Ulnar Nerve
Median Nerve
Flexor Carpi Radialis
Radialis Artery
Pronator Quadratus
Flexor Digitorum Profundus

LEFT WRIST
(Palm Up)

FIG. 5-14   Cross sectional anatomy of the wrist. Note the positions of the palmaris longus, flexor digitorum sublimus, and median nerve.

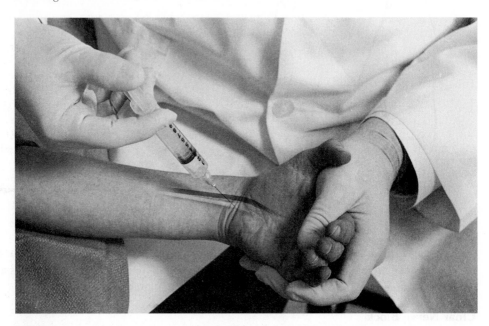

FIG. 5-15   Median nerve block. Note the position and path of the palmaris longus and median nerves. Immediately radial to the palmaris longus tendon, the needle is inserted throughout the flexor retinaculum towards the median nerve as described in the text.

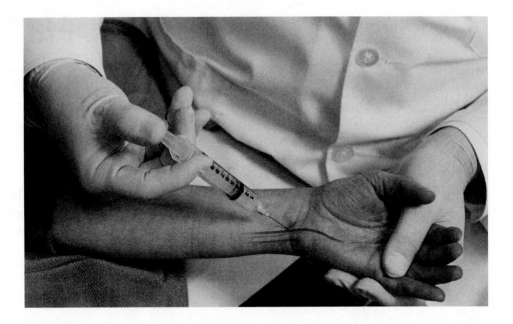

FIG. 5-16   Ulnar nerve block. The ulnar nerve lies deep to the flexor carpi ulnaris tendon as shown. The needle is inserted at the radial border of the tendon and directed toward the nerve. Because the nerve lies adjacent to the ulnar artery, great care is taken to aspirate before injection. See text.

Anatomy

The ulnar nerve has two branches that provide sensory innervation to the ulnar side of the hand. The palmar branch of the ulnar nerve is found immediately radial to the flexor carpi ulnaris tendon at the proximal wrist crease. It accompanies the ulnar artery. The dorsal branch of the ulnar nerve divides from the palmar branch approximately 4 to 5 cm proximal from the wrist and courses under the flexor carpi ulnaris tendon to the dorsal-ulnar side of the hand. Because of this division, both branches must be blocked to achieve successful anesthesia.

Technique for Ulnar Nerve Block

Using a 25-gauge 1¼- to 2-inch needle, attached to a 10- to 12-ml syringe, enter the wrist at the radial border of the flexor carpi ulnaris tendon (Fig. 5-16). Deposit anesthetic carefully and only after aspiration to prevent inadvertent ulnar arterial injection. If a paresthesia is elicited, deposit 3 to 5 ml. If no paresthesia occurs, in a small fanlike action, deposit the anesthetic. The nerve can also be approached from the ulnar aspect of the wrist. By inserting the needle lateral to the same tendon and slipping under it, the nerve can be blocked using the same amount of anesthetic. A block is achieved in 8 to 12 minutes. A separate branch, originating proximal to the wrist, of the ulnar nerve innervates the dorsum of the hand. To block that branch, a subcutaneous track of anesthetic is laid down from the dorsal midline of the wrist to the ulnar border of the flexor carpi ulnaris tendon.

Radial Nerve Block
Indications

Used for wounds located on the dorsum of the thumb, index, and middle fingers; and radial portion of the dorsum of the hand.

Anatomy

Approximately 7 cm proximal to the wrist a superficial cutaneous branch leaves the main radial nerve. At the level of the wrist, this branch begins to fan out into several rami that provide sensory innervation to the dorsal-radial aspect of the hand. These rami lie in the superficial fascia just deep to the skin.

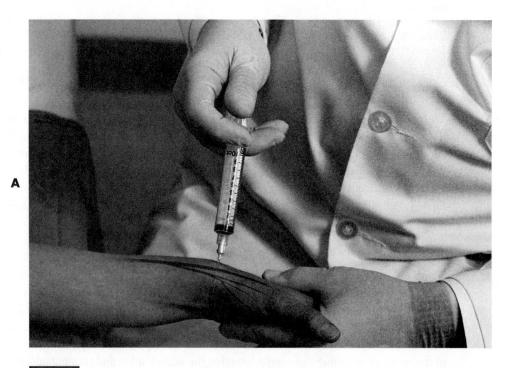

A

FIG. 5-17   Radial nerve block. **A,** Note location and branching of the radial nerve. The needle is introduced to its hub.

Technique for Radial Nerve Block

Starting at the dorso-radial aspect of the wrist, a continuous subcutaneous track of anesthetic is laid down to block all the sensory branches (Fig. 5-17). The technique is similar to that described for ulnar nerve blockade. Approximately 10 ml of anesthetic is required. Up to 8 to 12 minutes are necessary for this block to abolish sensation.

Sural and Tibial Nerve Block (Sole of Foot Blocks)
Indications

One of the most painful areas in which to inject local anesthetic is the sole of the foot. This area is commonly injured and subject to puncture wounds, lacerations, and the embedding of foreign bodies. Sural and tibial nerve blocks are recommended. These blocks are much less painful to the patient than direct infiltration.

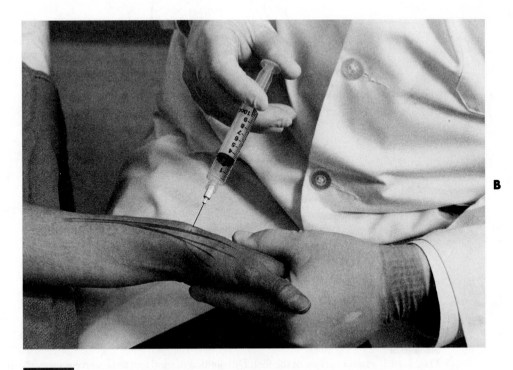

B

FIG. 5-17, *cont'd* **B,** A continuous track of anesthetic is laid down as the needle is withdrawn across the branches of the radial nerve.

Anatomy

The sural nerve courses behind the fibula and lateral malleolus to supply the heel and lateral aspect of the foot. The tibial nerve can be found between the Achilles tendon and the medial malleolus. It can be easily located because it accompanies the posterior tibial artery at that level. This nerve supplies a large portion of the sole and medial side of the foot. As denoted in Fig. 5-18, there is some overlap of distribution of these nerves, as well as some overlap of sensation with the anteriorly located saphenous and superficial peroneal nerves. Complete anesthesia is not always achieved by a single block. It can be supplemented by local infiltration with minimal discomfort to the patient because of the preexisting partial anesthesia from the block.

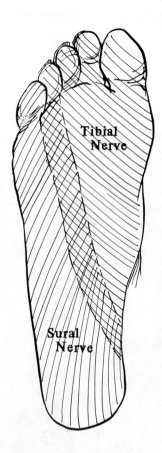

FIG. 5-18 Plantar surface of the foot. Distribution of sural and tibial nerve sensory component. Note that there is overlap between the two distributions.

Technique for Sural Nerve Block

The needle is introduced just lateral to the Achilles tendon approximately 1 to 2 cm proximal to the level of the distal tip of the lateral malleolus (Fig. 5-19). The needle is directed to the posterior medial aspect of the fibula, and 5 ml of anesthetic is deposited after aspiration of the syringe. To make sure all the branches of the sural nerve are properly infiltrated, a fan-shaped motion is made with the needle and multiple small boluses are delivered.

Technique for Posterior Tibial Nerve Block

The posterior tibial artery is palpated as a landmark. The needle is passed adjacent to the Achilles tendon toward the posterior tibial artery behind the medial malleolus (Fig. 5-20). Once the area of the artery is approximated, careful aspiration of the syringe is carried out. If there is no blood return, 5 ml of anesthetic is injected. Blocks of the posterior tibial and sural nerve take approximately 10 to 15 minutes to achieve appropriate anesthetic levels.

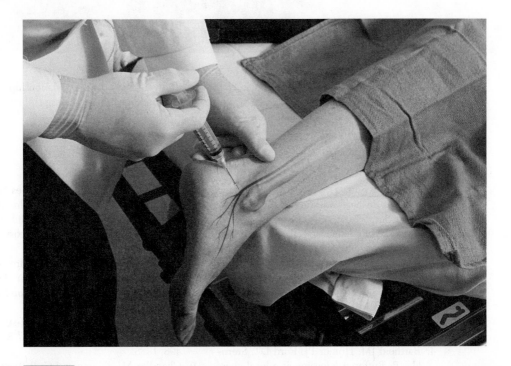

FIG. 5-19   Sural nerve block. Note the path of the sural nerve and its relationship to the tip of the fibula. Because of the branching of the nerve, the injection is carried out in a fanlike manner to create an effective block.

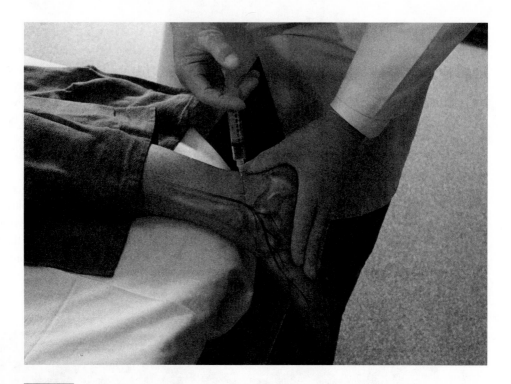

FIG. 5-20   Posterior tibial nerve block. Note the path of the nerve and its relationship to the tibial medial malleolus. Because the nerve travels in conjunction with the posterior tibial artery, care is taken to aspirate before injection.

REFERENCES

1. Arndt KA, Burton C, Noe JM: Minimizing the pain of local anesthesia, *Plast Reconstruct Surg* 72:676-679, 1983.
2. Barker W, Rodeheaver GT, Edgerton MT, et al: Damage to tissue defenses by a topical anesthetic agent, *Ann Emerg Med* 11:307-310, 1982.
3. Bartfield JM, Crisafulli KM, Raccio-Robak N, Salluzzo RF: The effects of warming and buffering on pain of infiltration of lidocaine, *Acad Emerg Med* 2:254-258, 1995.
4. Bartfield JM, Homer PJ, Ford DT, Sternklar P: Buffered lidocaine as a local anesthetic: an investigation of shelf life, *Ann Emerg Med* 21:16-19, 1992.
5. Berman D, Graber D: Sedation and analgesia, *Emerg Med Clinics N Am* 10:691-705, 1992.
6. Blackburn PA, Butler KH, Hughes MJ, et al: Comparison of tetracaine-adrenaline-cocaine (TAC) with topical lidocaine-epinephrine (TLE): efficacy and cost, *Am J Emerg Med* 13:315-317, 1995.
7. Bonadio WA, Wagner VR: Adrenaline-cocaine gel topical anesthetic for dermal laceration repair in children, *Ann Emerg Med* 21:1435-1438, 1992.
8. Bonadio WA, Wagner V: Half-strength TAC topical anesthetic, *Clin Ped* 27:495-498, 1988.
9. Chandler MJ, Grammer LC, Patterson R: Provocative challenge with local anesthetics in patients with a prior history of reaction, *J Allergy Clin Immunol* 79:883-886, 1987.

10. Dailey RH: Fatality secondary to misuse of TAC solution, *Ann Emerg Med* 17:159-160, 1988.

11. deJong R: Toxic effects of local anesthetics, *JAMA* 239:1166-1168, 1978.

12. Dire DJ, Hogan DE: Double-blinded comparison of diphenhydramine versus lidocaine as a local anesthetic, *Ann Emerg Med* 22:1419-1422, 1993.

13. Ernst AA, Marvez-Valls E, Nick TG, Wahle M: Comparison trial of four injectable anesthetics for laceration repair, *Acad Emerg Med* 3:228-233, 1996.

14. Ernst AA, Marvez-Valls E, Nick TG, Weiss SJ: LAT (lidocaine-adrenaline-tetracaine) versus TAC (tetracaine-adrenaline-cocaine) for topical anesthesia in face and scalp lacerations, *Am J Emerg Med* 13:151-154, 1995.

15. Fariss BL, Foresman PA, Rodeheaver GT, et al: Anesthetic properties of bupivacaine and lidocaine for infiltration anesthesia, *J Emerg Med* 5:275-282, 1987.

16. Hennes HM, Wagner V, Nonadio WA, et al: The effect of oral midazolam on anxiety of preschool children during laceration repair, *Ann Emerg Med* 19:1006-1009, 1990.

17. Knoop KJ, Trott AT, Syverud S: Comparison of digital versus metacarpal block for repair of finger injuries, *Ann Emerg Med* 23:1296-1300, 1994.

18. Mader TJ, Playe SJ, Garb JL: Reducing the pain of local anesthetic infiltration: warming and buffering have a synergistic effect, *Ann Emerg Med* 23:550-554, 1994.

19. Mather M, Cousins M: Local anesthetics and their current clinical use, *Drugs* 18:185-205, 1979.

20. McKay W, Morris R, Mushlin P: Sodium bicarbonate attenuates pain on skin infiltration with lidocaine, with or without epinephrine, *Anesth Analg* 66:572-574, 1987.

21. Murakami CS, Odland PB, Ross BR: Buffered local anesthetics and epinephrine degradation, *J Dermatol Surg Oncol* 20:192-195, 1994.

22. Norris RL: Local anesthetics, *Emerg Med Clinics N Am* 10:707-718, 1992.

23. Orlinsky M, Hudson C, Chan L, Deslauriers R: Pain comparison of unbuffered versus buffered lidocaine in local wound infiltration, *J Emerg Med* 10:411-415, 1992.

24. Pollack CV, Swindle GM: Use of diphenhydramine for local anesthesia in "caine"–sensitive patients, *J Emerg Med* 7:611-614, 1989.

25. Pryor G, Kilpatrick W, Opp D: Local anesthesia in minor lacerations: topical TAC versus lidocaine infiltration, *Ann Emerg Med* 9:568-571, 1980.

26. Qureshi FA, Mellis PT, McFadden MA: Efficacy of oral ketamine for providing sedation and analgesia to children requiring laceration repair, *Ped Emerg Care* 11:93-97, 1995.

27. Shane SA, Fuchs SM, Khine H: Efficacy of rectal midazolam for the sedation of preschool children undergoing laceration repair, *Ann Emerg Med* 24:1065-1073, 1994.

28. Singer AJ, Hollander JE: Infiltration pain and local anesthetic effects of buffered versus plain 1% diphenhydramine, *Acad Emerg Med* 2:884-888, 1995.

29. Terndrup TE, Dire DJ, Madden CM, et al: A prospective analysis of intramuscular meperidine, promethazine, and chlorpromazine in pediatric emergency department patients, *Ann Emerg Med* 20:31-35, 1991.

30. Todd K, Berk WA, Huang R: Effect of body locale and addition of epinephrine on the duration of action of a local anesthetic agent, *Ann Emerg Med* 21:723-726, 1992.

31. Vinci RJ, Fish SS: Efficacy of topical anesthesia in children, *Arch Ped Adolesc Med* 150:466-469, 1996.

32. Yealy DM, Ellis JH, Hobbs GD, Moscati RM: Intranasal midazolam as a desative for children during laceration repair, *Am J Emerg Med* 10:584-587, 1992.

6 *Wound Cleansing and Irrigation*

. . . .

Wound Cleansing Solutions
  Povidone-Iodine (Betadine)
  Chlorhexidine (Hibiclens)
  Nonionic Surfactants (Shur-Clens, Pharma Clens)
  Hexachlorophene (pHistlex)
  Quartenary Ammonium Compounds (Zephiran)
  Hydrogen Peroxide
Preparation for Wound Cleansing
  Hand Washing

Personnel Precautions
Wound Area Hair Removal
Anesthesia
Foreign Material
Wound Soaking
Wound Periphery Cleansing
Irrigation
Cleansing Setup and Procedures

Cleansing and irrigation are the foundation of good wound care. These steps can be time consuming and tedious. However, it is essential that all contaminants and devitalized tissue are removed before wound closure. If not, the risk of infection and a cosmetically poor scar are greatly increased. Neither clever suturing technique nor the use of prophylactic antibiotics can replace meticulous cleansing and irrigation, and, if needed, judicious debridement.

WOUND CLEANSING SOLUTIONS

Several skin-cleansing preparations are available commercially (Table 6-1). Most of the clinical data that compare the efficacy of these agents come from studies of elective surgery patients or experiments on laboratory animals.[2, 6, 18, 35] Only in recent years have there been reports detailing the use of skin-cleansing preparations in emergency department settings.[9, 13, 16] Based on these studies and the properties of the cleansing solutions, guidelines for use in emergency wound care can be suggested.

Povidone-Iodine (Betadine)

Povidone-iodine is a complex of the potent bactericidal agent iodine and the carrier molecule, povidone. On contact with tissues, the carrier complex slowly releases free iodine. Gradual release decreases tissue irritation and reduces potential toxicity while preserving its germicidal activity. Povidone-iodine is very effective against gram-positive

Table 6-1 *Summary of Wound Cleansing Agents*

Skin Cleanser	Antibacterial Activity	Tissue Toxicity	Systemic Toxicity	Potential Uses
Povidone-iodine surgical scrub	Strongly bactericidal against gram-positive and gram-negative bacteria	Detergent can be toxic to wound tissues	Painful to open wounds Other reactions extremely rare	Hand cleanser
Povidone-iodine solution	Same as povidone-iodine scrub	Minimally toxic to wound tissues	Extremely rare	Wound-periphery cleanser
Chlorhexidine	Strongly bactericidal against gram-positive organisms, less strong against gram-negative bacteria	Detergent can be toxic to wound tissues	Extremely rare	Hand cleanser Alternative wound periphery cleanser
Poloxamer 188	No antibacterial activity	None known	None known	Wound cleanser (particularly useful on face)
Hexachlorophene	Bacteriostatic against gram-positive, poor activity against gram-negative bacteria	Detergent can be toxic to wound tissues	Teratogenic with repeated use	Alternative hand cleanser
Hydrogen peroxide	Very weak antibacterial agent	Toxic to red cells	Extremely rare	Wound cleanser adjunct

and gram-negative bacteria, fungi, and viruses.[15] It is currently in widespread use for hand washing, preoperative skin preparation, and cleansing of traumatic wounds. When compared with other agents such as chlorhexidine, quarternary ammonium compounds, and hexachlorophene, povidone-iodine appears to have a greater bactericidal effect against gram-negative bacteria.[2, 8, 18, 32] However, unlike chlorhexidine and hexachlorophene, it has a shorter protective effect against bacterial buildup on the skin after hand washing and appears to be less effective than these agents for that purpose.[18]

Povidone-iodine is manufactured as a solution by itself (povidone-iodine solution) or in conjunction with an ionic detergent (povidone-iodine scrub preparation). The detergent in the scrub preparation appears to be toxic to several normal tissues, as well as to components of an open wound.[6, 12] Excessive exposure of open wounds to scrub solutions by wound scrubbing or soaking is not recommended. Scrub solutions were designed for preoperative preparation of intact skin before operative incisions.

Povidone-iodine, without the detergent, is most commonly distributed as a 10% solution. When diluted to a 1% concentration, or lower, it can be safely applied to wounds and retains its bactericidal activity.[1] The inherent lack of clinical toxicity of povidone-iodine without detergent was demonstrated with 225 patients undergoing ophthalmologic surgery.[4] Povidone-iodine 10% solution, diluted with saline, was used to prepare the eye and its surrounding structures for surgery. There was no reported corneal, conjunctival, or skin toxicity. Adverse and allergic reactions are extremely rare, even when the solution is used in known iodine-allergic patients.[29]

Chlorhexidine (Hibiclens)

Chlorhexidine is an antibacterial biguanide that is very effective against gram-positive bacteria. This agent is also effective against gram-negative bacteria, but slightly less so than povidone-iodine.[8] Its action against viruses is uncertain.[15] Repeated use can lead to buildup on the skin and prolonged suppression of hand bacterial count.[7] For this reason, it is an excellent hand washing preparation. Under normal conditions of use, it has an exceedingly low toxicity. The skin cleanser does, however, contain an ionic detergent like the povidone-iodine scrub preparation, and direct contact with an open wound is discouraged.[4]

Nonionic Surfactants (Shur-Clens, Pharma Clens)

Newer and potentially useful wound cleansers are the nonionic surfactants, pluronic F-68 (Shur-Clens) and poloxamer 188 (Pharma Clens).[3] They are surface-active agents with the cleansing properties of soap but virtually no tissue toxicity, including to the eye and cornea. There are no demonstrable adverse effects in wounds and lacerations. Poloxamer 188 has been used successfully in a trial of over 3000 patients without serious side effects.[10] The major drawback of the nonionic surfactants is that they have no antibacterial activity.[27] For this reason, alternative cleansing agents like povidone-iodine are preferable for contaminated wounds. Conversely, surfactants are well suited for use on the face because they are nontoxic to the eye, and the face is naturally resistant to infection.

Hexachlorophene (pHisoHex)

Hexachlorophene is a bacteriostatic agent with good activity against gram-positive bacteria, but it is not very effective against gram-negative organisms. Although this skin cleanser once enjoyed widespread popularity as a cleansing agent, it has been replaced by povidone-iodine and chlorhexidine. In recent years, new discoveries of its potential toxicity and teratogenicity have led to a further decline in its use.[18] Because hexachlorophene has a cumulative and protective buildup in the skin, it remains an alternative for hand washing before wound care procedures.

Quarternary Ammonium Compounds (Zephiran)

These compounds have characteristics that render them virtually useless in wound care.[11] They have a limited gram-negative spectrum and Pseudomonas can proliferate in stored solutions. Furthermore, they are inactivated by soap, blood, and organic matter. Once popular in the operative setting, these agents have no modern utility.

Hydrogen Peroxide

Without a clear scientific basis, as if by tradition alone, hydrogen peroxide is commonly used in emergency wound care. As it comes into contact with blood and tissue peroxidase, it makes visible bubbles from liberated oxygen. The reaction causes foaming that is thought to dislodge bacteria, debris, and other contaminants from small crevices in tissues. This effect gives the appearance of cleansing activity when, in fact, this agent has many drawbacks. It is naturally hemolytic, and the oxygen bubbles have been shown to separate new epithelial cells from granulation tissue.[14] The germicidal action of hydrogen peroxide is weak and brief at best.[15] In a controlled study of appendectomies, hydrogen peroxide topically applied to the incision site before suture closure did not reduce the infection rate when compared with the control.[20] Under experimental wound conditions, it can delay healing.[14] Because of its hemolytic effect, hydrogen peroxide is best limited to a role as adjunctive agent for wounds encrusted with blood.

PREPARATION FOR WOUND CLEANSING

Before actually cleansing and irrigating a laceration or wound, several issues have to be considered. These include hand washing, personnel precautions, hair removal, anesthesia, foreign material, and wound soaking.

Hand Washing

Because of the unsterile nature of traumatic wounds, fixed-time hand washing with preoperative scrubbing techniques is not necessary. Although a simple, brief hand washing will suffice before each procedure, it is necessary to make sure that the fingernails have been well cleaned because they harbor more bacteria than other parts of the hand.[11, 24] Chlorhexidine is a good choice for hand washing. As a skin cleanser it is well tolerated by users. With repeat washings, it builds up in the skin, with an accompanying prolonged antibacterial effect, and it does not stain clothing like povidone-iodine does. Compliance with hand washing among emergency personnel recently has been shown to be poor.[23] Nurses have been observed to comply (hand washing after patient contact before proceeding to the next contact) following 58.2% of patient contacts, residents after 18.6%, and faculty after 17%. Hand washing is just one of the defenses against the risks detailed in the following discussion.

Personnel Precautions

Because preparing and cleansing a wound brings wound care personnel into contact with blood and other secretions, it is recommended that appropriate protective gloves and eye wear be worn at all times. Gowns are also recommended but not always practical. The main infective agents that are of concern in the emergency department are hepatitis B and C and the human immunodeficiency virus (HIV). The prevalence of HIV in urban emergency department patients has been reported to be 4% to 5%.[30] More importantly, 25% of those patients are unknown positives on presentation.[17] It is common for practitioners to be diligent about protecting themselves during major trauma resuscitations. The bleeding laceration is no less of a threat when suture needles, tissue scissors, and scalpel blades are being used.

Wound Area Hair Removal

It is common practice to shave hair around lacerations and other wounds before repair. Although there are no studies of the wound care setting, shaving has the potential to increase the wound infection rate. Close shaving of intact skin can cause small dermal wounds that can act as portals of entry for bacterial invasion and possible infection.[11] Two studies of patients, shaved versus not shaved, for elective surgery have shown an increase in post-operative wound infection rates in the shaved groups.[5, 28] Although hair shafts harbor bacteria, structures such as roots, glands, and follicles do not contain high bacterial counts under normal conditions.[24] Hair can be easily and successfully cleansed using standard techniques for applying antiseptic solutions.[36]

A case for hair removal can be made on technical grounds. In areas like the scalp it is much easier to close lacerations without having the suture material become entangled with hair. Hair that is inadvertently buried in wounds can result in wound infection.[22] Clipping hair around the wound with scissors or shaving with a recessed blade razor are techniques for hair removal that avoid dermal damage.

The only site from which hair is absolutely not shaved or clipped is the eyebrow (Fig. 6-1). Hair regrowth of the brow is unpredictable in many patients, and return to the original appearance cannot be guaranteed. Eyebrow hair can be readily cleansed, and the brow borders provide excellent landmarks for laceration alignment during wound closure.

Anesthesia

Because wound cleansing can be uncomfortable if not outright painful, most wounds should be anesthetized before cleaning. Not only will the patient be more comfortable, but the cleansing can be more vigorous and effective. Techniques for administering anesthetics are discussed fully in Chapter 5.

An issue that often arises concerning the administration of anesthetics before wound cleansing is whether bacteria can be embedded further into a wound if a needle is passed through a contaminated surface. There is no clear scientific evidence that needles can spread bacteria beyond the wound margins.[19] In clean, sharp wounds this issue is of no concern and direct wound infiltration can be safely carried out. For wounds that are visibly and heavily contaminated, the parallel injection technique or an appropriate nerve block can be used, if need be, to avoid this hypothetical complication.

Foreign Material

As part of wound preparation it is very important to determine the presence or absence of foreign bodies in the wound. Foreign materials of all types should be considered harmful and as having the potential for causing infection if left in the tissues. Although

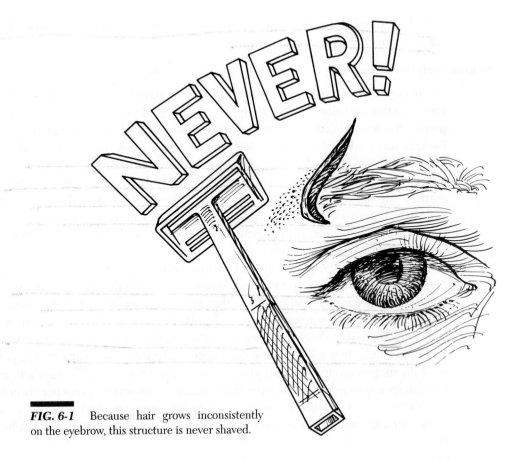

FIG. 6-1 Because hair grows inconsistently on the eyebrow, this structure is never shaved.

irrigation removes most debris, direct visualization and removal by instruments are often required. An alert patient can report the "sensation" of a foreign body still in the wound. Radiographs are particularly useful to find tooth fragments, metallic objects, and glass. It is a popular misconception that glass cannot be visualized by x-ray. In fact, 90% of all glass, even as small as 0.5 mm in size, can be detected by radiograph.[33] More detail on the removal of foreign bodies is contained in Chapter 15.

Wound Soaking

Wound soaking is a common practice in wound care. Soaking is believed to loosen debris, break up blood coagulum, and help sterilize the wound. However, under experimental conditions, povidone-iodine solution is unable to penetrate beyond 1.5 mm of tissue in spite of 20 minutes of wound soaking.[13] Although bacterial counts are lowered somewhat with soaking in povidone-iodine solution, significant contamination remains. Wound soaking has some value in loosening, softening, and removing gross contaminants from the skin surrounding the wound, but it is not a substitute for thorough mechanical skin cleansing and wound irrigation.

Wound Periphery Cleansing

The main purpose for periphery wound cleansing or "scrubbing" is to remove any visible contamination and dried blood. Periphery cleansing alone is insufficient for wound preparation without accompanying irrigation. The end point of skin cleansing is when the area surrounding the wound or laceration is visibly clean. There is no fixed scrubbing time. If the skin itself cannot be cleansed of all particulates then the risk for "tattooing" increases. Visible particulate matter "ground" into the skin can become permanently entrapped within the epidermis and dermis of the skin. These particulates need to be removed by sharp debridement. Because tattooing can have serious cosmetic consequences on the face, consultation and referral to a facial plastic surgeon should be considered if routine measures fail.

Scrubbing within the wound itself is controversial. In experimental wounds, scrubbing with surgical sponges has not been shown to decrease the incidence of infection but may produce mechanical trauma to the exposed tissues.[27] On the other hand, the mechanical action of a surgical sponge can be effective in removing gross contaminants and debris from within a wound. Because of the potential for tissue damage, scrubbing within a wound is best reserved for those wounds with visible contaminants. The porosity of the surgical sponges used for wound cleansing is also an issue. The standard, common, surgical sponge has 45 pores per linear inch. Sponges with 90 pores per linear inch (Optipore) are less irritating to tissues.[11] If handled gently, standard sponges are minimally traumatic, and the increased expense of higher porosity sponges may not justify their use.

Irrigation

"The solution to pollution is dilution" is an old maxim of wound care that still rings true today. Wound irrigation is the most effective way to remove debris and contaminants from within a laceration.[10] Irrigation is also the single most effective method of reducing bacterial counts on wound surfaces.[21, 26] In comparing methods of irrigation for highly contaminated wounds, high-pressure streams (5 to 70 psi) of saline are clearly superior to low-pressure streams such as those that might be obtained with a bulb-type syringe (0.5 to 1 psi).[31] Current practice is based on work done with a 35-ml syringe attached to a 19-gauge catheter.[31] This system develops 7 to 8 psi and is effective in reducing debris and bacterial contamination from the type of wound and laceration managed by emergency caregivers. Pulsatile lavage, which develops 50 to 70 psi, is very effective at lowering bacterial counts and wound infection rates.[25] However, significant amounts of irrigation fluid can dissect well beyond the wound margins.[34] Pulsatile lavage systems are suited for larger, heavily contaminated wounds best managed by surgical specialists in the operating room.

CLEANSING SETUP AND PROCEDURE

The following are suggested guidelines for wound cleansing and preparation:

Patient position: As in any procedure, proper preparation is essential. The patient is placed in a comfortable position, usually supine (see Fig. 1-1). It is impossible to predict how he or she will react to the discomfort of wound cleansing, the sight of blood, or the appearance of a wound. Vasovagal reactions (fainting) can occur if the patient is upright. Harmful injuries can be sustained by patients by falls to the floor during the procedure. It is also prudent to ask relatives to leave the area, or at least monitor their response to blood and the procedures that are being performed. They can sustain vasovagal syncope as well.

Anesthesia: For the most part, a wound or laceration should be anesthetized before periphery cleansing and irrigation. The pain of cleansing can inhibit the operator and lead to poor cooperation by the patient. The result is an incompletely cleansed wound.

Supplies and set-up:

- A single medium or large metal basin can be used for both periphery cleansing and irrigation.
- 10 to 20 parts saline and 1 part 10% povidone-iodine solution are mixed in the bowl.
- A packet of several 4×4 surgical sponges can be either placed directly in the solution or to the side of the bowl.
- A 20- to 35-ml syringe attached to a Zerowet splash shield is recommended for irrigation. This shield reproduces the 5 to 8 psi of an 18- or 19-gauge catheter. If the Zerowet shield is unavailable, a splash guard can be fashioned out of a 4×4 sponge pierced in the center by an intravenous catheter. Another option is to puncture the bottom of a plastic medicine cup and place it over the syringe and needle or catheter. The Zerowet has been shown to be very effective for caregiver protection from irrigant splatter.[24]

Cleansing technique: The sponges are used for periphery cleansing and discarded after use. Soiled sponges are never returned to the bowl. If there is significant contamination or debris within the wound itself, the sponges can be used for mechanical, in the wound, debridement. The actual technique for scrubbing the wound periphery is illustrated in Fig. 6-2. It is essential to be gentle and to start at the wound itself. The cleansing motion is circular, with gradually larger circles away from the wound. The sponge is then discarded. At no time should the sponge be brought from the periphery back toward the wound because this maneuver carries unwanted organisms from unsterile skin areas back to the area of the cleansed wound site. There is no specified amount of time for periphery cleansing. Scrubbing continues until the skin is visibly free from contaminants and dried blood.

Irrigation: Following periphery cleansing, the wound is irrigated with the syringe and splash shield (Fig. 6-3). Periphery cleansing and irrigation can be alternated until there are no visible skin or wound contaminants. The amount of irrigation fluid can vary from 100 ml to 250 ml or more, depending on the level of contamination of the

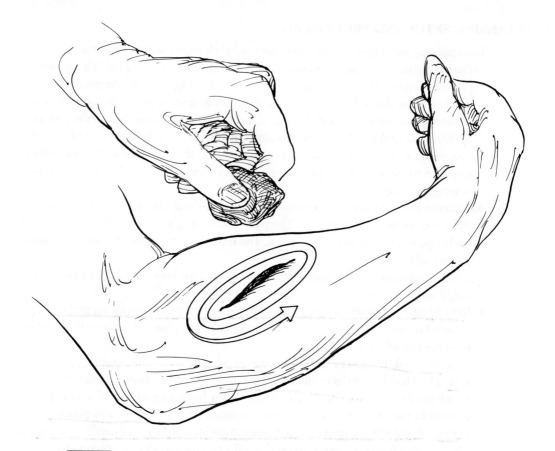

FIG. 6-2 Note the spiral technique of scrubbing a wound periphery by beginning at the center and moving away to the periphery without crossing back over the actual wound area.

wound. The syringe and splash shield are held close to the wound so that the force of the stream is not dissipated by distance. Whatever cannot be irrigated out of the wound is removed by mechanical scrubbing with a sponge or sharp debridement.

Debridement: If visible contamination remains, in spite of thorough cleansing and irrigation, sharp debridement is carried out with tissue scissors or a surgical scalpel with a #15 blade. Ultimately, other strategies, such as wound excision, might be necessary to handle wounds that cannot be managed with these steps. Strategies for the difficult wound are discussed in Chapter 8.

Cleansing is complete and a wound is ready to close when, literally, it looks clean to the eye. There should be no visible contaminants, and the tissue should appear pink and viable. Usually there is slight fresh bleeding. A sterile sponge can be laid over the wound until the operator is ready to proceed with repair.

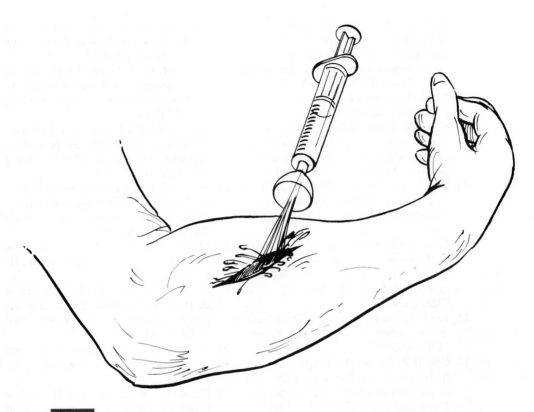

FIG. 6-3 Technique for wound irrigation. Note that the shield is held close to the wound.

REFERENCES

1. Berk WA, Welch RD, Bock BF: Controversial issues in clinical management of the simple wound, *Ann Emerg Med* 21:72-80, 1992.
2. Berry AR, Watt B, Goldacre MJ: A comparison of the use of povidone-iodine and chlorhexidine in the prophylaxis of postoperative wound infection, *J Hosp Infect* 3:55-63, 1982.
3. Bryant CA, Rodeheaver GT, Reem EM, et al: Search for a nontoxic surgical scrub solution of periorbital lacerations, *Ann Emerg Med* 13:317, 1984.
4. Caldwell DR, Kasti PR, Cook J, et al: Povidone-iodine: its efficacy as a preoperative conjunctival and periocular preparation, *Ann Ophthalmol* 16:577-588, 1984.
5. Cruse P, Foord R: A five-year prospective study of 23,649 surgical wounds, *Arch Surg* 107:206-209, 1973.
6. Custer J, Edlich RF, Prusak M, et al: Studies in the management of the contaminated wound, *Am J Surg* 121:572-575, 1971.

7. Cawthorn SJ, Parums DV, Gibbs NM, et al: Extent of mesorecta spread and involvement of lateral resection margin as prognostic factors after surgery for rectal cancer, *Lancet* 333:1055, 1990.

8. Dineen P: Hand washing degerming: a comparison of povidone-iodine and chlorhexidine, *Clin Pharmacol Ther* 23:63-67, 1978.

9. Dire DJ, et al: A comparison of wound irrigation solutions used in the emergency department, *Ann Emerg Med* 19:704, 1990.

10. Edlich RF, Rodeheaver GT, Morgan RF, et al: Principles of emergency wound management, *Ann Emerg Med* 17:1284-1302, 1988.

11. Edlich RF, Rodeheaver GT, Thacker JG, et al: *Technical factors in wound management: fundamentals of wound management in surgery*, South Plainfield, NJ, 1977, Chirurgecom, Inc.

12. Faddis D, Daniel D, Boyer J: Tissue toxicity of antiseptic solutions, *J Trauma* 17:895-897, 1977.

13. Gravett A, Sterner S, Clinton J, et al: A trial of povidone-iodine in the prevention of infection in sutured lacerations, *Ann Emerg Med* 16:167-171, 1987.

14. Gruber RP, Vistnes L, Pardoe R: The effect of commonly used antiseptics on wound healing, *Plast Reconstr Surg* 55:472, 1975.

15. Harvey S: Antiseptics and disinfectants; fungicides; ectoparasiticides. In Goodman A, Goodman L, Gilman A, editors: *The pharmacologic basis of therapeutics*, New York, 1980, Macmillan.

16. Howell JM, Stair TO, Howell AM, et al: The effect of scrubbing and irrigation with normal saline, povidone iodine, and cefazolin on wound bacterial counts in a guinea pig model, *Am J Emerg Med* 11:134-138, 1993.

17. Jue J, Stevens P, Hedberg K, Modesitt S: HIV seroprevalence in emergency department patients, *Acad Emerg Med* 2:773-783, 1995.

18. Kaul A, Jewett J: Agents and techniques for disinfection of the skin, *Surg Gynecol Obstet* 152:677-685, 1981.

19. Kelly AM, et al: Minimizing the pain of local infiltration anesthesia for wounds by injection into the wound edges, *J Emerg Med* 12:593, 1994.

20. Lau HY, Wong SH: Randomized, prospective trial of topical hydrogen peroxide in appendectomy wound infection, *Am J Surg* 142:393-397, 1981.

21. Madden J, Edlich RF, Schauerhamer R, et al: Application of principles of fluid dynamics to surgical wound irrigation, *Curr Top Surg Res* 3:85, 1971.

22. Mahlor D, Rosenberg L, Goldstein J: The fate of buried hair, *Ann Plast Surg* 5:131-138, 1980.

23. Meengs MR, Giles BK, Chisholm CD, et al: Hand washing frequency in an emergency department, *Ann Emerg Med* 23:1307-1312, 1994.

24. Pecora D, Landis R, Martin E: Location of cutaneous microorganisms, *Surgery* 64:1114-1117, 1968.

25. Pigman EC, Karch DB, Scott JL: Splatter during jet irrigation cleansing of a wound model: a comparison of three inexpensive devices, *Ann Emerg Med* 22:1563-1567, 1993.

26. Rodeheaver GT, Petrry D, Thacker JG, et al: Wound cleansing in high pressure irrigation, *Surg Gynecol Obstet* 141:357, 1975.

27. Rodeheaver GT, Smith SL, Thacker JG: Mechanical cleansing of contaminated wounds with a surfactant, *Am J Surg* 129:241, 1975.

28. Seropian R, Reyolds B: Wound infections after preoperative depilatory versus razor preparation, *Am J Surg* 121:251-254, 1971.

29. Shelanski H, Shelanski M: PVP-iodine: history, toxicity, and therapeutic uses, *J Int Coll Surg* 25:727-734, 1956.

30. Sloan EP, McGill BA, Zalenski R, et al: Human immunodeficiency virus and hepatitis B virus seroprevalence in an urban trauma population, *J Trauma* 38:736-741, 1995.

31. Stevenson TR, Thacker JG, Rodeheaver GT, et al: Cleansing the traumatic wound by high pressure syringe irrigation, *JACEP* 5:17, 1976.

32. Synder I, Finch R: Antiseptics, disinfectants, and sterilization. In Craig C, Stitzel R, editors: *Modern pharmacology*, Boston, 1982, Little, Brown.

33. Tandberg D: Glass in the hand and foot, *JAMA* 248:1872-1874, 1982.

34. Wheeler CB, Rodeheaver GT, Thacker JG, et al: Side effects of high pressure irrigation, *Surg Gynecol Obstet* 143:775, 1976.

35. White J, Duncan A: The comparative effectiveness of iodophor and hexachlorophene surgical scrub solutions, *Surg Gynecol Obstet* 135:890-892, 1972.

36. Winston KR: Hair and neurosurgery, *Neurosurg* 31:320-329, 1992.

7 *Instruments and Suture Materials*

Basic Instruments and Handling	Suture Materials
Needle Holders	Absorbable Suture Materials
Forceps and Skin Hooks	Nonabsorbable Suture Materials
Scissors	Needle Types
Hemostats	
Knife Handles and Blades	

It is not necessary to have large numbers of instruments and suture materials for emergency wound care. Wounds and lacerations can be managed with a few well-chosen instruments and a limited number of wound closure products. Although the type of instruments remains relatively constant, each wound has differing requirements for wound closure materials. Absorbable and nonabsorbable sutures, as well as a variety of wound tapes and staples, can be selected according to the specific patient problem. In the future, wound adhesives are likely to come into widespread use. The following are guidelines for the selection of suture materials, as well as the choice and proper handling of instruments. Tapes, staples, and adhesives are discussed in Chapter 13.

BASIC INSTRUMENTS AND HANDLING

Wound care can be carried out with the following set of instruments: needle holders, tissue forceps, skin hooks, suture scissors, iris (tissue) scissors, hemostats, a knife handle, and appropriate knife blades. For simple lacerations that do not require sharp debridement or revision, a needle holder, forceps, and suture scissors will suffice. There is a bewildering variety of instruments currently available through the major suppliers of surgical instruments, but only the types and configurations of instruments necessary to manage wounds and lacerations are covered here. There are also numerous disposable instrument sets that meet the needs of many emergency wound care problems.

Needle Holders

Because most lacerations are closed with relatively small suture materials, the needle holder need not be bulky or large. A 4½-inch Webster needle holder with serrated carbide-tipped jaws can accommodate most curved suture needles (Fig. 7-1). Occasionally, large needles are used and an instrument such as a 6-inch Webster needle holder is necessary.

Technique for Handling Needle Holder

Just as important as the choice of needle holder is the technique used for holding and arming it with the needle. Fig. 7-2 demonstrates the right and wrong way to hold the instrument during introduction of the needle into tissue for routine emergency laceration closure. The rings are only used to clamp and unclamp the jaws by closing and releasing the locking mechanism. When introducing the needle into the skin, better precision can be gained by grasping the needle holder close to the jaws in the manner illustrated. This precision is particularly important when closing lacerations on the face. The technique of maintaining the fingers in the ring is more common when closing cosmetically less important surgical incisions or large truncal and proximal extremity wounds.

The needle holder is armed with the needle by closing the very tip of the jaws onto the body of the needle (Fig. 7-3). If the needle is pushed farther back into the jaws of the instrument, the curve will be flattened, significantly weakening the needle and making it susceptible to breakage. The needle itself is grasped at right angles, approximately one third of the way down the body shaft from the end to which the suture is attached.

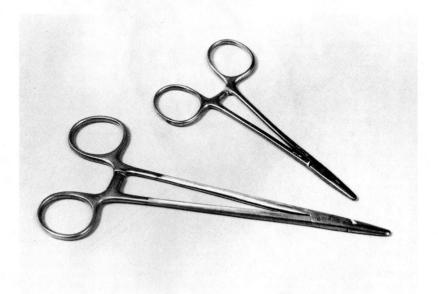

FIG. 7-1   Needle holders used in emergency wound care: 4½-inch and 6-inch Webster-style needle holders with serrated carbide tipped jaws.

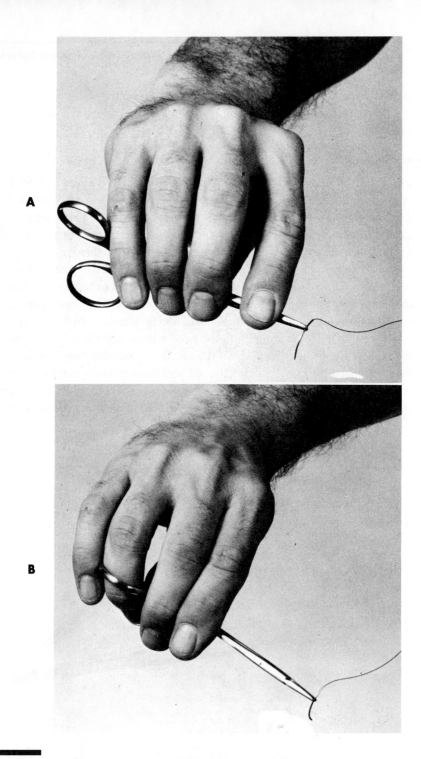

FIG. 7-2   Technique for properly holding the needle holder. **A,** The correct way allows for proper needle entry into the skin. **B,** The incorrect way—the finger holes are not used when introducing the needle holder into the skin.

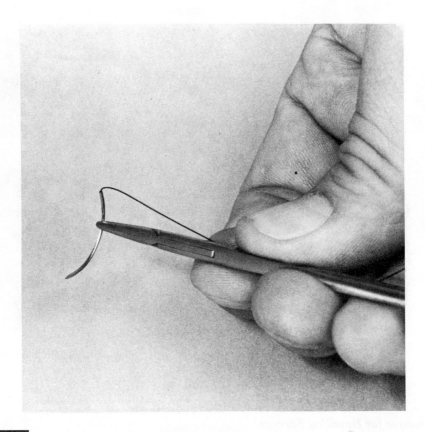

FIG. 7-3 Technique for arming a needle holder. Note that the needle is held approximately one third of the way from the swage and is grasped at the very tip of the needle holder. The angle of the needle to the holder is exactly 90 degrees.

Forceps and Skin Hooks

Grasping and controlling tissue with forceps or skin hooks during skin closure is essential to proper suture placement. However, whenever force is applied to skin or other tissues, inadvertent damage to cells can occur if an improper instrument or technique is used. Skin hooks are preferable to forceps because the "crushing" or "pincer" effect of forceps is eliminated. However, to use skin hooks properly, considerable skill and practice are required. Forceps are still widely used and are safe when proper technique is applied. The currently recommended forceps are 4¾-inch Adson's with small teeth (Fig. 7-4). Teeth decrease the need to apply excessive force to grasp and secure tissue. Forceps without teeth are to be discouraged because the flat surface of their jaws tends to crush tissue more easily.

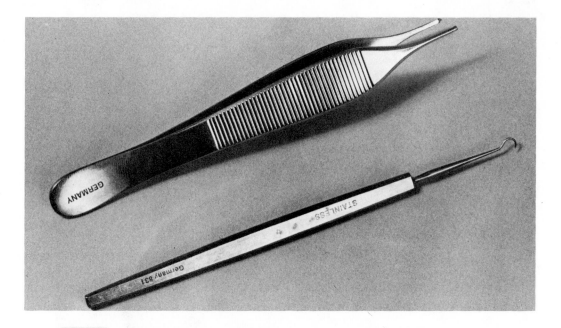

FIG. 7-4   Tissue grasping instruments: a 4¾-inch adson, a forceps with fine teeth, and a standard plastic skin hook.

Technique for Handling Forceps

When handling tissue, the jaws of the forceps are never closed on skin itself. The epidermis and dermis are avoided in favor of the superficial fascia (subcutaneous tissue). By grasping superficial fascia gently, the wound edge is stabilized for needle placement, and inadvertent damage to the dermis is avoided (Fig. 7-5). Forceps also can serve as a surrogate skin hook as illustrated. The needle entry point can be immobilized and supported without closing the jaws.

Fig. 7-6 illustrates the correct and incorrect methods for grasping forceps. The "pencil grasp" technique allows for better control of the forceps and tends to diminish the amount of force delivered to the tissue.

Skin hooks have the appearance of miniature retractors, but the hook portion has pointed tips to control dermis or superficial fascia. Piercing the epidermis is avoided because it can create an unnecessary puncture mark. Skin hooks are inserted directly into the wound, and the hook portion is used to gain purchase on the dermis or superficial fascia. In this manner the epidermis is avoided.

Scissors

Three types of scissors are useful in emergency wound care: iris or tissue scissors, dissection scissors, and suture scissors (Fig. 7-7). Four-inch iris scissors, both curved and

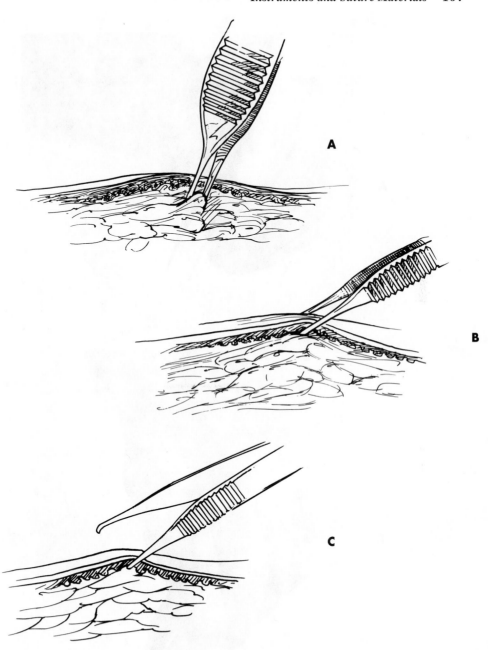

FIG. 7-5   The correct and incorrect way to grasp tissue with a forceps. **A,** The correct way is to grasp the tissue by the superficial fascia (subcutaneous tissue). **B,** The incorrect way to grasp tissue is by crushing the dermis and epidermis between the jaws of the forceps. **C,** Forceps can be used like a skin hook to retract or stabilize the wound edge for exploration or suture needle placement.

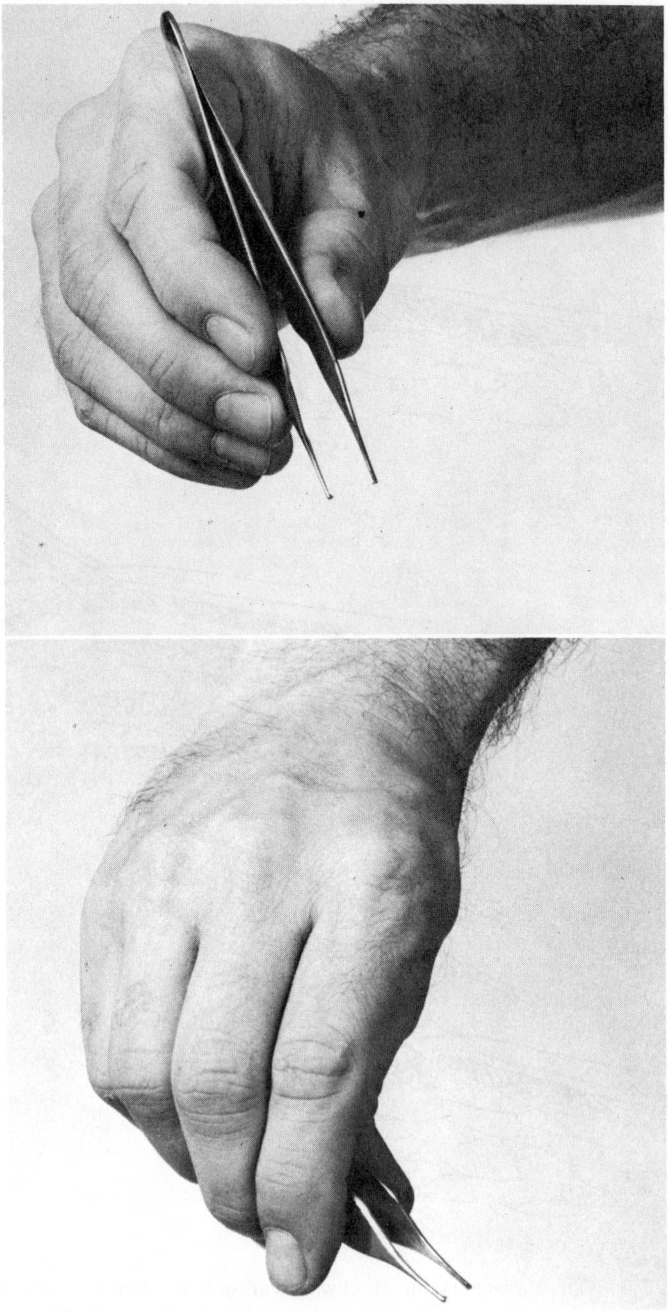

FIG. 7-6   The correct and incorrect way to hold the forceps manually. **A,** The forceps is held in the pencil grasp fashion as the correct technique. **B,** The incorrect technique is to grasp the forceps.

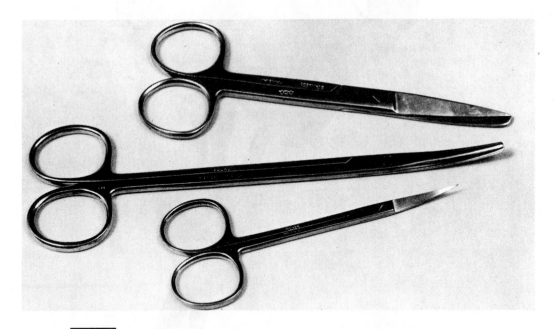

FIG. 7-7   Scissors. *Top,* All-purpose suture scissors; middle-Metzenbaum dissection scissors; *bottom,* curved iris or tissue scissors.

straight, are used to assist in debridement and wound revision. These scissors are very sharp and provide excellent precision in cutting tissue for whatever task. They are, however, very delicate and are not recommended for cutting sutures. Occasionally during suture removal, when very small sutures have been used in the face area, iris scissors can be used for their removal.

For heavier tissue revision, as might be necessary for wound undermining, blunt-tipped 6-inch Metzenbaum dissection scissors are recommended. Iris scissors are too small and delicate for this task and the larger Metzenbaums can overcome this shortcoming.

Standard 6-inch, single blunt-tip, double-sharp suture scissors are most useful for cutting sutures, adhesive tape, sponges, and other dressing materials. Because of their size and bulk, these scissors are very durable and practical.

Technique for Scissor Tip Control

Whenever scissor tip control is essential, such as cutting close to the knots of deep or dermal closures with absorbable sutures, the technique illustrated in Fig. 7-8 is recommended. The tips of the scissors are brought gently down to the knot. Just before cutting, the tips are rotated slightly to avoid cutting the knot itself.

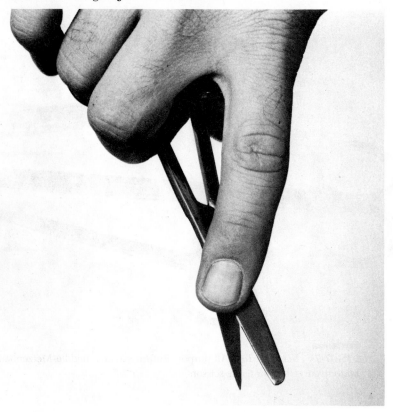

FIG. 7-8   Proper technique for tip control for scissors.

Hemostats

Hemostats have three functions in emergency wound care. Originally, hemostats were designed to clamp small blood vessels for hemorrhage control. Another use is to grasp and secure superficial fascia during undermining and debriding wounds. Finally, this instrument is an excellent tool for exposing, exploring, and visualizing the deeper areas of a wound. Two types of hemostats are commonly used in wound care (Fig. 7-9). For general use, the standard hemostat is recommended. Finer work in small wounds is often best served by the 5-inch curved mosquito hemostat with fine serrated jaws.

Knife Handles and Blades

The choice of a knife handle can be limited to the #3 standard Bard/Parker-style knife handle. Generally three blade configurations are necessary for a variety of tasks (Fig. 7-10). The #10 blade is not commonly needed in emergency wound care but occasionally is helpful for larger excisions during wound revision. Very commonly used and quite ver-

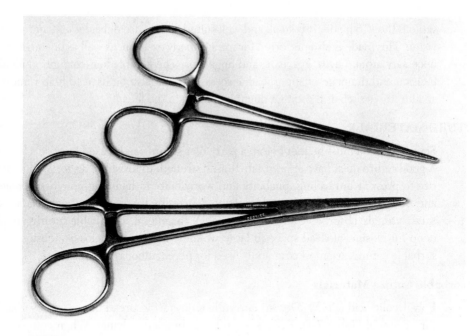

FIG. 7-9   Hemostats. *Top*, Mosquito hemostat; *bottom*, standard hemostat.

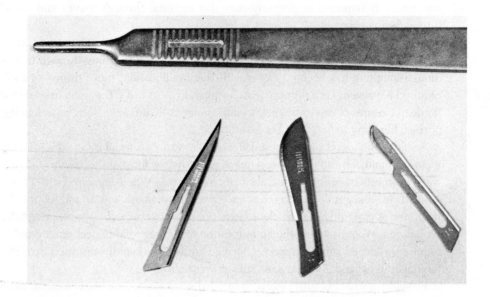

FIG. 7-10   Knife handle and #11 (*left*), #10 (*middle*), #15 (*right*) knife blades.

satile is the #15 blade. It is small and well suited for precise debridement and wound revision. This blade is also preferred for foreign-body excision, as well as the intricate work necessary around eyes, lips, ears, and fingertips. The #11 blade is configured ideally for incision and drainage of superficial abscesses. It can also be used to help remove very small sutures such as those that might be placed in the face.

SUTURE MATERIALS

Several criteria must be met before a particular suture can be used to close a laceration. A good suture must have appropriate tensile strength to resist breakage, good knot security to prevent unraveling, pliability and workability in handling, low tissue reactivity, and the ability to resist bacterial infection. Currently there are two main classes of suture materials: absorbable and nonabsorbable. In general, absorbable sutures are placed deep for closure of dead space in large wounds or to reduce closure tension. Nonabsorbable sutures are most commonly used for percutaneous or skin closure.

Absorbable Suture Materials

Polyglycolic acid (PGA) (Dexon) currently enjoys widespread use as an absorbable suture material (Table 7-1). PGA is a synthetic, braided polymer. When compared with plain or chromic catgut, PGA is much less reactive and is experimentally better able to resist infection from contaminating bacteria.[4] PGA has excellent knot security and maintains at least 50% of its tensile strength for 25 days.[8] The main drawback of PGA is that it has a high friction coefficient and "binds and snags" when wet. For this reason, some experience is required to properly pass this material through tissues and "seat" the throws during knotting.

Recently, the manufacturer has modified PGA (Dexon Plus) by coating it with poloxamer 188, an agent that significantly reduces the friction and drag through tissues. Although handling has become easier with this modification, more throws (4 to 6) are required to prevent knot slippage than for plain PGA (3 to 4). The main uses of PGA are for deep closures of superficial fascia (subcutaneous tissue) in wounds, as well as ligature of small bleeding vessels to effect hemostasis.

An older and less commonly used absorbable suture material is gut. Gut is an organic material manufactured from sheep intestines. A newer form of this suture is gut treated with chromium trioxide to retard absorption in tissues. When compared with PGA, plain gut and chromic gut appear to have inferior tensile strength and wound security.[6,8] The main use of chromic gut is to close lacerations within the oral mucosa, perineum, and scrotal skin. Wounds within the bounds of the oral cavity tend to heal rapidly and do not require prolonged suture support. Chromic gut is more rapidly absorbed than PGA on the oral mucosa and does not need suture removal.[5]

Polyglactin-910 (PG 910) (Vicryl) is braided synthetic polymer also used for deep closures. It has similar dry tensile strength when compared with PGA, but maintains in vivo strength somewhat longer. On the other hand, PGA has greater knot security.

Table 7-1 *Absorbable Suture Materials*

Material	Structure	Tissue Reaction	Tensile Strength	Tissue ½ Life (Days)	Uses and Comments
Gut	Natural	++++	++	5-7	For mucosal closures, rarely used
Chromic gut	Natural	++++	++	10-14	For oral mucosa, perineal, and scrotal closures; can be annoying to patients because of stiffness
Polyglyolic acid-PGA (Dexon)	Braided	++	+++	25	For subcutaneous closure; coated version easier to use but requires more knots (Dexon-Plus)
Polyglactin 910 (Vicryl)	Braided	++	++++	28	Comes dyed and undyed; do not use dyed on face; irradiated polyglactin excellent for mucosal closures
Polyglyconate (Maxon)	Monofilament	+	+++++	28-36	For subcutaneous closure; less reactive and stronger than PGA and polyglactin
Polydioxanone (PDS)	Monofilament	+	++++	36-53	For subcutaneous closures that need high degree of security; stiffer and more difficult to handle than PGA or maxon

(Rapide?)

Polyglactin-910 can be modified by irradiation, which greatly increases its tissue absorption.[9] This quality makes PG 910 ideal for closure of oral mucosa, scrotal skin, scalp, and perineum. The suture can be placed, and because of rapid absorption, no return visit is necessary for removal.

Two monofilament absorbable suture materials, polyglyconate (Maxon) and polydioxanone (PDS) have some advantages over PGA and polyglactin-910. The main advantage of these suture materials is that they maintain their in vivo tensile strength longer than PGA and the other absorbables.[3, 7] They also appear to have greater knot security and lower friction coefficients. Polyglyconate is less stiff and easier to handle than polydioxanone. Because they are monofilaments, they enjoy the theoretic advantage of creating a lower potential for infection. These new materials have excellent characteristics and have the potential to replace older, braided sutures provided cost becomes comparable.

Nonabsorbable Suture Materials

Of all the nonabsorbable suture materials, monofilament nylon (Ethilon, Dermalon) is most commonly used for surface, percutaneous closure (Table 7-2). The monofilament configuration makes it minimally tissue reactive and able to resist infection from experimental wound contamination when compared with braided suture material.[4] Nylon has tensile strength that ensures wound security. The main disadvantage of nylon is the difficulty in achieving good knot security. Because monofilaments have greater memory (the tendency to return to their packaged shape) than braided sutures, they tend to unravel if not tied correctly. Therefore at least 4 to 5 carefully fashioned "throws" or knots are required to achieve a secure final knot.

The polymer polypropylene (Prolene) is another nonabsorbable monofilament. Polypropylene appears to be stronger than nylon and has better overall wound security.[8] It is also less reactive and is able to resist infection at least as well as nylon.[4] However, it has greater memory than nylon and is somewhat more difficult to work with. The main uses of polypropylene are for percutaneous and subcuticular pull-out closures.

A newer monofilament suture material is polybutester (Novafil).[2] Polybutester appears to be stronger than other monofilaments. This material does not have significant memory and therefore does not maintain its packaging shape like nylon and polypropylene do. For this reason it is reported to be easier to work with and has greater knot security. A unique feature of polybutester is that it has the capacity to adapt or "stretch" with increasing wound edema. Once the edema subsides, polybutester resumes its original shape. When compared with nylon, this suture material has a lower risk of causing hypertrophic scarring.[10] The ability to adapt to the swelling and changing configuration of a healing wound is credited for this reduction in risk.

Less commonly used for minor wound care problems are the braided, nonabsorbable suture materials. These include cotton, silk, braided nylon, and multifilament Dacron. Until the advent of synthetic fibers, silk was the mainstay of wound closure. It is the most workable of sutures and has excellent knot security. However, the usefulness and popularity of silk have declined because of its propensity for causing tissue reactivity and infection.[4, 8] Research has shown that like silk, the braided synthetics have a greater tendency to cause wound infection when exposed to contaminating bacteria.[1, 4] These materials, however, have excellent workability and knot security. Because of the latter properties, braided sutures have some usefulness on the face where maximal control and precision are needed. The earlier removal time of facial sutures and the natural resistance of the face to infection make the chance of inflammation and infection developing almost negligible.

NEEDLE TYPES

Like instruments and suture materials, there is a bewildering variety of needles manufactured for wound closure. However, the vast majority of wound closures can be accomplished with a limited number of needles. Curved needles have two basic configurations: tapered and cutting (Fig. 7-11). For wound and laceration care, the cut-

Table 7-2 *Nonabsorbable Suture Materials*

Material	Structure	Tissue Reaction	Tensile Strength	Knot Security	Uses and Comments
Silk	Braided	++++	++	++++	Easy to handle but has increased potential for infection
Nylon (Ethilon, Dermalon)	Monofilament	++	+++	++	Commonly used in skin closure but high degree of memory; requires several throws for secure closure
Polypropylene (Prolene)	Monofilament	+	++++	+	High degree of memory, low tissue adhesion; good for subcuticular pull-out technique
Dacron (Mersilene)	Braided	+++	++	++++	Easy to handle, good knot security; like silk but less risk to tissue for inflammation and infection
Polybutester (Novafil)	Monofilament	+	++++	++++	Excellent handling, strength, and security; expands and contracts with changes in tissue edema

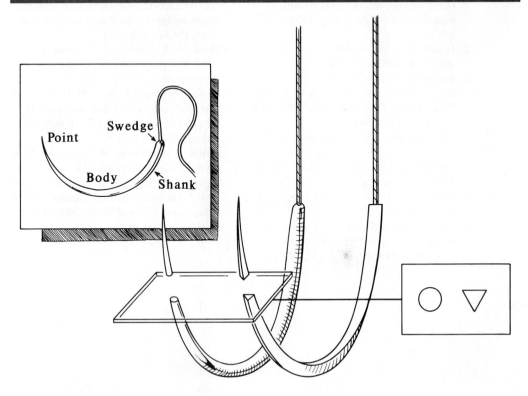

FIG. 7-11   Basic needle configurations: *Left,* The standard round, tapered needle; *right,* the reverse cutting needle. Note that the sharp edge is on the convex portion of the needle.

ting needle is used almost exclusively. What are now commonly referred to as cutting needles are in fact reverse cutting needles. The needle is made in such a way that the outer edge is sharp so as to allow for smooth and atraumatic penetration of the skin, and the inner portion is flattened so that the needle puncture wound is not inadvertently enlarged as the suture passes through the hole and the knot is tied.

Needles come in two grades, cuticular and plastic. These differ significantly in their usefulness for wound care. Cuticular needles are less expensive but noticeably less sharp than plastic grade needles. The increased sharpness of plastic needles allows the operator to better control entry and passage of the needle through tissues. Plastic needles are also less traumatic. Although they are more expensive, these needles are recommended for emergency wound and laceration repair. There is a bewildering number of code designations for needles. Cuticular needles can be recognized by the letters C (cuticular) or FS (for skin). Plastic grade needle codes usually start with the letter P.

REFERENCES

1. Alexander J, Kaplan J, Altemeier W: Role of suture materials in the development of wound infection, *Ann Surg* 165:192-199, 1967.

2. Bernstein G: Polybutester suture, *J Dermatol Surg* 14:615-616, 1988.

3. Bourne RB, Bitar H, Andreae PR: In vivo comparison of four absorbable sutures: Vicryl, Dexon Plus, Maxon, and PDS, *Can J Surg* 31:43-45, 1988.

4. Edlich R, Panek PH, Rodeheaver GT, et al: Physical and chemical configuration of sutures in the development of surgical infection, *Ann Surg* 177:679-687, 1973.

5. Holt G, Holt J: Suture materials and techniques, *Ear Nose Throat J* 60:23-30, 1981.

6. Howes E: Strength studies of polyglycolic acid versus catgut sutures of the same size, *Surg Gynecol Obstet* 137:15-20, 1973.

7. Rodeheaver GT, Powell TA, Thacker TJ, et al: Mechanical performance of monofilament synthetic absorbable sutures, *Am J Surg* 154:544-547, 1987.

8. Swanson N, Tromovitch T: Suture materials 1980s: properties, uses, and abuses, *Int J Dermatol* 21:373-378, 1982.

9. Tandon SC, Kelly J, Turtle M, Irwin ST: Irradiated polyglactin 910: a new synthetic absorbable suture, *J Royal Coll Surg Edinburgh*, 40:185-187, 1995.

10. Trimbos JB, Smeets M, Verdel M, Hermans J: Cosmetic result of lower midline laparotomy wounds: polybutester and nylon skin suture in a randomized clinical trial, *Obstet Gynecol* 82:390-393, 1993.

8 Decisions Before Closure-Timing, Debridement, Consultation

Timing of Closure
    Primary Closure (Primary Intention)
    Secondary Closure (Secondary Intention)
    Tertiary Closure (Delayed Primary Closure)
Wound Exploration

Hemostasis
Tissue Debridement and Excision
Surgical Drains
Immediate Antibiotic Therapy
Guidelines for Consultation

Before proceeding with definitive management, such as suture placement, several issues have to be considered and decisions made that are separate from the choice of closure method. Time from the injury; tissue condition; level of contamination; potential for foreign material, etc., all factor into the total care. The following questions capture this phase of emergency wound care:

- What is the proper timing of wound closure—primary, open, or delayed?
- Which wounds need invasive exploration?
- What are the appropriate measures to achieve wound hemostasis to facilitate exploration and repair?
- When and how is a wound debrided?
- Under what conditions is a drain placed?
- What are the indications for immediate intravenous antibiotic administration?
- When should consultation be obtained?

TIMING OF CLOSURE

Determining the time of injury is important to wound repair. The chance of developing a wound infection increases with each hour that elapses from the time of injury.[12] It has been traditionally taught that there is a "golden" period within which a wound or laceration can be safely closed primarily (primary intention). The exact length of that period is influenced by such factors as the mechanism of injury, anatomic location, and level of contamination. As a rough guideline, 6 to 8 hours from the time of injury has been considered to be a safe time interval within which to repair the average uncomplicated laceration. However, this period can vary from as little as 3 hours for heavily contaminated wounds of the foot to 24 hours or more for clean lacerations of the face. A complete dis-

117

cussion of primary, secondary, and tertiary (delayed) closure is in Chapter 3. The following is a summary with recommendations for delayed wound closure.

Primary Closure (Primary Intention)

Lacerations that are relatively clean and uncontaminated, with minimal tissue loss or devitalization, are considered for primary closure. Repair of these wounds is usually necessary within 6 to 8 hours from the time of injury on most regions of the body. Wounds of the highly vascular face and scalp can often be sutured up to 24 hours after injury.[9] Because there are no hard and fast rules that govern every possible situation, the following recommendation is offered: any injury, irrespective of the time from injury, that can be converted to a fresh-appearing, slightly bleeding, nondevitalized wound, with no visible contamination or debris after aggressive cleansing, irrigation, and debridement, can be considered for primary closure.

Secondary Closure (Secondary Intention)

Skin infarctions, ulcerations, abscess cavities, punctures, small cosmetically unimportant animal bites, and partial-thickness (abrasions, second-degree burns) tissue losses are often better left to heal by secondary intention. Wound care consists of thorough cleansing, irrigation, and debridement of devitalized or contaminant-impregnated tissue. These wounds are not closed with sutures and are allowed to gradually heal by granulation and eventual reepithelialization.

Tertiary Closure (Delayed Primary Closure)

Some wounds are candidates for delayed closure. Patients with lacerations occasionally present to the emergency department well after the time period in which primary closure is safe. Even though there are no technical contraindications to sutures or staples, this wound will have a high bacterial count and excessive devitalized tissue. The wound can be "converted" to a "fresh" one by cleansing, irrigation, and debridement followed by a 4- to 5-day period during which the natural host defenses reduce the bacterial load to acceptable, minimal levels (Fig. 8-1).[2, 8] Antibiotics can aid these defenses. Other wounds that are candidates for delayed closure include animal bites and bullet wounds.

Technique for Delayed Primary Closure

Cleanse, irrigate, and debride as much as possible during the initial encounter. Pack the wound with saline-moistened, fine-mesh gauze or gauze sponges. The wound is covered with a bulky, absorbent gauze dressing. Oral antibiotics are administered after initial care before delayed closure. Dicloxacillin or one of the first-generation cephalosporins are appropriate choices. Erythromycin can be given to patients who have a significant history of allergy to the penicillins.

If no signs of infection or excessive discomfort develop beforehand, have the patient return in 4 to 5 days. If the wound appears clean and uninfected, then it can be closed

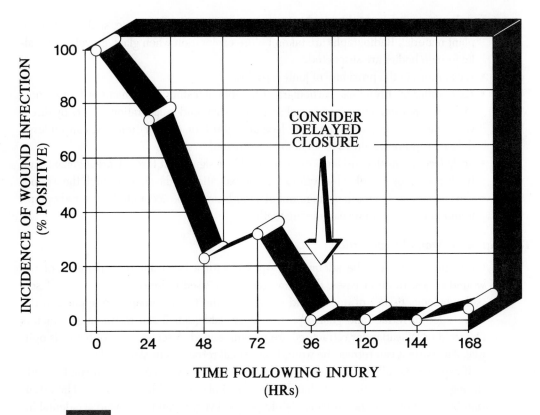

FIG. 8-1   Graph illustrating the incidence of wound infection risk after injury and optimal timing of tertiary or delayed wound closure. (Adapted from Edlich R, et al: *A manual for wound closure*, St Paul, Minn, 1979, Surgical Products Division, 3M.)

with sutures, tapes, or staples. Dermal (deep) or subcutaneous sutures are avoided in this setting. These wounds can accumulate excessive granulation tissue during the 4- to 5-day period. This tissue can be judiciously excised to permit better wound edge apposition. The intervals for suture or staple removal are the same as for primary closure starting at the time of closure. Delayed closure is associated with a low (3%) infection rate.[14]

WOUND EXPLORATION

Surface wounds and lacerations require thorough inspection and direct exploration if necessary. It is important to always evaluate the functional status of the relevant nerves, tendons, arteries, joints, or other related structures of the wounded area and to remain alert for potentially occult, serious underlying structural damage. Although more specific information is included in other chapters and sections specific to special anatomic sites and problems, the following guidelines are offered for wound exploration:

- Suspicion of a foreign body, particularly if it is potentially organic, such as wood or plant material. Radiographs are taken before exploration when glass, gravel, or metallic foreign bodies are suspected.
- Lacerations in the proximity of joint capsules.
- Lacerations over tendons, particularly if functional testing of the hand or foot is "normal." It is not uncommon to reveal serious partial tendon lacerations solely by direct visualization. Unrepaired, partially lacerated (50% or greater) tendons can undergo delayed rupture within 12 to 48 hours if untreated.
- Scalp lacerations that are large or are caused by a significant force. Unrecognized skull fractures can be revealed by exploration and palpation of the skull through the wound.
- Lip lacerations, if a tooth or fragment of a tooth cannot be accounted for. A radiograph is another method to reveal missing teeth.

Techniques for Wound Exploration

Often the wound can be adequately exposed with a hemostat by separation of the wound edges. In other cases, the hemostat can be used to grasp the superficial fascia (subcutaneous tissue) of one wound edge while the tissue forceps are applied to the other edge to retract and gain exposure. If available, small self-restraining retractors (Mastoid or Wheatlander retractors) are recommended. A second pair of hands is optimal. An assistant can retract the wound with small retractors or skin hooks.

If exposure is still not adequate, then a small wound extension incision can be made through the dermis with a knife handle and a #15 blade or with iris scissors. The extension begins at one wound end and should proceed very carefully to avoid accidental injury to underlying structures (Fig. 8-2). On the face, extension incisions are made parallel to the skin tension lines discussed in Chapter 2. Once the epidermis and dermis are divided, the superficial fascia (subcutaneous tissue) is not incised but is gently spread apart with forceps or tissue scissors to reveal any suspected foreign body, or tendon or joint capsule injury.

HEMOSTASIS

Wounds often bleed actively, particularly during assessment and exploration. In addition to the problem of adequate wound visualization with active bleeding, hematomas can cause an increase in the rate of wound infection and delay the healing process.[1]

The simplest and most effective way to stop bleeding is by applying direct pressure to the wound with hand-held surgical 4 × 4 sponges. Continuous pressure has to be applied for a minimum of 10 minutes. Because of the time involved, sponges secured with an Ace wrap can be substituted if the wound is in an anatomic area that lends itself to wrapping.

An epinephrine (1:100,000) moistened sponge applied for 5 minutes, also with pressure, to the wound will often suffice in cases where direct pressure fails. However, epinephrine is contraindicated for use on the fingers, toes, ears, penis, and tip of the nose.

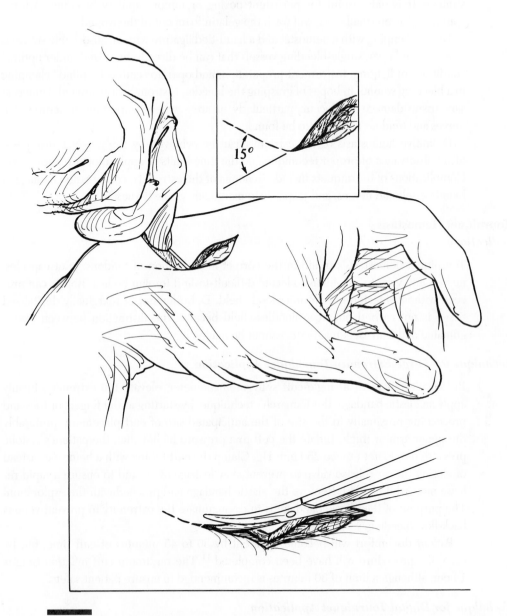

FIG. 8-2 Illustration of a technique to extend a wound for better deep-structure exploration and evaluation. Note that the incision is at a slight angle from the original axis of the wound and parallel to underlying structures.

Packing the wound with the hemostatic gelatin foam, Gelfoam, is another hemostatic strategy. It is only useful for persistent oozing or minor capillary bleeding. Arterial "pumpers," even small ones, will wash the gelatin foam out of the wound.

Direct clamping with a hemostat and a hand-tied ligature with an absorbable suture is reserved for larger, single-bleeding vessels that can be directly visualized under optimal conditions of lighting, instrument preparation, and operator comfort. "Blind" clamping in a bleeding wound, in hopes of grasping the bleeder, is strongly discouraged. Unnecessary tissue damage can occur, particularly in areas where important structures like nerves and tendons are likely to be found.

Definitive hemostasis of the extremity can be achieved by the use of tourniquets. Strict observance of proper technique and the time limits of application are imperative. Complications of tourniquets include ischemia of the extremity, compression damage of blood vessels and nerves, and jeopardy to marginally viable tissues.[8]

Tourniquet Hemostasis
Indications

Tourniquet hemostasis can aid in the correct identification of tendons, joint capsules, nerves, and vessels, as well as to locate difficult-to-find foreign bodies. Repair can proceed without interference from a bloody field. Debridement of marginally devitalized tissue is not carried out in a bloodless field because the distinction between exsanguinated and truly ischemic tissue cannot be made.

Technique for Large-Extremity Tourniquet Application

Before placement of a single-cuff sphygmomanometer, elevate the extremity. Firmly apply an elastic bandage, the Esmarch's technique, by starting at the fingers or toes and proceeding proximally to the site of the anticipated site of cuff placement, preferably the upper arm or thigh. Inflate the cuff to a pressure higher than the patient's systolic pressure but do not exceed 250 mm Hg. Clamp the cuff tubing with a hemostat instead of closing the air release valve to prevent slow leakage of air and to ensure a rapid release method if needed. Remove the elastic bandage and proceed with the exploration. The purpose of the elastic bandage is to exsanguinate the extremity to prevent venous back-flow bleeding.

Patient discomfort will become apparent by 30 to 45 minutes of cuff time, but by then, the procedure will have been completed.[11] The maximum cuff inflation time is 1 hour, although a limit of 30 minutes is recommended to ensure patient safety.

Technique for Digital Tourniquet Application

Unfold a 4 × 4 gauze sponge to its fullest length and fold it in half so it appears to be an 8-inch band. Moisten that band with saline. Wrap the band firmly around the finger, starting at the tip and proceeding to the base. Stretch a Penrose drain around the base of the finger in a slinglike fashion and apply a hemostat to the drain to form a tight "ring" at

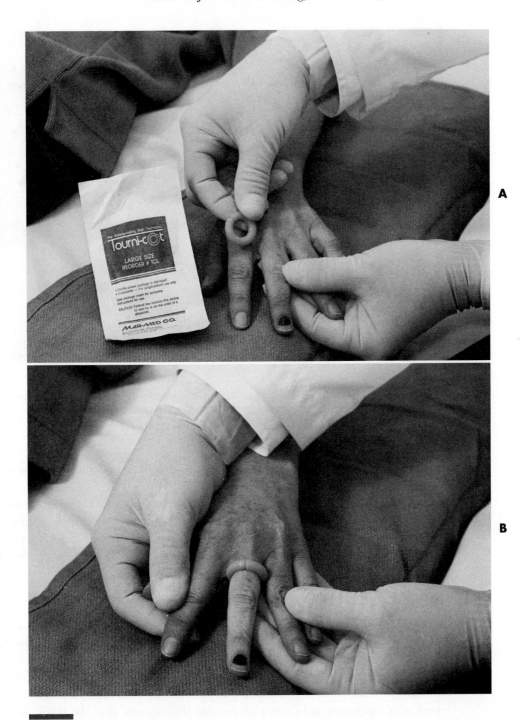

A

B

FIG. 8-3 Tourniquet hemostasis for finger injuries. **A,** Example of rubber digital tourniquet. Available in different sizes. **B,** The tourniquet is placed on the finger by rolling it from nail to base of digit.

Continued

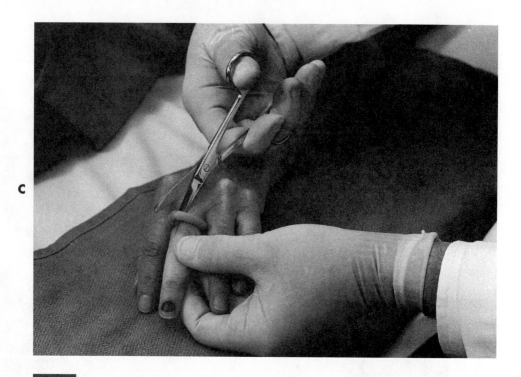

FIG. 8-3, cont'd   **C,** To avoid disturbing the repaired wound, the tourniquet is removed by cutting it off with scissors.

the base of the finger. Remove the sponge wrapping. A Penrose drain can also be substituted for the gauze sponge wrap.

There are preformed rubber disposable tourniquets (Tourni-Cot) that "roll" onto the finger and exsanguinate it before coming to rest at the digit base (Fig. 8-3). After use, they can be easily cut off with scissors. These tourniquets are easier to apply and effective in most cases where the digit circumference can accommodate them. The maximum allowable tourniquet time for a finger is 20 to 30 minutes.

TISSUE DEBRIDEMENT AND EXCISION

Before actual suturing and knot-tying, the wound has to be made free of contaminants and devitalized tissue. Devitalized tissue can be recognized by its shredded, ischemic, or blue/black appearance. Occasionally, these appearances can be misleading and true demarcation between viable and devitalized skin cannot be made until 24 hours following wounding.[3] Therefore one overriding principle of wound debridement is to spare as much skin, epidermis and dermis, as possible immediately after the injury. Subcutaneous fat, on the other hand, can be liberally debrided. Revision of the complex wound

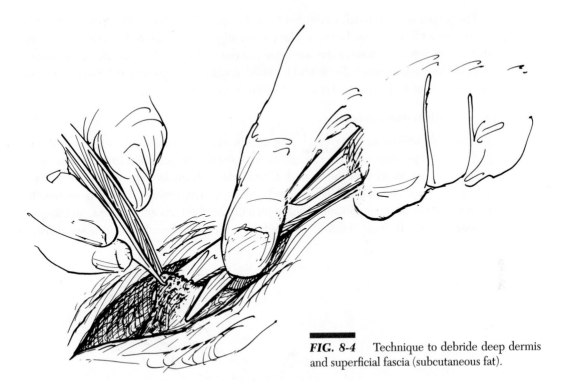

FIG. 8-4   Technique to debride deep dermis and superficial fascia (subcutaneous fat).

can be made at later interventions by consultant surgeons. They will be grateful for as much preserved skin as is possible to leave at the wound site.

Static skin tension plays an important role in wound edge debridement and revision. It is tempting to want to excise jagged wound edges to convert an irregular laceration into a straight one. If the wound is already gaping because of static tension, debridement of tissue increases the tension necessary to pull the new edges together. The resulting scar might be wider and more noticeable than it would have been by piecing together the original irregular edges.

Technique for Simple Excision and Wound Edge Revision

Most debridement can be carried out by simple, minimal excision of debris-laden tissue bits, using tissue forceps and iris scissors (Fig. 8-4). Superficial fascia (subcutaneous fat) under the skin can be freely excised without concern for deleterious cosmetic results. Soiled, devitalized fatty tissue is a fertile substrate for the growth of bacteria with subsequent development of infection.[6] More care has to be taken in debriding and excising epidermis and dermis. The best principle is to trim as little skin as possible, particularly on the face. It is preferable to repair wound edges in a jigsawlike pattern than to excise the irregular edges only to be left with a wound under excessive tension.

The proper method to trim a dermal wound edge is illustrated in Fig. 8-5. Iris (tissue) scissors or a #15 blade can be used. The wound edge is cut or incised at a slight angle so that the epidermal surface of the skin edge juts out slightly farther than the dermal portion. In this manner, when the wound is closed, it will naturally evert with the proper suture placement technique and resulting suture loop configuration.

Technique for Full Wound Excision

Full wound excisions are reserved for injuries in which all wound edges are devitalized and are obviously impossible to salvage. There must also be sufficient tissue redundancy in the anatomic location of the wound. If redundancy is inadequate, then excision creates a gap or defect that can only be closed under excessive tension. Areas where there is sufficient tissue to accommodate excision include the chest, abdomen, arms, and thighs. Whenever there is doubt about this procedure, it is best to consult a surgical specialist.

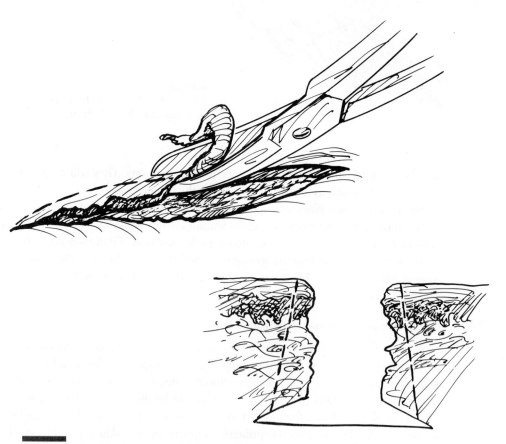

FIG. 8-5   Technique for excision by careful tissue scissor trimming of devitalized epidermis and dermis. Note the angle of excision that will facilitate wound-edge eversion during percutaneous closure.

Use the scalpel with a #15 blade to outline the tissue to be removed by partially incising or "scoring" the dermis (Fig. 8-6). Generally the excision is lenticular, that is shaped like an ellipse. To achieve proper closure without excessive tension or creating tissue "humps" at either end of the wound, the length of the ellipse should exceed the width by at least a 3:1 ratio. Once the ellipse is defined, use the scalpel or iris scissors or both in combination, to complete the excision (Fig. 8-7). The wound edges are incised at the same angle as described for dermal edge trimming. Not only do the edges have to be excised, but the excised tissue has also to be released from its base in the superficial fascia (subcutaneous tissue). Considerable bleeding often ensues and hemostatic measures

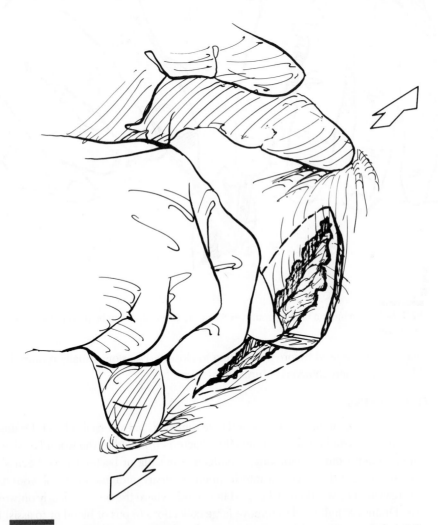

FIG. 8-6 Technique for initiating or "scoring" the epidermis and dermis before full wound excision. Note that the fingers are used to provide tension to the skin and the axis of the wound. This facilitates easier application of the scalpel to the skin.

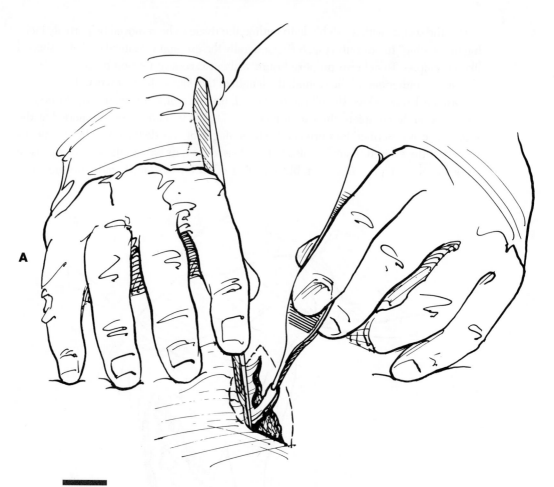

FIG. 8-7 Technique for full wound excision. **A,** The scalpel can be used to excise the wound in its entirety.

may have to be used before proceeding to closure. Excisions usually require both deep (dermal) and percutaneous sutures for closure.

SURGICAL DRAINS

Surgical drains for emergency wound care remain a controversial subject. Drains can act as retrograde conduits for contaminating bacteria from either the wound or skin. Under experimental wound conditions, subinfective inocula of bacteria have been shown to greatly increase the infection rate in drained versus undrained control wounds.[10] For this reason, they should only be used in wounds where the benefit clearly outweighs the risk. Drains are indicated to remove large collections of pus or blood or to assist in eliminating large pockets of dead space. As a general rule, wounds that can be managed in an emergency department setting do not need drains.

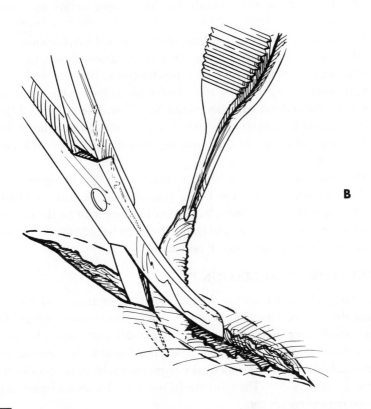

FIG. 8-7, *cont'd* **B,** Tissue scissors can be used to follow the original wound outline created by the "scoring" of the epidermis and dermis with the scalpel blade.

IMMEDIATE ANTIBIOTIC THERAPY

For simple, uncomplicated wounds and lacerations, there is no good clinical or investigative evidence that systemic antibiotics provide protection against the development of wound infection.[4, 5, 7, 13, 15] Occasionally, however, the physician is faced with a wound or laceration that necessitates the consideration of immediate antibiotic coverage during or even before wound management itself. Under these conditions, there is experimental evidence that antibiotic action rapidly decreases in effectiveness if it is not initiated within 3 to 4 hours of the injury.[12] Therefore, if intravenous antibiotics are thought necessary by the physician, they need to be administered without delay. The following are situations in which the immediate administration of intravenous antibiotics should be considered:

- Complex or mutilating wounds, especially of the hand or foot (e.g., lawn-mower or chain-saw injuries)
- Grossly contaminated wounds with penetrating debris and "ground-in" foreign material
- Lacerations in areas of lymphatic obstruction and lymphedema
- Extensive lacerations of the ear and its cartilaginous skeleton
- Suspected penetration of bone (open fractures), joints, or tendons
- Amputation injuries, especially where replantation is a consideration
- Extensive or distal extremity animal-bite wounds (see Chapter 14)
- Significant lacerations in patients with preexisting valvular heart disease
- Presence of disease or drugs causing immunosuppression or altered host defenses (e.g., diabetes)

The initial intravenous antibiotic of choice is usually a first-generation cephalosporin such as cefazolin (Kefzol, Ancef). For penicillin-allergic patients, clindamycin is a reasonable alternative. For animal bites, refer to Chapter 14 for the recommended agents. It is recommended that a wound culture be taken before initiation of antibiotics to assist in later modification of therapy if necessary.

GUIDELINES FOR CONSULTATION

Inevitably, physicians are faced with wounds, lacerations, and related problems that cause them to consider consulting a specialist. There are no hard and fast rules governing consultations. Because there are many different circumstances under which a consultation might be considered, it is impossible to make comprehensive recommendations. Additionally, each emergency physician has his or her own level of expertise, experience, and comfort. Therefore the following guidelines are based on practice realities governing emergency care.

Standard of Care: Driven largely by the legal system, medical care is often defined in terms of some standard. In the case of wound care, emergency physicians are often held to the same "standard of care" as might be practiced by a surgical specialist. In reality, there is no fixed standard for any specialty or type of care. Through board certification, emergency physicians are clearly qualified to provide emergency wound care. However, the "practice" line between an emergency physician and a surgical specialist is blurred. Each practitioner of wound care has to understand his or her strengths and limitations and act accordingly. It is also important to have knowledge of community defined patterns of care. For example, in some locales, only specialists perform tendon repairs, whereas, in others, emergency physicians comfortably treat extensor tendons lacerations.

Logistics of Care: Certain wounds can be technically managed by emergency physicians, but the time necessary to close the wound would significantly impede the operation of the emergency department. If direct physician involvement time exceeds 30 minutes, then consultation might be considered.

Cosmetics/Patient Expectation: Patients or family members often have expectations that "specialists" need to be involved in the care and repair of wounds. Parents frequently request a "plastic" surgeon for their child's facial laceration. If the laceration can be confidently repaired by the emergency caregiver, most parents can be made comfortable with a clear explanation of the actual repair needed and the skills of the caregiver. However, there are patients or relatives who are fixed on the need for a specialist. Usually, it is best to accede to those wishes.

Continuity of Care: Certain wounds, particularly those of the hand, require close follow-up and rehabilitation. It may be best to involve a specialist in the initial care to ensure continuity. It is a common arrangement between emergency physicians and hand specialists to have the emergency physician do the primary closure with follow-up care going to the specialist. Specific circumstances include uncomplicated injuries to tendon or digital nerves. The emergency physician does the initial injury assessment and skin closure. The specialist can follow the patient and schedule a delayed repair of the tendon or nerve. This collaboration can be very successful and is built on trust between the different caregivers.

REFERENCES

1. Altemeier W: Principles in the management of traumatic wounds and infection control, *Bull NY Acad Med* 55:123-138, 1979.
2. Dimick AR: Delayed wound closure: indications and techniques, *Ann Emerg Med* 17:1303-1304, 1988.
3. Edlich RF, et al: Principles of emergency wound management, *Ann Emerg Med* 17:1284-1302, 1988.
4. Grossman J, Adams J, Kunec J: Prophylactic antibiotics in simple hand lacerations, *JAMA* 245:1055-1056, 1981.
5. Haughey R, Lammers R, Wagner D: Use of antibiotics in the initial management of soft tissue hand wounds, *Ann Emerg Med* 10:187-192, 1981.
6. Haury B, et al: Debridement: an essential component of wound care, *Am J Surg* 135:238-242, 1978.
7. Hutton P, Jones B, Law D: Depot penicillin as prophylaxis in accidental wounds, *Br J Surg* 65:549-550, 1978.
8. Lammers RL: Principles of wound management. In Roberts JR, Hedges JR, editors: *Clinical procedures in emergency medicine*, Philadelphia, 1985, WB Saunders.
9. Losken HW, Auchinloss JA: Human bites of the lip, *Clin Plast Surg* 11:159-161, 1984.
10. Magee C, et al: Potentiation of wound infection by surgical drains, *Am J Surg* 131:547-549, 1976.
11. Roberts JR: Intravenous regional anesthesia, *J Am Coll Emerg Phys* 6:261-264, 1977.
12. Robson M, Duke W, Krizek T: Rapid bacterial screening in treatment of civilian wounds, *J Surg Res* 14:426-430, 1973.
13. Rutherford W, Spence R: Infection in wounds sutured in the accident and emergency department, *Ann Emerg Med* 9:350-352, 1980.
14. Smilanich RP, Bonnet I, Kirkpatrick JR: Contaminated wounds: the effect of initial management on outcome, *Am Surg* 61:427-430, 1995.
15. Thirlby R, Blair A: The value of prophylactic antibiotics for simple lacerations, *Surg Gynecol Obstet* 156:212-216, 1983.

9 Basic Laceration Repair Principles and Techniques

Definition of Terms
Basic Knot-Tying Techniques
Principles of Wound Closure
    Layer Matching

Wound-Edge Eversion
Wound Tension
Dead Space
Closure Sequence and Style

Each wound and laceration has different technical requirements that have to be met to properly effect closure. By understanding the basic principles that underlie the technical requisites of wound care, lacerations and wounds can be closed with the best chance for an optimal result. During actual closure, every attempt is made to match each layer evenly and produce a wound edge that is properly everted. Of paramount importance is proper knot-tying technique to facilitate eversion and to prevent excessive tension on the wound edge. When necessary, dead space is closed and finally, sutures are spaced and sequenced to provide the best and most gentle mechanical support.

DEFINITION OF TERMS

Several techniques and maneuvers used in wound care are referred to by terms that can be confusing. These terms are defined in the following discussion so that the reader thoroughly understands the material contained in this chapter.

Bite

A bite is the amount of tissue taken when placing the suture needle in the skin or fascia. The farther away from the wound edge that the needle is introduced into the epidermis, for example, the bigger the bite.

Throw

Each suture knot consists of a series of throws. A square knot is fashioned with two throws. Because of its tendency to unravel, several additional throws are necessary to secure the final knot when nylon is being used.

Percutaneous closure (Skin closure)

Sutures, usually of a nonabsorbable material, that are placed in skin with the knot tied on the surface are called percutaneous closures. They are also referred to as skin closures.

Dermal closure (Deep closure)

Sutures, usually of an absorbable material, that are placed in the superficial (subcutaneous) fascia and dermis with the knot buried in the wound are called deep closures.

Interrupted closure

Single sutures, tied separately, whether deep or percutaneous, are called interrupted sutures.

Continuous closure (Running suture)

A wound closure accomplished by taking several bites that are the full length of the wound, without tying individual knots, is a continuous or running suture. Knots are tied only at the beginning and end of the closure to secure the suture material. Continuous closures can be percutaneous or deep.

BASIC KNOT-TYING TECHNIQUES

There are several knots that can be used to tie sutures during wound closure. The most common is the surgeon's knot (Fig. 9-1). The advantage of this knot is that the double first throw offers better knot security and there is less slipping of the suture material as the wound is gently pulled together during tying. The wound edges will remain apposed while the second and subsequent single throws are accomplished. The knot-tying sequence shown in Fig. 9-1 illustrates the proper instrument technique required to obtain a surgeon's knot. The instrument tie can be used for almost all knots, whether for deep or superficial closures.

Occasionally it is necessary to perform a hand tie. Hand ties in emergency wound care are most useful for ligating vessels to achieve hemostasis. After a small bleeding vessel is clamped with the tip of a hemostat, an absorbable suture is brought around the vessel held by the hemostat and tied in the manner illustrated in Fig. 9-2. Because two hands are necessary for this tie, an assistant is often required to hold the hemostat and display the tie so that the vessel can be easily encircled with the suture.

PRINCIPLES OF WOUND CLOSURE
Layer Matching

When closing a laceration it is important to match each layer of a wound edge to its counterpart. Deep fascia, when opened traumatically, is closed to deep fascia. Superficial fascia has to meet superficial fascia. Finally, dermis to dermis will necessarily bring

Text continues on p. 143

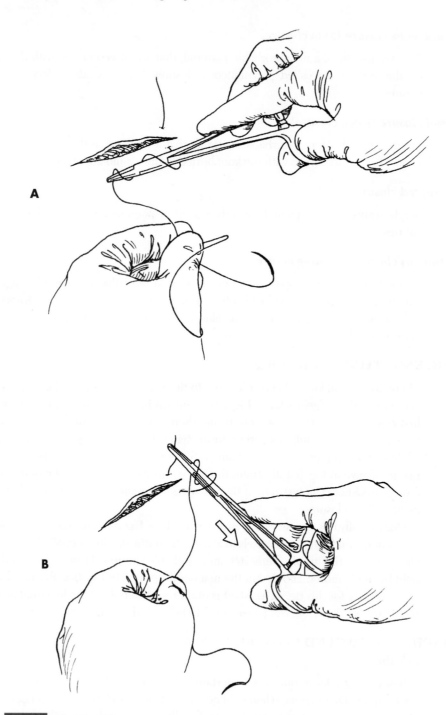

FIG. 9-1   For legend see opposite page.

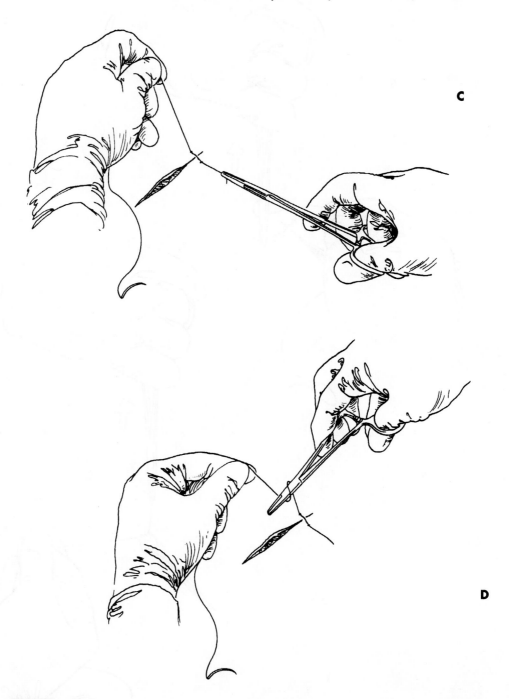

C

D

FIG. 9-1, cont'd   Sequence for instrument tie of a standard percutaneous suture closure. Note in the boxed illustration in **G,** the surgeon's knot and final square knot configuration.

Continued

136

E

F

FIG. 9-1, cont'd For legend see p. 135.

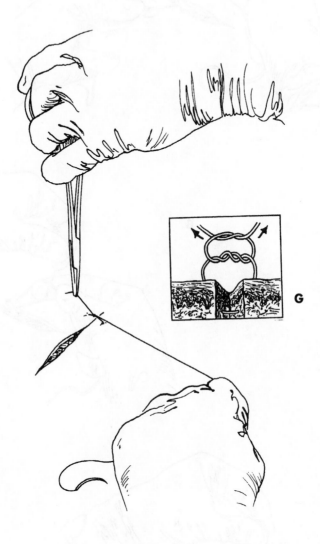

G

FIG. 9-1, cont'd   Note in the boxed illustration in **G**, the surgeon's knot and final square knot configuration.

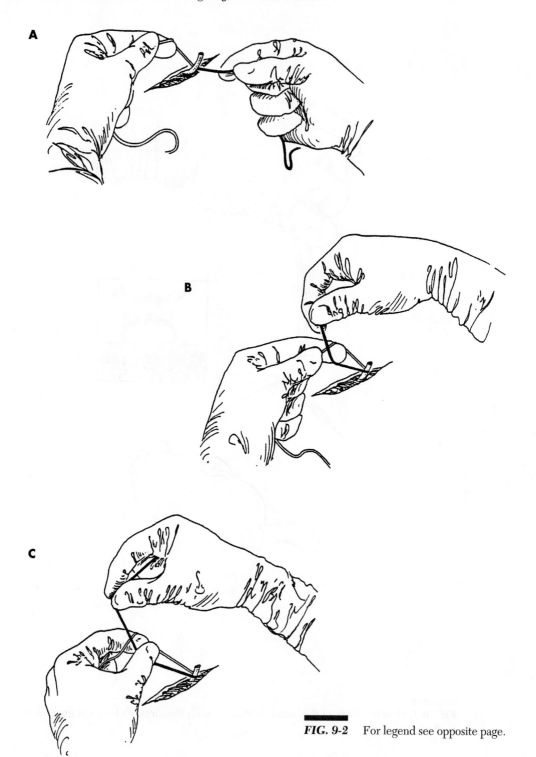

FIG. 9-2 For legend see opposite page.

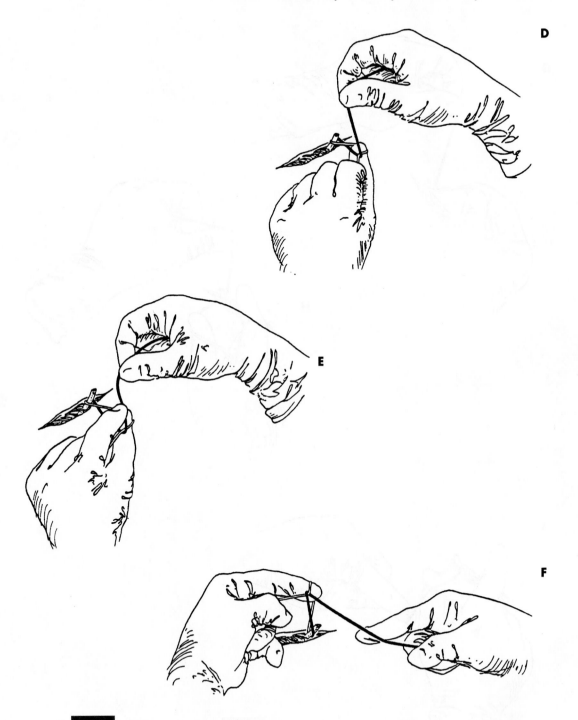

FIG. 9-2, *cont'd*   Sequence for a two-handed tie of hemostat-clamped vessels for hemostasis.

Continued

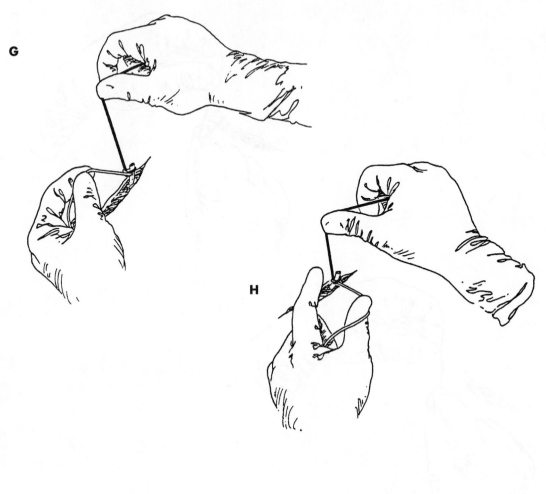

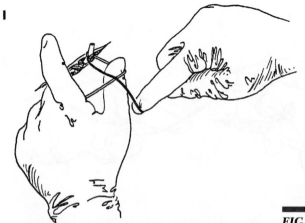

FIG. 9-2, *cont'd*   For legend see opposite page.

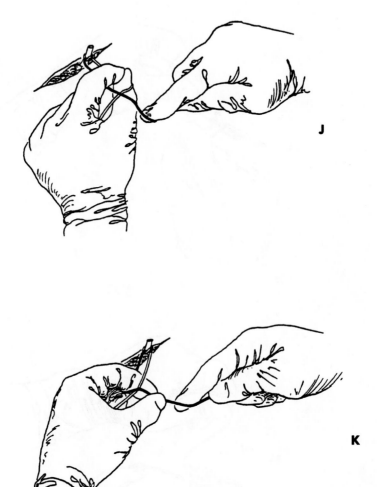

FIG. 9-2, cont'd   Sequence for a two-handed tie of hemostat-clamped vessels for hemostasis.

Continued

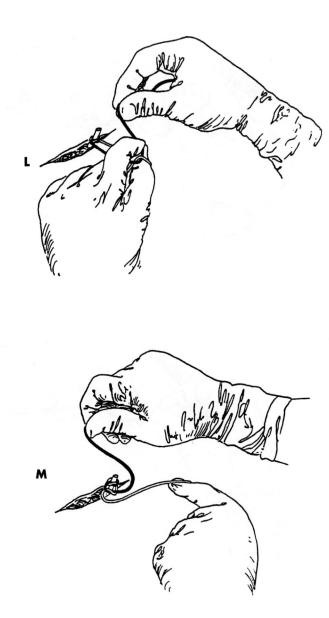

FIG. 9-2, cont'd   Sequence for a two-handed tie of hemostat-clamped vessels for hemostasis.

epidermis to epidermis. Failure to appose layers meticulously can cause improper healing with an unnecessarily large scar (Fig. 9-3).

Wound-Edge Eversion

Just as important as layer matching is proper wound-edge eversion during the initial repair. Because of the normal tendency of scars to contract with time, a slightly raised wound edge above the plane of the normal skin will gradually flatten with healing and have a final appearance that is cosmetically acceptable (Fig. 9-4). Wounds that are not everted contract into linear pits that become noticeable cosmetic defects because of their tendency to cast shadows.

Techniques for Wound-Edge Eversion

The key to achieving proper wound-edge eversion is to use the correct technique for introducing the needle into the skin and producing the proper suture configuration. As illustrated in Fig. 9-5, the point of the needle should pierce the epidermis and dermis at a 90-degree angle before it is curved around through the tissues. To ensure a 90-degree angle, the needle holder has to be held in the manner described in Chapter 7. It is me-

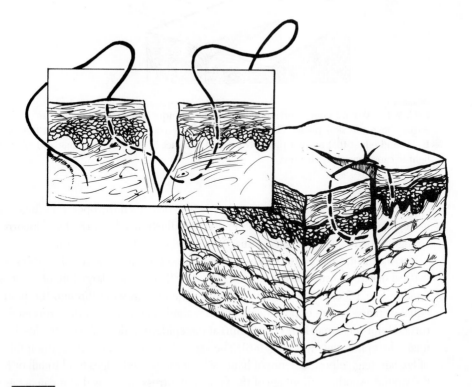

FIG. 9-3   Illustration of the incorrect technique to provide for layer matching.

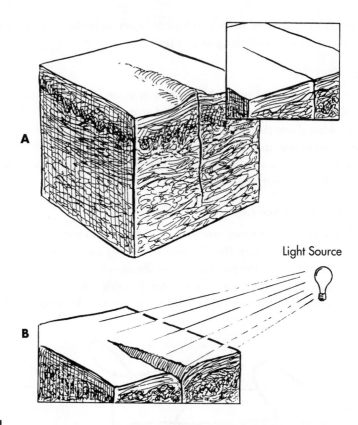

FIG. 9-4 Wound edge eversion. **A,** Correct technique allows for a slight rise of the wound edges above the skin plane. These edges eventually contract to flatten out at the skin plane. **B,** Wound edges that are not properly everted contract below the skin plane and allow incident light to cause unsightly shadows.

chanically very difficult to maneuver the needle correctly if the operator's fingers remain in the finger rings of the needle holder. Fig. 9-5 illustrates the correct and incorrect final configuration of an interrupted suture to achieve wound-edge eversion.

Vertical Mattress Suture. Another useful method for wound-edge eversion is the vertical mattress suture. This suture is placed by first taking a large bite of tissue approximately 1 to 1.5 cm away from the wound edge and crossing through the tissue to an equal distance on the opposite side of the wound. The needle is then reversed and returned for a very small bite (1 or 2 mm) at the epidermal/dermal edge to closely approximate the epidermal layer (Fig. 9-6). The vertical mattress suture is very helpful in areas of lax skin (e.g., elbow, dorsum of hand) where the wound edges tend to fall or fold into the wound. Another advantage of the vertical mattress suture is that it can act as a deep and a superficial closure all in one suture. Some wounds are not deep enough to accom-

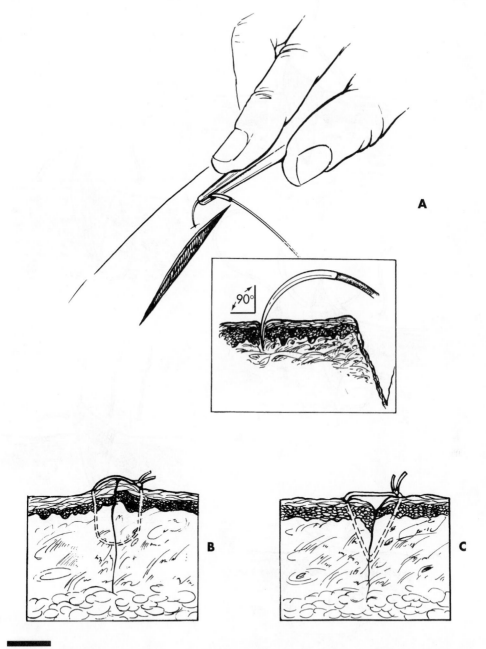

FIG. 9-5 Technique for proper wound-edge eversion. **A,** The suture needle is introduced at a 90-degree angle to the epidermis. **B,** The proper configuration of the suture should be square or bottle shaped. It is recognized that this configuration is difficult to achieve in actuality; however, this figure illustrates the correct principle. **C,** The incorrect technique of needle placement and suture configuration leads to wound edge inversion, which leads to "pitting" of the eventual scar.

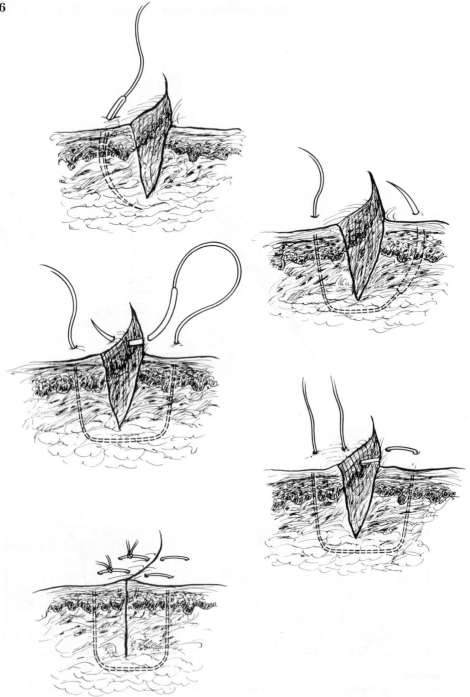

FIG. 9-6 Technique for a vertical mattress suture. Note that the second bite barely passes through the dermis to provide meticulous apposition of the epidermal edges.

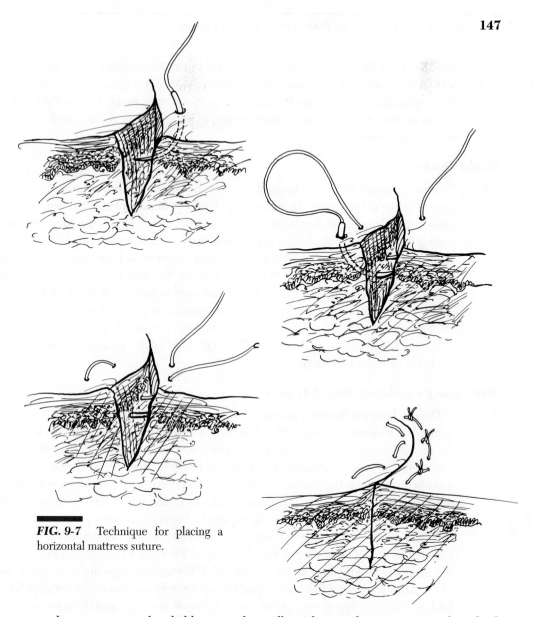

FIG. 9-7 Technique for placing a horizontal mattress suture.

modate a separate, absorbable suture but still need some deep support to close dead space. This technique can meet that need.

A modification of the vertical mattress suture, the shorthand technique, allows the suture to be placed more rapidly.[3] Instead of taking the large bite first, as described earlier, take the small bite, then the large one. By placing simultaneous traction on the trailing and leading portion of the suture after the small bite, the wound edges are elevated so that the needle easily takes the large bite.

Horizontal Mattress Suture. Another technique, the horizontal mattress suture, can also be used to achieve wound edge eversion (Fig. 9-7). The needle is introduced into the skin in the usual manner and is brought out at the opposite side of the wound. A second bite is taken approximately 0.5 cm adjacent to the first exit and is brought back to the original starting edge, also 0.5 cm from the initial entry point. The knot is tied leaving an everted edge. This is a suture technique often used in closing hand (palm and dorsum) lacerations.

Wound Tension

Whenever wound edges are brought together by suturing, there is inevitable tension created in the tissue within the suture loop. It is very important to minimize tension to preserve capillary blood flow to the wound edge. Excessive force exerted on the tissue leads to ischemia and can possibly cause some degree of cellular necrosis.[1] Necrosis provokes a more intense inflammatory response with the eventual formation of an irregular, cosmetically unacceptable scar. When tying knots, the first throw is crucial. As the wound edges are brought together, they are allowed to just barely touch. Bringing the edges together more forcibly by making the first throw too tight promotes ischemia. Wound edges tend to become slightly edematous after repair; therefore a small amount of slack between them will disappear. The addition of edema to a suture line that is already too tight can be disastrous.

Techniques for Reducing Wound Tension

Deep Closures. Proper placement of deep closures to bring the dermis close together before suture closure will reduce final wound edge tension. Fig. 9-8 illustrates the method for placing and tying deep closures. To start this suture, the needle is introduced into the superficial fascia, close to the underside of the dermis. The needle is then brought up through the dermis. At this point, the needle has to be rearmed with the needle holder. The needle is then introduced into the dermis of the matching opposite wound edge and carried down into the superficial fascia to complete the second bite.

Crucial to this technique is that both the trailing and leading portions of the suture remain on the same side of the portion of the suture that crosses from dermis to dermis. In this manner, when the knot is tied, it is buried. If the trailing edges are on opposite sides of the dermal crossing, the knot is pushed superficially and interferes with epidermal healing. Three or four throws are adequate to secure the knot, and the suture ends are cut close to the knot itself, leaving no more than 2-mm "tails." The temptation to place numerous deep closures must be resisted. These sutures act as foreign bodies and become a nidus for wound infection.[2] They also provoke a greater healing response and can increase the total bulk of a scar. Therefore place only as many sutures as are necessary to accomplish the task of reducing wound tension.

Wound Undermining. Another technique for reducing tension is wound undermining. Undermining releases the dermis and superficial fascia from their deeper attachments, allowing the wound edge to be brought together with less force. Anatomic areas where undermining is useful include the scalp, forehead, and lower legs, particularly

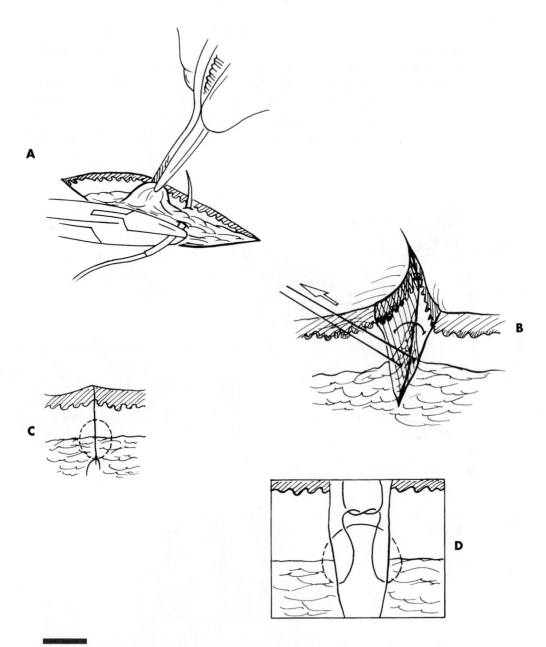

FIG. 9-8   Technique for placing a deep suture. **A,** Suture placement is initiated by driving the needle from deep in the wound to superficial. **B,** The needle is then driven superficial to deep on the opposite side of the wound. Note that the leading and trailing suture come out on the same side of the cross suture. **C,** This same-side technique allows for the knot to be tied deep and away from the wound surface. **D,** If the same-side technique is not followed, the knot is forced to the wound surface by the cross suture and may possibly protrude out of the wound.

over the tibia where the skin is under a great deal of natural tension. Caution has to be exercised in deciding to undermine because this procedure can spread bacteria into deeper tissues, as well as create a deeper, larger dead space.

The technique for undermining is illustrated in Fig. 9-9, A. For most minor wound care problems, the proper tissue plane is between the superficial fascia (subcutaneous tissue) and deep fascia overlying the muscle. Staying in this plane maintains the integrity of the blood and nerve supply to the skin (dermis and epidermis). Metzenbaum dissec-

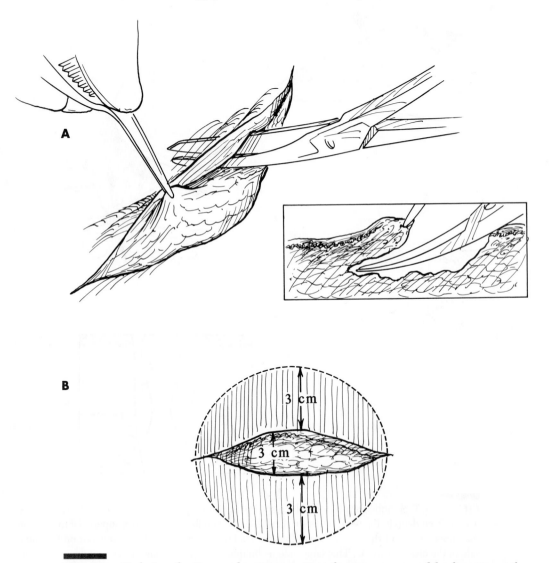

FIG. 9-9 Technique for tissue undermining. **A,** Note that scissors are used for dissection at the dermal superficial fascia level. Tissue spreading is preferred to cutting the sharp edges. **B,** The zone of undermining is illustrated.

tion scissors (or for smaller wounds, iris scissors) can be inserted parallel to the deep fascia where it joins the superficial fascia. The instrument is gently spread to create a plane of dissection. Undermining also can be carried out with a #15 blade on a standard knife handle. The blade is rotated away from the deep fascia and used as a combination cutting instrument and probe. Actual cutting is kept to a minimum to prevent excessive bleeding.

Wounds are undermined from end to end, to a distance from the wound edge that approximates the extent of "gapping" of the wound edges. In other words, if a wound gaps open 3 cm from edge to edge, then undermining is carried out to 3 cm under the der-

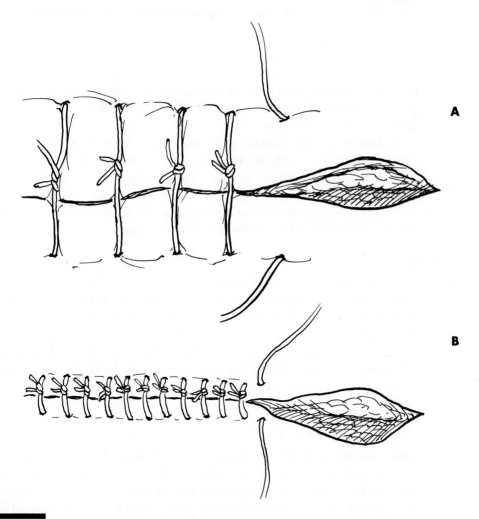

FIG. 9-10   A technique for reducing wound tension. **A,** A few sutures, placed far apart and far from the wound edges, increase wound tension. **B,** More sutures placed closer together and closer to the wound edges reduce tension.

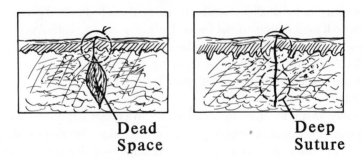

Dead
Space

Deep
Suture

FIG. 9-11   Example of dead space and a two-layered closure to obliterate that space.

mis, perpendicularly away from the wound edge. A common mistake in using this technique is to fail to include the wound ends. Fig. 9-9, *B*, illustrates the proper zone of undermining during dissection.

Additional Suture Placement. Placing more sutures closer together also reduces wound tension (Fig. 9-10). Mechanically, a greater number of sutures lessens the total force exerted on each suture, thereby reducing potential tissue compression. The caregiver has to keep in mind, however, that sutures act as foreign bodies and can potentiate infection. Therefore when closing a wound a balance has to be struck between the number of sutures used and the desired tension reduction.

Dead Space

In the past it was axiomatic that no open or dead spaces should be left behind during wound closure. These spaces tend to fill with hematoma and can act as potential sites for wound infection (Fig. 9-11). Hematoma formation in these areas can also delay wound healing. However, there is experimental evidence that suture closure of these spaces, when they are contaminated with bacteria, increases the chance of wound infection.[2] Therefore it is recommended that deep closures only be used to close dead space in clean, minimally contaminated wounds. Even in these cases, as few sutures as possible should be used.

Closure Sequence and Style

Students learning wound care often ask how close together sutures should be placed. As a general rule, sutures are placed just far enough from each other so that no gap appears between the wound edges. As a general guideline, the distance between sutures is equal to the bite distance from the wound edge (Fig. 9-12). The great variability of lacerations, however, dictates that experience rapidly teaches the practitioner the proper distances at which sutures should be placed to close the wound.

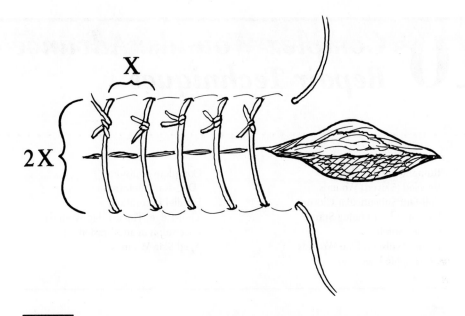

FIG. 9-12 Example of closure style and sequence. Note that the knots should be placed evenly on one side of the wound. Knots directly over the wound increase inflammation and scar tissue formation.

The final appearance of a suture line should be neat and organized. The knots are aligned to one side of the laceration. In addition to appearing orderly, knots are placed away from the wound edge to prevent a further inflammatory response that can be provoked by an increased amount of foreign material directly over the healing surface. Aligning of the knots to one side or the other contributes to wound edge eversion.

REFERENCES

1. Crikelair G: Skin suture marks, *Am J Surg* 96:631-639, 1958.
2. Edlich RF, Panek PH, Rodeheaver GT, et al: Physical and chemical configuration of sutures in the development of surgical infection, *Ann Surg* 177:679-687, 1973.
3. Jones SJ, Gartner M, Drew G, et al: The shorthand vertical mattress stitch: evaluation of a new suture technique, *Am J Emerg Med* 11:483-485,1993.

10 *Complex Wounds: Advanced Repair Techniques*

Running Suture Closure
Beveled (Skived) Wounds
Pull-Out Subcuticular Closure
Subcuticular Running Suture
Corner Stitch
Partial Avulsion, Flap Wounds
Geographic Lacerations

Complete Avulsions
"Dog-Ear" Deformities
Parallel Lacerations
Thin-Edge, Thick-Edge Wounds
Laceration in an Abrasion
Aged Skin Wounds

The majority of lacerations and wounds are straightforward and can be closed with the basic techniques (Chapter 9). On the other hand, some wounds are more complicated and present with a variety of technical challenges. The following are descriptions of some of the more complicated wound problems that can be encountered in a wound care setting. Techniques for "solving" these "puzzles" are suggested in the following discussions.

RUNNING SUTURE CLOSURE
Description

Lacerations, usually caused by simple shearing forces, can be quite long and therefore time-consuming to close. They are often caused by slash wounds from a knife or piece of glass. The continuous "over-and-over" (running) suture technique can be used when time is a factor.[5] Wounds over 5 cm in length can be considered for this technique. The time saved is beneficial to the person repairing the wound, because he or she can return quickly to other emergency department duties. There are drawbacks to this technique. If one loop of the suture breaks or is imperfectly positioned, then the whole process has to be repeated. Wound edge eversion can be difficult to control with this technique. Continuous sutures are reserved for straight lacerations in healthy, viable skin that will not collapse in with suturing. If this technique is applied to curved lacerations, it can create a "purse string" effect that bunches up the wound. Another technique that can be used for long, straight lacerations is wound stapling (see Chapter 13).

Technique for the Continuous Over-and-Over (Running) Suture

The technique for continuous over-and-over suturing is demonstrated in Fig. 10-1, *A*. The closure is started with the standard technique of a percutaneous interrupted suture, but the suture is *not* cut after the initial knot is tied (Fig. 10-1, *A*). The needle is then used to make repeated bites, starting at the original knot by making each new bite, through the skin, at an angle of 45 degrees to the wound direction (Fig. 10-1, *B* through *F*). The cross-stays of suture, on the surface of the skin, are at an angle of 90 degrees to the wound direction. The final bite is made at an angle of 90 degrees to the wound direction to bring the suture out next to the previous bite exit (Fig. 10-1, *G*). The final bite is left in a loose loop. The loop acts as a free end of suture for knot tying. The first throw of the final knot is made by looping the suture end held in the hand around the needle holder, then grasping the free loop (Fig. 10-1, *H*). The first throw is snugged down to skin level (Fig. 10-1, *I*). The knot is completed in the standard instrument-tie manner with several more throws at skin level (Fig. 10-1, *J* and *K*).

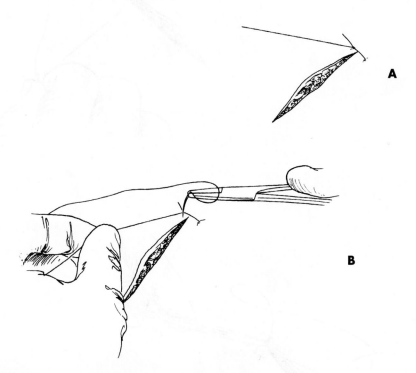

A

B

FIG. 10-1   Technique for continuous over-and-over suture (running suture). Note that the needle bites are made at an angle of 45 degrees to the axis of the wound. By taking bites at this angle, the cross stay of the suture at the skin surface is at an angle of 90 degrees to the wound axis. See text for complete description of technique.   *Continued*

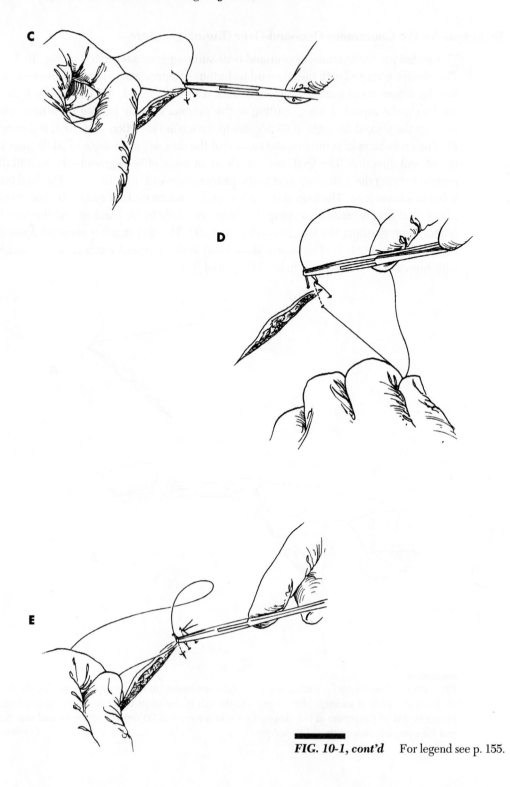

FIG. 10-1, cont'd   For legend see p. 155.

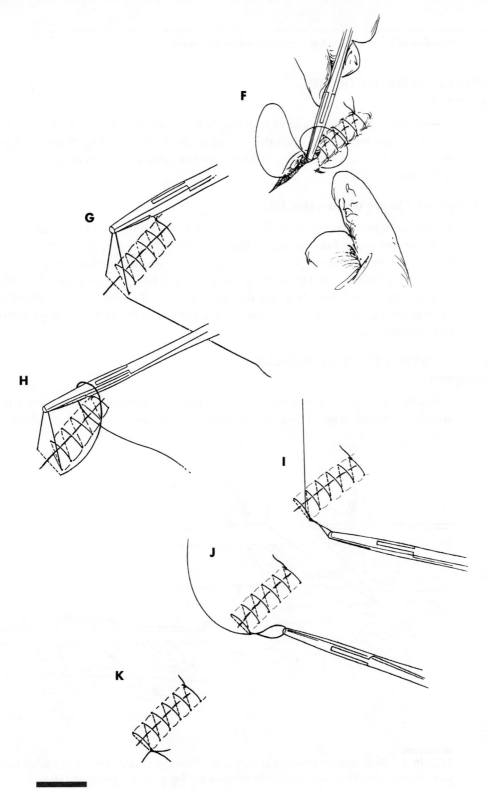

FIG. 10-1, cont'd   For legend see p. 155.

BEVELED (SKIVED) WOUNDS
Description

A very common problem in layer matching is the beveled-edge or "skived" laceration. Beveled edges are created when the striking angle of the wounding object is not perpendicular. The angle and force, however, are not acute enough to create a true flap deformity.

Technique for Closure of a Beveled Edge

A common misconception about the repair of this wound is that a larger bite is taken from the thin edge of the laceration than from the bigger edge. In fact, the opposite technique is the solution to proper layer matching. The technique for closing a beveled laceration is illustrated in Fig. 10-2. By taking unequal bites as shown, the edge will be brought into correct apposition with the opposite edge. If sufficient tissue redundancy exists in the wound area, excision of the edges can equalize the wound so simple sutures can close the wound.

PULL-OUT SUBCUTICULAR CLOSURE
Description

A favorite technique of plastic surgeons is the pull-out subcuticular stitch using a nonabsorbable suture material such as polypropylene (Prolene). This suture material is

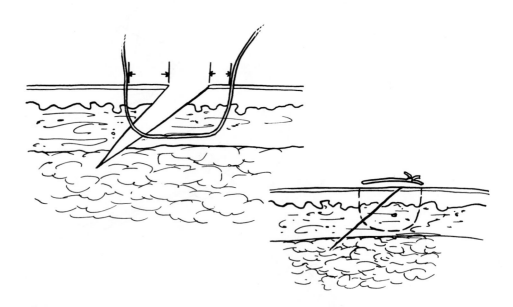

FIG. 10-2 Technique for closing a beveled edge. Note that there is a larger bite taken on the larger wound edge. There is a smaller bite taken on the flap portion of the wound edge.

stiffer and stronger than nylon and allows for easier removal.[3] The newer, nonabsorbable suture material, polybutester (Novofil), is also useful for this technique.[1] The pull-out is limited to straight lacerations less than 4 cm long because the suture would be too hard to extract at removal time. Children have naturally higher skin tension, so this technique is thought by some to be superior for that age group because it prevents suture marks. In spite of this fact, the pull-out subcuticular closure has no distinct advantage over percutaneous closure when final wound and scar appearance is compared.[4] Another use for this technique is for closure of lacerations over which splinting materials or plaster will be placed. It can also be used in patients who are at risk for keloid formation to prevent keloid formation at the needle puncture sites.

Technique for the Pull-Out Subcuticular Closure

Before placement of a pull-out subcuticular closure the superficial fascia (subcutaneous tissue) has to be adequately apposed with absorbable suture to bring the dermis close to approximation. The actual closure is begun by passing the needle of 4-0 or 5-0 nylon or polypropylene 1 to 1.5 cm from the wound end through the dermis layer and bringing it out the wound parallel to and through the plane of the dermis. Subsequent bites are made (Fig. 10-3) parallel to the dermis at a depth of 2 to 3 mm into the dermis. Each bite should "mimic" the other with regard to bite size and dermal depth on each side of the wound until the "tail" is brought out at the opposite end of the wound. The begin-

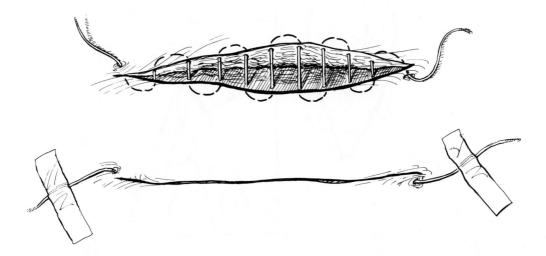

FIG. 10-3   Technique for pull-out dermal closure. See text for complete description of technique.

ning and final tail can be secured by wound tape. In the face this suture can remain in place for up to 7 days. This technique is often used in conjunction with wound taping to accurately match dermal and epidermal layers.

The suture is removed merely by pulling on one end with forceps or a needle holder and sliding the suture out of the dermal layer.

SUBCUTICULAR RUNNING CLOSURE
Description

This technique is often used by surgeons to close straight incisions. It can suffice to close the wound alone or can be supplemented with interrupted skin sutures. In wound care, it should be reserved for straight, clean lacerations with sharp, nondevitalized wound edges. It can be used to close wounds that have been excised or trimmed where the edges are left fresh and straight.

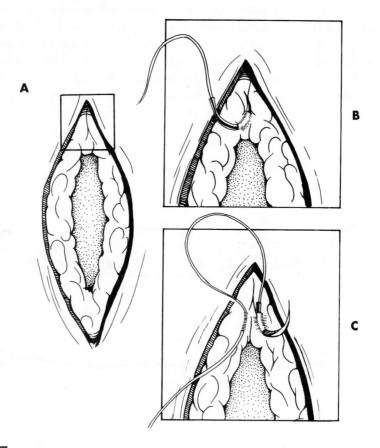

FIG. 10-4   Technique for running subcuticular suture. See text for complete description of technique.

Technique for the Subcuticular, Running Suture

An absorbable suture material, such as Dexon, Vicryl, PDS, or Maxon can be used. As for other running sutures, one strand is used, without interruption, for the entire laceration. As demonstrated in Fig. 10-4, the suture is anchored at one end of the laceration. The plane chosen is either the dermis or just deep to the dermis in the superficial subcutaneous fascia. While maintaining this plane, "mirror image" bites are taken horizontally the full length of the wound. The final bite leaves a trailing loop of suture, as shown, so that the knot can be fashioned for final closure. This technique is commonly supplemented with wound tapes, particularly if there remains some degree of gapping of the edges.

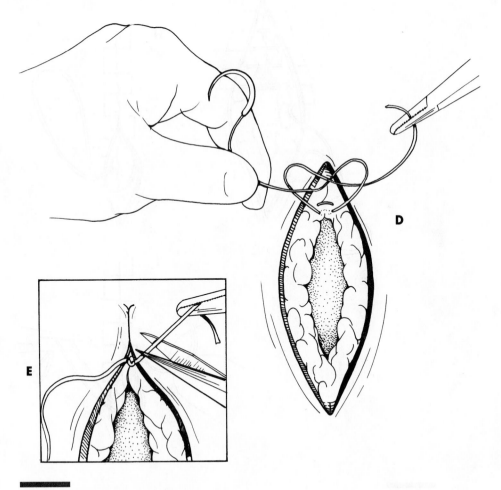

FIG. 10-4, cont'd   For legend see opposite page.
Continued

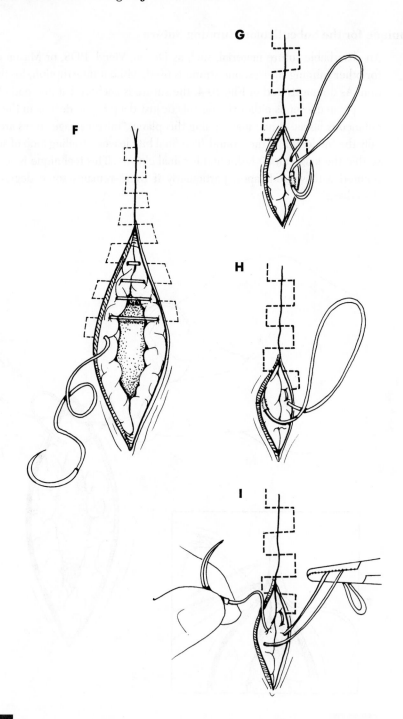

FIG. 10-4, cont'd   For legend see p. 160.

CORNER STITCH
Description

Many wounds are irregular and jagged, with corners that need to be secured during closure. Corners and flaps are particularly vulnerable because they receive their blood supply only from an intact base. Improper suturing of the tip of a corner can compromise an already tenuous vascularity.

Technique for Closing a Corner

A simple technique to secure a corner without interrupting the small capillaries at the tip is demonstrated in Fig. 10-5. The technique used is the half-buried horizontal mattress suture. The suture is introduced percutaneously, through the skin in the noncorner portion of the wound. The needle is brought through the dermis and then passed *horizontally* through the corner dermis and brought back to the same plane of dermis on the opposite side of the noncorner portion. Finally, it is led out through the epidermis.

The key to this suture is that the flap portion of the suture passes horizontally through the dermis and not vertically through both the epidermis and dermis. Once the tip is in place with the corner stitch, then the remainder of the flap can be closed with interrupted percutaneous or half-buried horizontal mattress sutures, which should be placed far enough from the tip to allow for unrestricted dermal circulation.

A single corner stitch can encompass several corners of stellate lacerations by capturing all of the corners of flaps (Fig. 10-6) until the final percutaneous reexposure is completed to tie the knot. The corner suture is one of the most useful suture techniques in emergency wound and laceration care for complex wound closure.

PARTIAL AVULSION, FLAP WOUNDS
Description

Flap lacerations are the result of forces that tear up, or avulse, a flap skin from the subcutaneous tissue. The vascular supply of a complicated flap is even more tenuous because it derives blood from only its intact dermal attachment. A general rule for viability is that the flap base should exceed flap length by a ratio of 3:1.[2] Flaps with lower ratios are less likely to survive. The rule varies according to anatomic site and other considerations. Obviously, a long, narrow-based flap is in greater jeopardy than a short, broad-based flap.

Flaps that are distally based have the tip pointing opposite to the natural cutaneous arterial flow. They rely solely on venous backflow for oxygen and nutrients. The repair technique has to be meticulous; gentle; and dictated by the condition of the flap, the width of the total wound, and the anatomic location. Flaps that are proximally based usually have adequate perfusions, but the repair has to be no less careful.

Technique for Preparing and Repairing a Complicated Flap

Excessive fatty superficial fascia (subcutaneous tissue) on the underside or dermal part of the flap can impair healing when it is secured with sutures. A raw dermal surface is

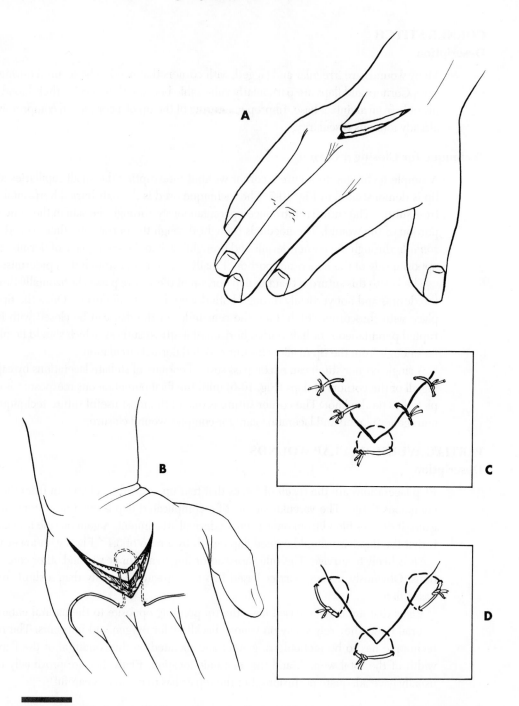

FIG. 10-5 Technique for closing a corner (flap stitch). See text for complete description of technique.

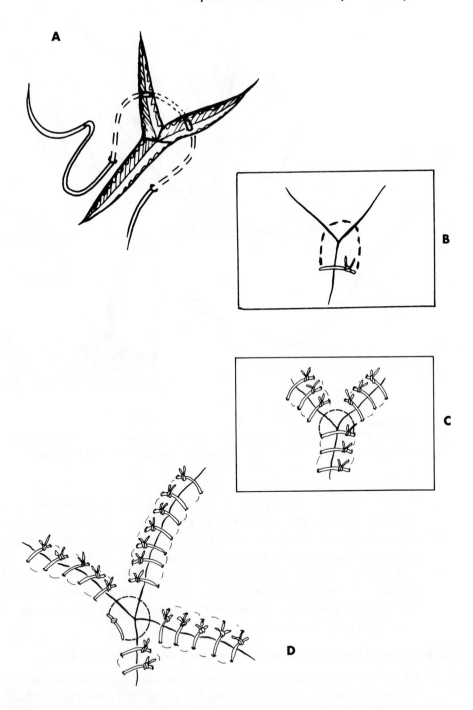

FIG. 10-6 Technique for using the corner stitch to close a stellate or multi-flap laceration.

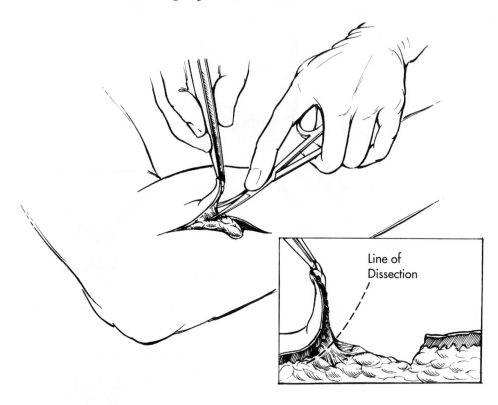

Line of
Dissection

FIG. 10-7 Technique for defatting the base of a flap for better union and vascularization to occur after suture anchoring. Fat is removed at the dermal-superficial fascia plane.

preferable to damaged fat when the flap is replaced in the laceration defect. In this sense, flaps are similar to grafts. To improve the chance of flap survival during early healing, it is best to remove the excessive fat from the flap before suturing (Fig. 10-7). Iris scissors can be used to trim the fat until only a fresh tissue surface remains.

If the flap is otherwise in good condition with viable edges, then the initial suture is the half-buried mattress suture described earlier for corner closure. The remainder of the flap can be closed with the same suture technique for the corner closure with simple interrupted percutaneous sutures.

Technique for Closure of Flaps with Nonviable Edges: the V-Y Closure

Often flaps will have damaged edges that are not viable, in which case the edges can be excised to create a smaller but more viable flap. Fig. 10-8 illustrates how this flap is then secured by converting a **V**-closure to a **Y**-closure to accommodate the smaller amount of tissue available. With iris scissors, the edges of the flaps are trimmed back to viable tis-

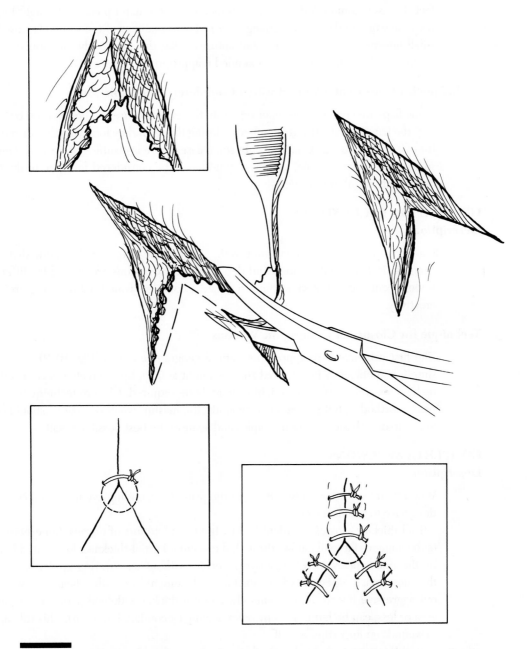

FIG. 10-8   Technique for closure of flaps with nonviable edges: the V-Y closure. Note that the edges of the flap are excised. The remaining flap is not large enough to fill the defect; therefore a corner stitch is placed to close the wound as a Y instead of its original V configuration.

sue. The remaining flap, however, is not large enough to accommodate the resultant defect. By using a modified corner stitch technique, the flap tip can be brought together with the wound edges in a Y configuration. The remainder of the wound is closed with small-bite percutaneous interrupted sutures. Like the previously mentioned complicated flap, defatting is also recommended if appropriate.

Technique for Closure of a Wound with a Completely Nonviable Flap

Some flaps are beyond revision or repair. In this case, closure can be achieved by "ellipsing" the flap (Fig. 10-9) and completely closing the wound by following the 3:1 ratio rule for ellipse closure (see Chapter 8). In some cases there is insufficient tissue redundancy so ellipsing is not feasible, and the wound has to be considered for open healing (secondary intention) or grafting.

GEOGRAPHIC LACERATIONS
Description

One of the most challenging wounds is the "geographic laceration," a wound that can be irregular in both configuration and depth. These lacerations are caused by differential forces occurring at the same time to create a complex wound. Closure requires some creativity.

Technique for Closure of Geographic Wounds

The first principle is to appose the natural geographic points (Fig. 10-10). After that, simple percutaneous interrupted sutures might suffice, but a creative mix of different techniques and suture sizes might ultimately be required. Closure techniques may appear unorthodox, but for traumatic wounds, the maxim "whatever works" should be followed to obey basic closure principles and achieve the best possible result.

COMPLETE AVULSIONS
Description

When tissue is lost or avulsed through the primary wounding event, several considerations have to be addressed.

Full-thickness losses are identified by the complete loss of dermis. Superficial fascia (subcutaneous fat) will "show" through the wound. Partial-thickness losses are identified by the raw appearance of underlying dermis without its covering epidermis. Partial-thickness losses, especially when intact dermal elements are visible, heal quite well without aggressive intervention. Generally, any full-thickness defects 1 to 2 cm square in area or less, can be left to heal by open healing (secondary intention). This rule applies to wounds on fingertips as well.

Full-thickness gaps or defects that are greater than 2 cm square in area need to be considered for grafting. Whenever questions about the possibility of grafting arise, a

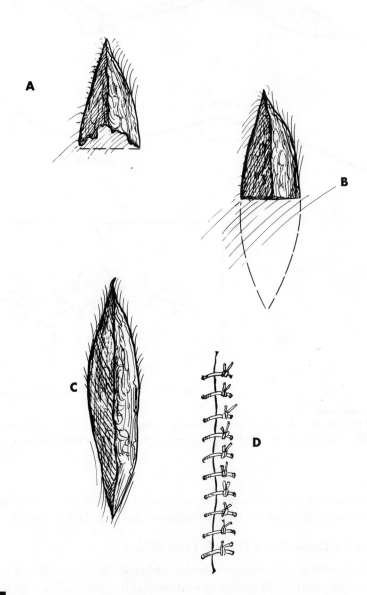

FIG. 10-9 Technique for closure of the wound with a completely nonviable flap. In this case, a complete ellipse can be fashioned and then closed primarily.

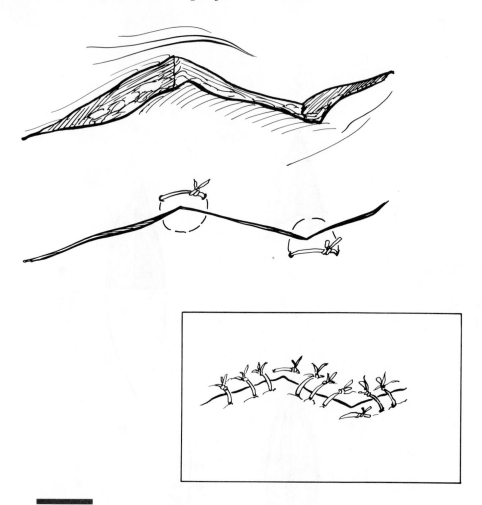

FIG. 10-10 Technique for closure of geographic wounds. Note that obvious geographic points are apposed first with either simple percutaneous sutures or corner sutures.

consultation with a specialist is recommended. Some defects can be closed primarily, without grafting, and suggested techniques are described in the following material.

Technique for Converting a Triangle to an Ellipse

If the avulsion defect is configured as a triangle, then conversion of that defect to an ellipse can be made by extending with excision the "defect" (see Fig. 10-9, *B* to *D*). If the basic 3:1 length-to-width rule (see Chapter 8) can be maintained during this process, then the whole defect can be closed with a few dermal (deep) supporting sutures and a line of percutaneous sutures with the result of a simple, single suture line. Undermining

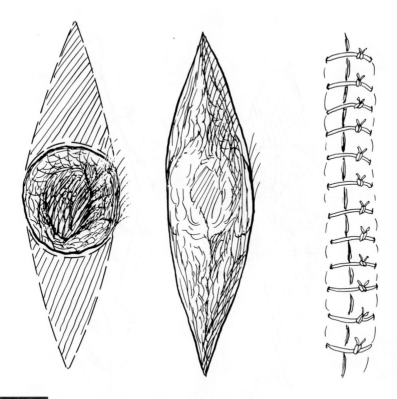

FIG. 10-11   Technique for closure of a circular defect by the ellipse method.

may be required to bring the wound edges together to reduce wound-edge tension. Again, there must be sufficient tissue redundancy to perform this closure successfully.

Technique for Closing a Circular or Irregular Defect

The simplest way to close this defect is to turn it into an ellipse as illustrated in Fig. 10-11. If the defect is too great, the technique of a double V-Y closure can be used. In this case, the defect is covered by two sliding pedicle flaps created by a #15 blade (Fig. 10-12). It is crucial not to disturb the fascial attachments of the flaps and interrupt the blood supply. Incise the dermis without including the subcutaneous tissue to allow the flaps to move forward on their vascular base into the gap.

"DOG-EAR" DEFORMITIES
Description

Trying to evenly close a laceration, particularly if it has a curving configuration, can lead to bunching of one or both of the wound edges as the suture closure proceeds. One edge of the wound can become redundant and can lead to the creation of a dog ear.

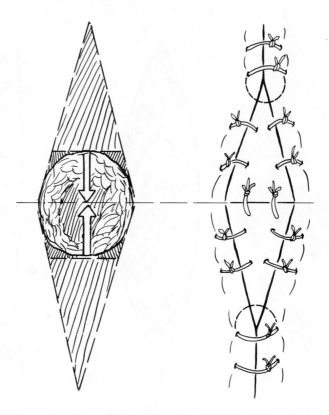

FIG. 10-12   Technique for closure of a circular or irregular defect by advancing flap pedicles to effect a double V-Y closure. (Adapted from Zukin D, Simon R: *Emergency wound care: principles and practice*, Rockville, Md., 1987, Aspen Publishers.)

Technique to Close a Dog Ear

To correct this problem, an incision is made with a #15 blade, beginning at the end of the wound and at a 45-degree angle from the direction of the laceration on the side of the redundancy (Fig. 10-13). The redundant tissue flap is excised along an imaginary line that directly corresponds with the incision. The remaining portion of tissue then fits the new configuration of the laceration incision and is appropriately sutured. The final outcome is a slightly angulated wound with a "hockey-stick" appearance.

PARALLEL LACERATIONS
Description

Two or more parallel lacerations that are in close proximity are often the result of self-inflicted wounds on the wrists or forearms. They are usually superficial but because of the nature of the anatomic site, these wounds can result in significant injuries to the un-

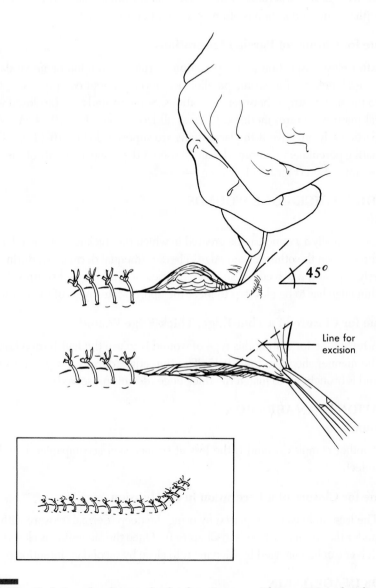

FIG. 10-13 Technique for closure of redundant tissue or a "dog ear." Note that the incision is made approximately at an angle of 45 degrees from the original axis of the wound. See text for complete description of technique.

derlying flexor structures of the wrist. Careful functional testing of nerves and tendons with wound exploration is often necessary before closure.

Technique for Closure of Parallel Lacerations

After close inspection and exploration to rule out tendon or nerve damage, there are several methods for closing parallel lacerations without compromising the blood supply to the tissue "strips" between lacerations. Some wounds can be closed with the horizontal mattress suture, modified to cross all lacerations (Fig. 10-14, *A*). Wound tapes are particularly effective if the lacerations are superficial (Fig. 10-14, *B*). Finally, the alternating percutaneous approach can be used if the vascular supply of the tissue will not be compromised (Fig. 10-14, *C*).

THIN-EDGE, THICK-EDGE WOUNDS
Description

Occasionally a wound can be created in which the thickness of one edge is markedly different from the other wound edge. There is unequal dermal loss during injury. To properly appose the two edges, simple percutaneous interrupted sutures do not suffice. The thin edge has to be elevated to meet the appropriate layers of the full-thickness edge.

Technique for Closure of a Thin-Edge, Thick-Edge Wound

A technique for closing this type of wound is to use the half-buried horizontal suture in the manner shown in Fig. 10-15. The thin edge (dermis lost) is captured by the suture and is brought up to match the thick edge (dermis preserved).

LACERATION IN AN ABRASION
Description

Another complex wound is the loss of surface skin accompanied by a laceration in the defect.

Technique for Closure of a Laceration in an Abrasion

The laceration can be repaired by using the deep (dermal) closure with the knot buried under the wound surface (see Chapter 9). Once the laceration is closed (Fig. 10-16), the defect can be managed by allowing it to close by secondary intention or grafting.

WOUNDS IN AGED SKIN
Description

People with older, thinner skin are subject to large partial avulsions of skin even if the traumatic forces involved are minor. In addition to the laceration, the skin separates at the dermal/superficial fascia (subcutaneous layer) resulting in a flap. The skin is thin, friable, and does not hold sutures well. Patients taking large chronic doses of corticosteroids have altered skin biomechanics that result in similar disruptions.

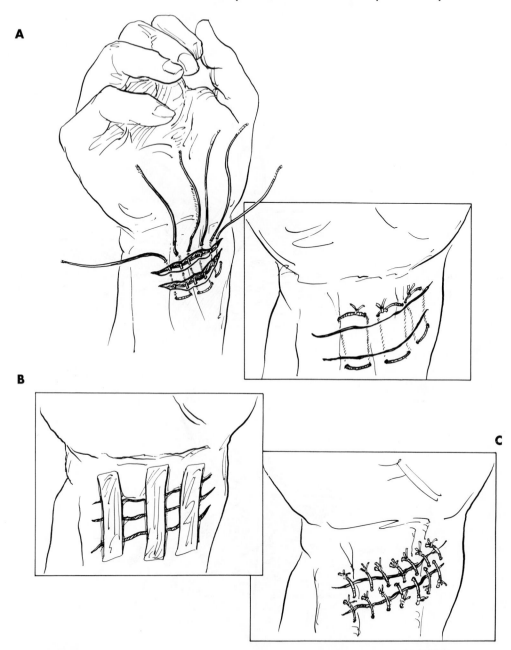

FIG. 10-14   Note the three techniques for closure of parallel lacerations. **A,** The horizontal mattress technique is used to cross all lacerations for closure. **B,** Wound tapes can be used to close these lacerations. **C,** If the island of tissue is wide enough, alternating sutures can be used on each laceration. However, it is necessary to be very careful not to compromise vascular supply when using this technique. (Adapted from Zukin D, Simon R: *Emergency wound care: principles and practice*, Rockville, Md., 1987, Aspen Publishers.)

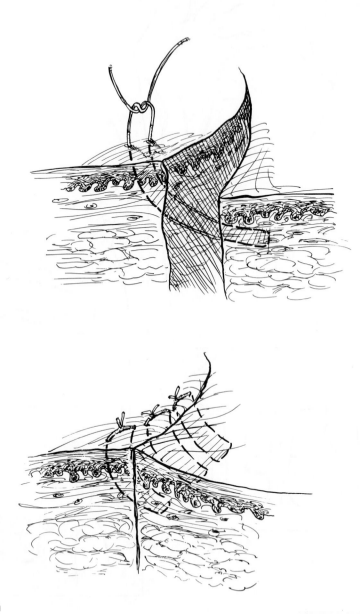

FIG. 10-15   Technique for closure of a thin-edge, thick-edge laceration. Notice that the horizontal mattress technique is used; however, one portion is buried and not brought through the opposite side of the wound surface.

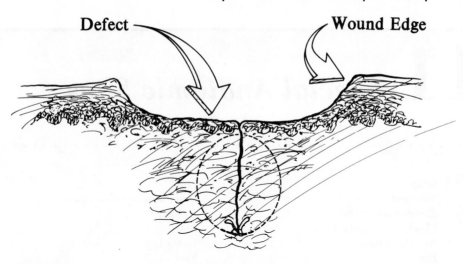

Defect · Wound Edge

FIG. 10-16 Technique for closure of a laceration within a deep abrasion. Note that the deep-suture technique is used and the abraded surface is avoided.

Techniques for Closing Wounded Aged Skin

It is very important not to close aged, friable skin under tension. Attempts to do so can risk the already tenuous vascularity of the skin and result in a large area of tissue loss. If the wound cannot be properly brought back together without undue tension, it is best to leave a gap for later grafting. Under these conditions a consultation with a specialist is recommended.

If the wound edges can be apposed easily, the simplest method to close friable, elderly skin is to use wound tapes. Applying the tapes is technically not difficult. But, because of their adherence, they are allowed to fall off on their own or removed very carefully to not disrupt the delicate, early, collagenous bonds of healing.

Another closure method is to appose the edges with horizontal mattress sutures (see Fig. 9-7). The configuration of this suture allows for maximal "gathering" of tissue and minimal "tearing" forces are applied.

REFERENCES

1. Bernstein G: Polybutester suture, *J Dermatol Surg* 14:615-616, 1988.
2. Grabb WC: Introduction to the clinical aspects of flap repair. In Grabb WC, Myers MB, editors: *Skin flaps*, Boston, 1975, Little, Brown.
3. Swanson NA, Tromovitch TA: Suture materials, 1980s: properties, uses, and abuses, *Int J Dermatol* 21:373-378, 1982.
4. Winn HR, Jane JA, Rodeheaver GT: Influence of subcuticular sutures on scar formation, *Am J Surg* 133:257-259, 1977.
5. Wong NL: Review of continuous sutures in dermatologic surgery, *J Dermatol Surg Oncol* 19:923-931, 1993.

11 *Special Anatomic Sites*

. . . .

Scalp	Lips
Forehead	Oral Cavity
Eyebrow and Eyelid	Perineum
Cheek or Zygomatic Area	Knee
Nasal Structures	Lower Leg
Ear	Foot

Although the wound closure principles and suture techniques discussed in Chapters 9 and 10 can be applied to all lacerations and wounds, several areas of the body have unique anatomic considerations that require special attention. Particular emphasis is placed on the face because of cosmetic concerns. Initial management and wound closure are crucial to eventual scar formation and the final appearance of the injury. Table 11-1 is a reference guide for choice of suture material and size for each anatomic region of the body.

SCALP

The scalp extends anteriorly from the supraorbital ridges to the external occipital protuberance posteriorly (Fig. 11-1). Laterally the boundaries are the temporal lines. There are five layers of the scalp: skin (epidermis, dermis), dense superficial fascia, galea aponeurotica, loose areolar connective tissue, and periosteum. The skin is densely covered with hair. Ragged lacerations are often closed without regard to cosmetics under the assumption that hair will hide the scar. However, the majority of males experience some balding in their lifetime, a fact that must be taken into consideration during wound closure.

Underlying the skin is a dense layer of connective tissue that corresponds to the superficial fascia. This layer is richly invested with arteries and veins. Although this profuse vascularity protects against the development of infection, the denseness of the connective tissue tends to hold vessels open when the scalp is lacerated. For this reason, even small lacerations can cause considerable bleeding, even leading to hypovolemia and hypotension.

Table 11-1 *Suggested Guidelines for Suture Material and Size for Body Region*

Body Region	Percutaneous (Skin)	Deep (Dermal)
Scalp	5-0/4-0 Monofilament[1]	4-0 Absorbable[2]
Ear	6-0 Monofilament	—
Eyelid	7-0/6-0 Monofilament	—
Eyebrow	6-0/5-0 Monofilament	5-0 Absorbable
Nose	6-0 Monofilament	5-0 Absorbable
Lip	6-0 Monofilament	5-0 Absorbable
Oral mucosa	—	5-0 Absorbable[3]
Other parts of face/forehead	6-0 Monofilament	5-0 Absorbable
Trunk	5-0/4-0 Monofilament	3-0 Absorbable
Extremities	5-0/4-0 Monofilament	4-0 Absorbable
Hand	5-0 Monofilament	5-0 Absorbable
Extensor tendon	4-0 Monofilament	—
Foot/Sole	4-0/3-0 Monofilament	4-0 Absorbable
Vagina	—	4-0 Absorbable[3]
Scrotum	—	5-0 Absorbable[3]
Penis	5-0 Monofilament	—

1. Nonabsorbable monofilaments
   Nylon: Ethilon, Dermalon
   Polypropylene: Prolene
   Polybutester: Novafil
2. Absorbable materials for dermal and fascial closures
   Polyglycolic acid: Dexon, Dexon Plus
   Polyglactin 910:   Vicryl
   Polydioxanone: PDS (monofilament absorbable)
   Polyglyconate: Maxon (monofilament absorbable)
3. Absorbable materials for mucosal and scrotal closure
   Chromic Gut
   Polyglactin 910:   Vicryl

The next layer is the galea aponeurotica. It is a dense, tendonlike structure that covers the skull and inserts into the frontalis muscle of the forehead anteriorly and into the occipitalis muscle posteriorly. Failure to repair large, horizontal lacerations of the aponeurosis can cause the frontalis muscle to contract asymmetrically, which can cause a significant cosmetic deformity of the forehead. Closure of galea lacerations is also important for protection of the loose connective tissue that is vulnerable to infection.

Blood and bacteria can easily spread from a laceration of the skin through the injured galea to the loose connective tissue. Within this layer are emissary veins that drain into the skull and intracranial veins. Infection of this space can lead to osteomyelitis or brain abscess. Beneath the loose connective tissue layer is the periosteum of the skull itself.

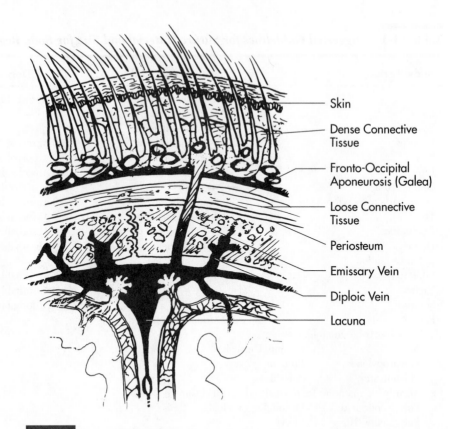

Skin

Dense Connective Tissue

Fronto-Occipital Aponeurosis (Galea)

Loose Connective Tissue

Periosteum

Emissary Vein

Diploic Vein

Lacuna

FIG. 11-1   Cross-sectional anatomy of the scalp. Note the emissary vein. It can act as a conduit for bacteria to brain tissues should the scalp wound become infected.

The periosteum can be mistaken for the galea but is not as dense, nor does it readily accept sutures without the risk of tearing.

Preparation for Closure

Because of the propensity of the scalp to bleed profusely, hemorrhage control is necessary before attempts at closure. Hemorrhage is worsened if alcohol is present, a finding in as many as 50% of patients with scalp lacerations.[7] Trying to suture a bleeding scalp wound can be difficult and frustrating. The vessels do not lend themselves to easy clamping or ligation because they are encased in the dense connective tissue. Direct pressure, applied in the manner described, is the most efficacious way to gain hemostasis. First, gross contaminants, if present, are removed immediately with a brief cleansing or irrigation. The wound is then covered with sterile, saline-moistened sponges and compressed with an elastic bandage. This bandage can be left in place for 30 to 60 min-

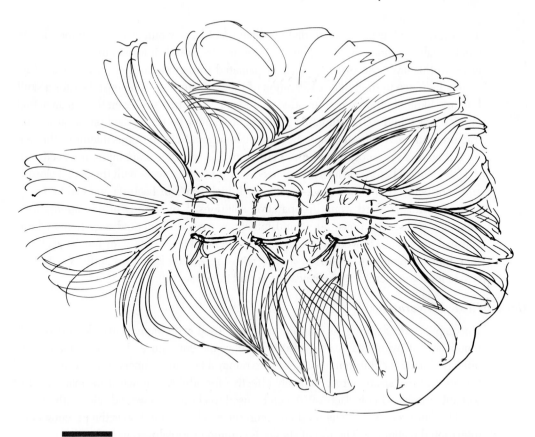

FIG. 11-2   Horizontal mattress suture technique for closure of scalp wounds with uneven or macerated edges.

utes. After compression, significant bleeding will usually have been brought under control.

After pressure bandage removal and wound evaluation have been performed, an anesthetic can be administered. Repair can then take place under more controlled conditions. Because scalp lacerations frequently occur in intoxicated patients, the strategy of waiting for hemostasis has the added benefit of allowing the patient to "settle down" before any attempts at intervention are made. Another solution to profuse bleeding is to just proceed with wound closure using the horizontal mattress technique with large bites (Fig 11-2). Under these conditions, an assistant can temporarily control the bleeding by putting upward traction on hemostats fixed to the galea. Once closed, the bleeding usually ceases.

Anesthesia for scalp wounds can be accomplished by the direct or parallel wound technique using lidocaine with epinephrine. This solution further controls bleeding if necessary. Visual inspection and digital palpation of large wounds are recommended to identify galeal or bone injuries. The periosteum is frequently injured during trauma. Injuries to this layer can often be seen or palpated through a laceration. Because of its close adherence to the bone, a laceration of the periosteum can be mistaken for a skull fracture. Skull films are recommended to rule out a true fracture, even though an actual break is not found.[7] Unfortunately, radiographs cannot be fully relied on because true fractures, not seen on radiographs, are not uncommon. In spite of this dilemma, the real issue is not the presence or absence of a fracture but whether brain injury has occurred.

Hair removal before closure is only necessary if hair interferes with the actual closure and knot tying. Hair is not contaminated with high levels of bacteria and can be easily cleansed with standard wound-preparation solutions.[11] In a study of 68 patients with traumatic scalp lacerations, no wound infections were documented in patients whose hair had not been removed before closure.[9] If removal is necessary for mechanical reasons, then clipping with scissors or shaving with a recessed blade razor suffices.[6] Shaving at skin level can increase the chance for wound infection.[3, 13]

Uncomplicated Lacerations

Uncomplicated, shearing lacerations can be closed with nonabsorbable 5-0 or 4-0 monofilament nylon, staples, or absorbable chromic gut suture. The latter material is often preferred for children because suture removal becomes unnecessary. Some practitioners find this strategy to be equally effective for adults. A new suture material, absorbable irradiated polyglactin-910, can be used to close scalp wounds also without the need for later removal.[15] The most common suture closure method is the percutaneous interrupted technique. The use of staples is common for scalp wounds. Stapled wounds heal the same as those treated with standard closure methods.[8, 12]

Galeal Lacerations

Because the galea is a key anchoring structure for the frontalis muscle, large frontal galeal lacerations need to be separately repaired with 3-0 or 4-0 absorbable sutures to prevent a serious cosmetic deformity from developing. If the frontalis muscle loses its anchoring point at the muscle-galeal junction along the frontal scalp line, then facial expressions dependent on that muscle will appear distorted and asymmetric. Closure of large galeal lacerations in other areas of the scalp is also recommended to protect the loose connective tissue layer from infection.

Compression Lacerations with Irregular Margins

Often lacerations of the scalp are caused by blunt rather than sharp shearing forces. The wound and its edges are irregular and macerated. Simple closure with percutaneous, interrupted sutures can be difficult under these conditions. The scalp does not have excessive tissue redundancy, so debridement has to be kept to a minimum or else the wound cannot be approximated without abnormally high tension. Fortunately, the rich vascularity of the scalp allows for eventual successful healing even if less than optimal tissues are brought together. Therefore, after judicious wound-edge trimming, the horizontal mattress suture technique is recommended to approximate the remaining edges (see Fig. 11-2). This technique is also useful for closing the excessively bleeding wound.

Compression injuries can result in complex, stellate lacerations. Once again, judicious debridement is advised. The corner closure (flap) technique described in Chapter 10 often approximates all of the corners and flaps in one suture. The remainder of the repair is carried out with simple percutaneous or half-buried mattress sutures.

Avulsion or "Scalping" Lacerations

High-speed forces that are delivered in a tangential manner to the scalp can cause large flaps or complete loss of portions of the scalp. Associated intracranial injury can also occur. These wounds are best managed by a consultant. Preserved portions of complete scalp avulsions, like other amputated parts, are wrapped in saline-moistened gauze, placed in a plastic bag, and cooled over ice. It is possible that they might be reimplanted in the defect by using grafting or microvascular anastomoses techniques.

Aftercare

After repair, it is sometimes necessary to place a temporary (24-hour) light-pressure compression wrap with an elastic bandage over the scalp dressing of large lacerations to prevent formation of wound hematoma. The patient can be instructed to remove the bandage after the recommended compression period.

Most scalp lacerations do not require dressing, just a thin layer of an antibacterial ointment. Scalp sutures are left in place for 7 to 9 days for adults and 5 to 7 days for children. Gentle bathing of the scalp can commence 24 hours after closure. Daily application of ointment following cleansing is recommended.

FOREHEAD

The forehead is a common site of injury in both children and adults. It is also of paramount cosmetic importance because of its visibility. Three principles govern the initial repair of a forehead injury:

- Skin tension lines that parallel skin creases play a major role in the outcome of any laceration. A laceration that is perpendicular to dynamic skin tension lines tends to heal with a more visible scar than one that is parallel to these lines (see Chapter 2).
- The forehead has little excess tissue to permit extensive revisions and excisions. The temptation to excise ragged wounds has to be carefully assessed or resisted. A small defect can inadvertently become larger by overaggressive repair efforts.[4] It is often best to preserve as much tissue as possible just by "tacking down" ragged tissue tags so that later cosmetic revisions can be made when conditions are more favorable.
- Whenever possible, few dermal (deep) absorbable sutures should be placed. Excessive tissue reaction with increased scar size can result from deep sutures.

Preparation for Closure

Anesthesia for small or single lacerations of the forehead can be accomplished by the direct or parallel injection techniques, using an anesthetic with adrenaline to decrease bleeding. Large or multiple lacerations often are best managed by the forehead block (see Chapter 5). This block reduces the number of needlesticks and prevents distortion of the tissues to allow for more accurate wound edge approximation.

Once anesthesia is achieved, the wound can be explored for any bony abnormality or foreign body. Radiographs are recommended when the suspicion for either is raised. Surprisingly large pieces of glass can be discovered under small and innocuous-appearing wounds. After gentle scrubbing with a sponge, irrigation, and debridement with the tip of a #11 blade, most foreign material should have been removed. Any remaining permanent material can be surgically removed. Every effort is made to remove potential tattooing objects at the time of the first repair. When in doubt, consultation with a specialist should be considered.

Uncomplicated Lacerations

Most lacerations can be closed with the simple percutaneous technique using a 6-0 monofilament nonabsorbable suture. Deeper lacerations may require placement of a few supporting dermal (deep) 5-0 absorbable sutures. The percutaneous technique in any laceration should be performed by taking small bites (close to the wound edge) with several sutures rather than large bites with few sutures. This technique reduces wound-edge tension and allows for more accurate wound edge apposition.

Complex Lacerations: Multiple Small Flaps, Lacerations, and Abrasions ("Windshield" Injury)

One of the most daunting wounds is the windshield injury, characterized by multiple lacerations, abrasions, gouges, and small flaps. The anesthetic technique of choice is the forehead block. Flaps that are smaller than 5 mm in width and length are tacked down with single 6-0 percutaneous nonabsorbable sutures (Fig. 11-3). Larger flaps can be closed by using the corner technique. Partial-thickness abrasions and shallow gouges (less than 5 to 10 mm wide and 1 to 2 mm deep) can be left to heal by secondary intention. Other lacerations are closed as necessary with percutaneous sutures. A petroleum-based antibiotic ointment applied 3 times a day will suffice as a dressing. Again, because of cosmetic concerns, a consultant might be helpful, especially if the wounds are severe. Consultation is also appropriate if the estimated time of repair will interfere with an emergency physician's other duties, even if there is little technical challenge.

Complex Lacerations: Ragged-Edge Lacerations, Large Flaps, and Tissue Defects

Lacerations with ragged and macerated edges can be trimmed as described in Chapter 8. If the unevenness or maceration is not extensive, then complete excision is an option if the laceration is parallel to the skin tension lines and there is sufficient tissue redundancy.

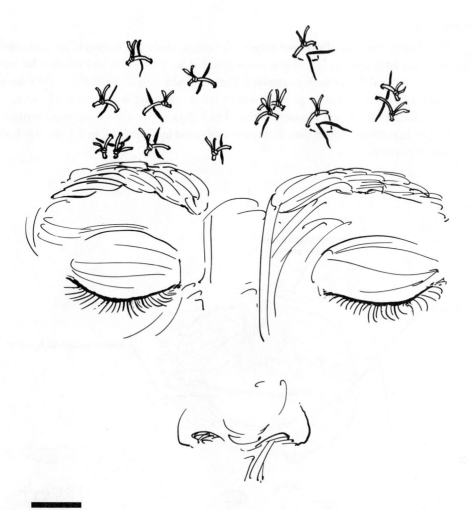

FIG. 11-3 Small abrasions/lacerations, caused by the "windshield" injury, can often be closed by using simple, single, percutaneous sutures or single corner sutures.

Lacerations perpendicular to skin tension lines have less tissue redundancy and cannot tolerate wide excision. Once again, the principle of tissue preservation has to be kept in mind when considering excision. When there is any doubt about tissue availability for excision, try to preserve what is viable, or obtain a consult.

Large avulsion flaps and near scalping injuries are prone to what is known as the "trap-door" phenomenon in which congestion and lymphedema lead to unsightly bulging of the flap after repair. These flaps are U-shaped with the base in a superior position on the forehead. These injuries are best managed by a consultant.

Aftercare

Facial lacerations usually do not require dressings. Daily application of an antibacterial ointment after gentle cleansing is recommended for protection and to allow for easier suture removal (by reducing crusting). Cotton swabs moistened with a mild soap and water solution or hydrogen peroxide are useful for cleaning in and around facial lacerations. Facial sutures are removed within 3 to 5 days to prevent suture mark formation. Larger lacerations (larger than 2 cm) are supported by wound tapes for one week after suture removal.

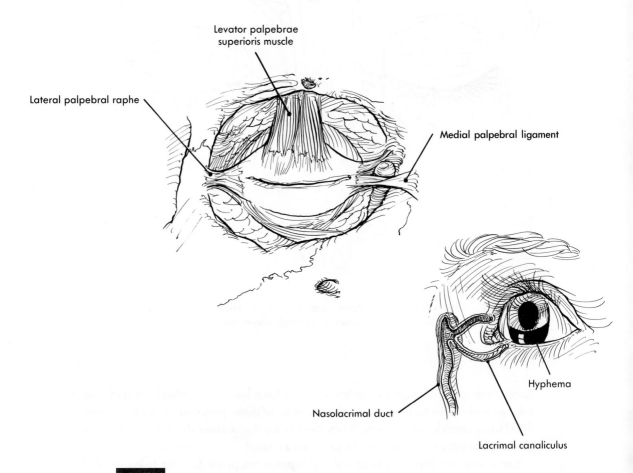

FIG. 11-4   Important anatomic structures that can be injured during eye trauma. The integrity of these structures must be confirmed before the closure of any laceration (see text).

EYEBROW AND EYELID

The eye and periorbital tissues are susceptible to serious injury by relatively minor trauma. Fig. 11-4 illustrates various structures that must be checked for damage before repair proceeds. Should any of the important anatomic parts in the following discussion be involved, immediate referral to a consultant is recommended.

Lacerations of the medial lower lid can injure the tear duct apparatus (lacrimal canaliculus and nasolacrimal duct) or the medial palpebral ligament at the medial canthus. Copious tears running down the cheek of the patient is a sign of possible tear duct injuries. A laceration of the medial palpebral ligament displaces the lid apparatus laterally, giving the appearance that the patient is "cross-eyed."

The levator palpebrae muscle is responsible for maintaining the eyelid in its normal position when open. Interruption of the muscle causes traumatic ptosis. Injury to the muscle is suspected when periorbital fat can be seen to extrude from a laceration of the upper lid. Periorbital fat signifies that the orbital septum has been violated. The levator muscle originates from the septum; therefore any septum injury will risk this muscle.

Close inspection of the eye itself is necessary to rule out a hyphema, corneal abrasions, and foreign bodies. Of these injuries, hyphema is the most serious. It is caused by a direct blow to the eye and is recognized by a blood layer in the anterior chamber of the eye in patients in the upright position. In patients who are supine, blood distributes evenly in the anterior chamber over the iris and gives the iris a different color from the opposite iris. The patient will also complain of decreased vision in the affected eye. Having the patient sit up reveals the hyphema as the blood settles with gravity.

Preparation for Closure

It is best to deliver an anesthetic to the eyelid by direct wound infiltration, using a small 27- or 30-gauge needle. Adrenaline-containing anesthetics are not necessary. For the eyebrow, the same technique is used, but adrenaline in the anesthetic can be useful to control minor bleeding. Special care is taken to minimize spillage of cleansing agents into the eye to prevent unnecessary corneal irritation. Povidone-iodine solution (not a detergent-containing solution) diluted 1:10 with saline and nonionic surfactants (Shur-Clens) are the cleansing agents of choice.[5] Inadvertent spilling of these preparations can be prevented by holding a folded 4 × 4 sponge over the closed eyelid margin to absorb free solution.

One important point to remember is never to shave the hair from the lid margin or brow because of the unpredictability of hair regrowth in these locations.

Closure of Extramarginal Lid Lacerations

Extramarginal lacerations are usually horizontal and occur most commonly in the upper lid. If extramarginal lacerations are simple and superficial, they can be repaired with a single layer of 6-0 nonabsorbable suture material (Fig. 11-5). No dressing is ap-

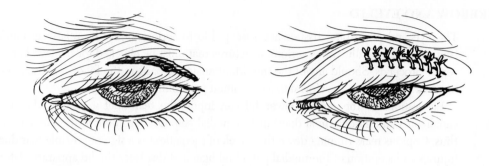

FIG. 11-5   Extramarginal lacerations of the upper lid are usually horizontal and can be closed with a simple row of percutaneous closures.

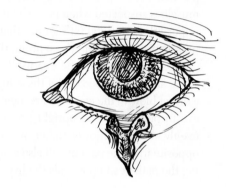

FIG. 11-6   A vertical, intramarginal lid laceration is best left to a consultant to repair.

plied. These lacerations heal well enough so that scars become virtually unnoticeable with time.

Closure of Intramarginal Lid Lacerations

Intramarginal lacerations involve the lid margin and, like lip lacerations, require extremely precise repair to ensure proper alignment. Abnormal eversion (ectropion) or inversion (entropion) is a complication of improper alignment. Intramarginal injuries are probably best left to a consultant for repair (Fig. 11-6).

Closure of Eyebrow Lacerations

Simple, uncomplicated eyebrow lacerations can be closed with a 5-0 nonabsorbable monofilament. As previously mentioned, the eyebrow is never shaved or trimmed. Occasionally one or two dermal (deep) closures are necessary to approximate the superficial fascia. Great care is taken to properly align the brow margins to prevent a cosmetic deformity. Alignment sutures at the superior and inferior margins of the brow hair are

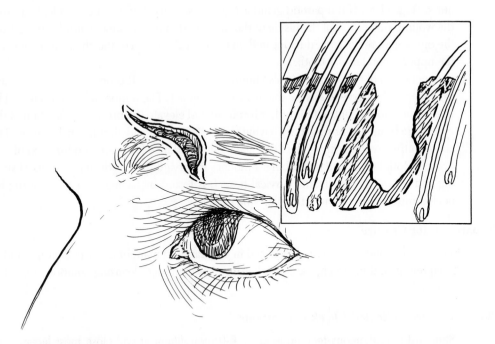

FIG. 11-7 Most eyebrow lacerations can be closed without tissue debridement. However, if macerated or devitalized tissue must be removed, it is important to excise this tissue parallel to the hair shaft. This excision technique prevents an unsightly cosmetic defect.

placed to initiate closure. Deep sutures, if required, can be placed after the alignment ones.

If the laceration has particularly ragged or macerated edges, then trimming or careful excision can be carried out. A basic principle to observe is that any debridement has to be parallel to the brow hair shafts (Fig. 11-7). Failure to observe this principle can lead to an unnecessary defect following the repair.

Aftercare

No dressing is necessary for lid or brow lacerations. Daily cleansing followed by application of an antibacterial ointment is recommended. Sutures are removed in 3 to 5 days in both children and adults.

CHEEK OR ZYGOMATIC AREA

There are two major structures underlying the cheek area, just anterior to the ear, that can be injured by penetrating lacerations. These are the parotid gland and the facial nerve (Fig. 11-8). If the parotid gland is injured, salivary fluid can be seen leaking from the wound. Inspection of the inside of the mouth often reveals bloody fluid coming from the opening of the parotid duct located on the buccal mucosa of the cheek at the level of the upper second molar tooth.

Lacerations of this region can also injure the facial nerve. It is necessary to test all five branches of the nerve to ensure that each one is intact. The temporal branch is tested by having the patient contract his or her forehead and elevate the brow. The function of the zygomatic branch is observed by having the patient open and shut his or her eyes. The act of sniffing with flaring of the nasal alae is also evidence for preserved function of that branch. Both buccal and mandibular branches innervate the lips during the acts of smiling and frowning. Finally, the cervical branch is tested by having the patient shrug his neck through contraction of the platysma muscle.

Preparation for Closure

The cheek is anesthetized and cleansed in the standard manner described earlier and in Chapters 5 and 6. Again, care is taken to avoid spilling cleansing solutions onto the eye itself.

Closure of Uncomplicated Cheek Lacerations

Standard percutaneous technique using 6-0 monofilament will close most lacerations. One important point to remember is that many people have natural creases in the skin of the cheek and face. These creases have the same importance cosmetically as the vermilion border of the lip. Proper alignment of them has to be given special attention. Often the initial percutaneous suture is placed to align with the crease before proceeding with the remainder of the closure.

Deep or Through-and-Through Lacerations

Complex lacerations that travel deep into the soft tissues of the cheek or those that penetrate the oral cavity are at risk for injuring the parotid gland or facial nerve as mentioned earlier. If neither of these structures is injured, repair can proceed. If there is any doubt, then a consultant is required. The oral cavity portion of a penetrating laceration is left open unless it is large (greater than 3 to 5 cm). Large mucosal lacerations are closed with 5-0 chromic gut suture. The external wound is irrigated and closed with 6-0 monofilament.

Aftercare

Dressings are usually unnecessary for lacerations in this area. Daily cleansing and application of an antibacterial ointment allow for easier suture removal at the 3 to 5 day interval for children and adults.

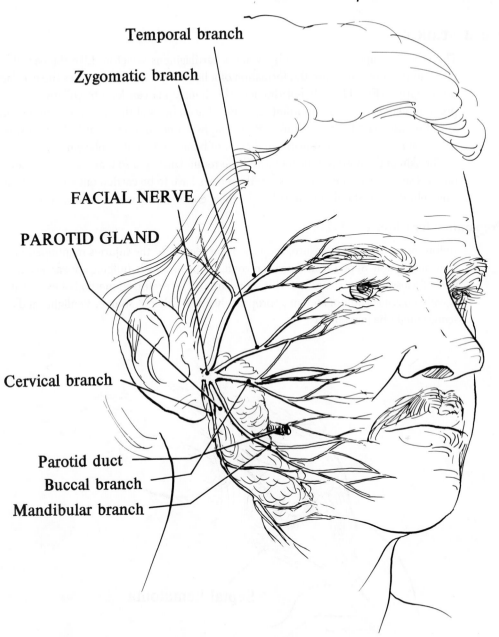

FIG. 11-8 The parotid gland and facial nerve underlie the zygomatic and cheek areas. Any lacerations anterior to the ear must be carefully assessed for injuries to the various branches of the facial nerve, parotid gland, or parotid duct.

NASAL STRUCTURES

The nose is composed of both a bony and a cartilaginous skeleton. Like the ear, direct blows to the nose can cause the formation of a hematoma that compresses the cartilaginous septum (Fig. 11-9). If not drained, this hematoma can lead to collapse through pressure necrosis of this important structure. Lacerations of the nose are common and are often associated with fractures. Radiographs do not always identify fractures, and palpation remains a more sensitive indicator of bone injury and displacement.

The skin of the nose is inflexible with little redundancy. It also tears easily with percutaneous suture placement. Consequently, repairs have to be carried out with great care. Any debridement should be considered only in consultation with a facial specialist.

Preparation for Closure

Before preparation and closure, the nose is inspected for the injuries mentioned in the previous section. Septal hematoma is recognized by its bluish, bulging appearance in the area of Kiesselbach's plexus (anterior septal area). The preferred method of examination is with a nasal speculum and an appropriately powerful light source. Penlights and otoscopes might be inadequate.

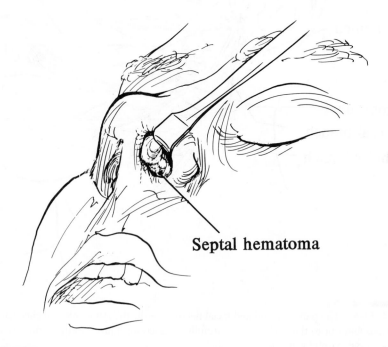

Septal hematoma

FIG. 11-9   The septal hematoma in the area of the anterior nasal septum. Failure to drain this hematoma will lead to septal necrosis and collapse.

Anesthesia of the nose is best accomplished by the direct wound infiltration technique with a 27- or 30-gauge needle, using an agent without adrenaline. Nasal blocks are difficult to achieve and are usually reserved for major repairs. Cleansing of the nose is carried out by using povidone-iodine solution and saline irrigation.

Skin Lacerations

Most skin lacerations can be repaired with 6-0 nonabsorbable percutaneous monofilament sutures. Sutures are placed with small bites because nasal skin tends to invert. The skin is also easily torn, so great care has to be taken to avoid creating excessive tension. If tension is present, the placement of 1 or 2 deep 6-0 or 5-0 absorbable sutures will support the percutaneous sutures. Complex and irregular skin wounds have to be handled carefully. Since there is little redundancy of nasal skin, debridement has to be minimal. The best strategy is to "tack down" small tags or flaps percutaneously or obtain consultation.

Nostril and Cartilage Wounds

Nostril lacerations involve the rim with skin, cartilage, and mucosal injuries. Alignment of the rim is crucial to prevent "notching." The skin is closed with 6-0 nonabsorbable suture, and the mucosa is sutured with 5-0 or 6-0 absorbable. Placement of sutures in the cartilage is not necessary during repair. Closing the skin and mucosa over the cartilage ensures adequate healing. Complete coverage of cartilage is mandatory because of its tendency to develop chronic chondritis if exposed. Avulsion and mutilating injuries of either the skin or cartilage are best managed by a consultant.

Septal Hematoma

A hematoma over the septal cartilage is drained with a hockey-stick or crescent-shaped incision (Fig. 11-10). The incision is always made in the dependent portion of the hematoma. To prevent reaccumulation, an anterior nasal pack is placed with Vaseline gauze, and the patient is referred to a consultant within 24 to 48 hours for follow-up. When packing is placed, antibiotics are often recommended to prevent sinus infection. Amoxicillin or Bactrim are reasonable choices.

Lacerations With Bone Involvement

Uncomplicated lacerations of the skin over nondisplaced nasal fractures can be closed using the previously described techniques. Complex lacerations with fracture displacement, mucosal injury from bone fragmentation, or extensive cartilage involvement are best managed by a consultant.

Aftercare

Dressings are optional for nasal lacerations. Often a simple Band-Aid will suffice. The percutaneous sutures are removed in 3 to 5 days in both children and adults. The value

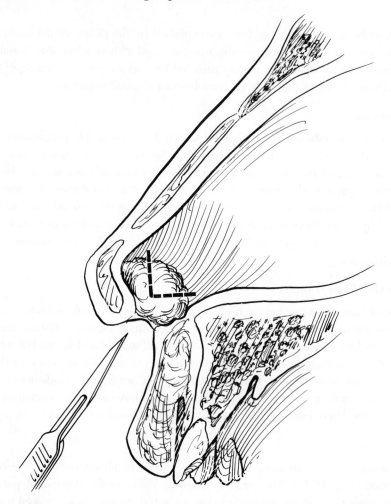

FIG. 11-10   Technique to drain a septal hematoma. A #11 blade is used to create a "hockey-stick" incision. Following drainage, the nose is packed with Vaseline gauze. (Adapted from Zukin D, Simon R: *Emergency wound care: principles and practice*, Rockville, Md., 1987, Aspen Publishers.)

of antibiotics for nasal lacerations is unclear. The natural vascularity of the face is protective against infection. Any decision to use antibiotics is based on the circumstances of individual cases.

EAR

The ear consists of a cartilaginous skeleton covered by tightly adherent skin with little intervening superficial fascia (subcutaneous tissue). A direct blow to the ear can cause a

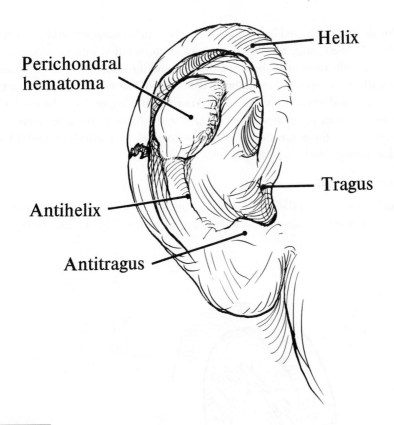

Helix

**Perichondral
hematoma**

Tragus

Antihelix

Antitragus

FIG. 11-11   Anatomy of the external ear. Note the presence of perichondral hematoma. Perichondral hematoma formation can occur following blunt trauma to the ear and can accompany lacerations.

hematoma to form, usually in the area of the antihelix, with a resultant breakdown of the cartilage caused by pressure between the skin and cartilage (Fig. 11-11). The eventual result is the well-known "cauliflower" ear. The most important objective for repair of open wounds is coverage of any exposed cartilage. Failure to do so leads to chondritis and breakdown.

Preparation for Repair

In addition to inspecting the external ear for hematoma formation and cartilage injury, the internal canal and tympanic membrane are visualized to complete the examination. Blunt injuries to the ear can cause perforations of the tympanic membrane. The most significant injury that can accompany lacerations to the ear is a basilar skull fracture, which can be recognized by hemotympanum or Battle's sign (ecchymosis of the mastoid area).

Small, uncomplicated lacerations to the ear can be anesthetized by direct infiltration with a 27- or 30-gauge needle using an anesthetic solution without adrenaline. The needle is carefully introduced between the skin and the cartilage, and only a small amount of anesthetic is deposited to minimize distortion of the wound edges. For large, complex lacerations and wounds, the ear block described in Chapter 5 can be used. Cleansing is carried out with povidone-iodine solution and irrigation. Because of the complicated topography of the ear, cotton-swab applicators can be particularly useful for cleansing and removing dried blood in crevices.

Uncomplicated Lacerations

Simple lacerations of the helix and lobule that do not involve cartilage can be closed with interrupted 6-0 nonabsorbable monofilament suture (Fig. 11-12). To prevent wound-

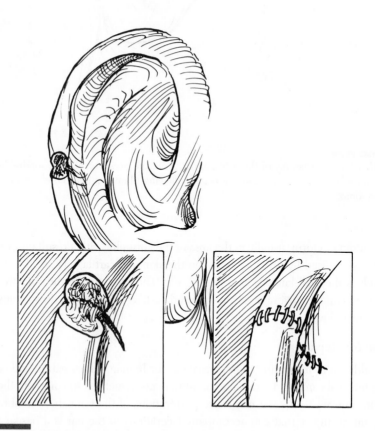

FIG. 11-12   Simple noncartilaginous lacerations of the ear are closed with either interrupted or running percutaneous skin sutures.

edge inversion, small 1 to 2 mm bites are taken. If debridement is necessary, it should be kept to a minimum to prevent exposure of the cartilage. Sutures are removed 4 to 5 days after repair.

Lacerations Involving Cartilage

Sharp, shearing lacerations that penetrate cartilage can be managed by carefully apposing the skin overlying the cartilaginous interruption. The skin is sufficiently adherent and supporting so that sutures do not have to be placed through the cartilage itself to bring together the lacerated cartilage edges. Additionally, cartilage tears easily and does not hold sutures well. Sharp, through-and-through lacerations can be managed by suturing the anterior and posterior portions of the laceration. The cartilage will come together without sutures. Care is taken to ensure that the skin over the helix rim is everted so scar contraction will not cause notching.

Irregular wounds that involve cartilage have to be managed with two principles in mind: debridement must be kept to a minimum, and no cartilage must be left exposed. If cartilage is exposed and the skin cannot be brought together over it without undue tension, then it can be debrided conservatively to match the skin and cartilage edges. A total of 5 mm of cartilage can be sacrificed without deforming the cartilaginous skeleton. No sutures are placed in the cartilage (Fig. 11-13). Complex cartilage injuries require consultation.

Perichondral Hematoma

When a perichondral hematoma is present, it has to be adequately drained. There is a 72-hour window for hematoma drainage beyond which the risk of cauliflower ear increases.[2] A small incision is made over the hematoma, and the hematoma is evacuated from the space between the perichondrium and the cartilage. Placement of a small rubber drain is optional. After drainage, a mastoid dressing is placed as described in Chapter 17. The dressing is removed in 24 hours and is inspected for reaccumulation. More often than not, complex lacerations and hematomas of the ear are best cared for by or under the guidance of a consultant.

Aftercare

Because the ear is difficult to dress it is often left open. Daily, gentle cleansing is recommended followed by application of an antibacterial ointment. If there is any question of possible perichondral blood accumulation after the patient is discharged, then a mastoid dressing is recommended (see Chapter 17). Sutures are removed after 4 to 5 days for adults and 3 to 5 days for children. When cartilage is involved or a septal hematoma has been drained, antibiotic prophylaxis is recommended. Choices include dicloxacillin, a first-generation cephalosporin, or amoxicillin with clavulanate. Erythromycin or clindamycin can be used in the penicillin-allergic patient. Uncomplicated, noncartilaginous injuries do not require antibiotics.

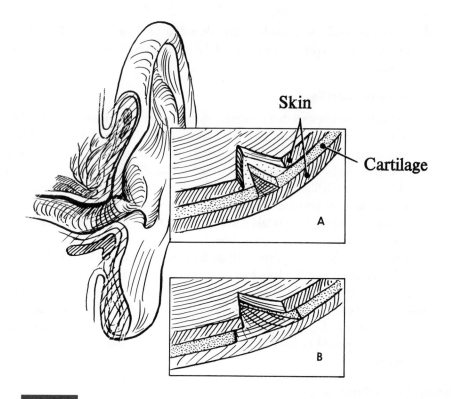

FIG. 11-13   **A,** Cartilage that extends beyond the margins of the skin injury can be trimmed back, by using tissue scissors, to ensure complete coverage both anteriorly and posteriorly by skin. **B,** Skin is closed with simple percutaneous sutures. No sutures are necessary for the cartilage. (Adapted from Zukin D, Simon R: *Emergency wound care: principles and practice*, Rockville, Md., 1987, Aspen Publishers.)

LIPS

Lacerations of the lip can cause devastating cosmetic defects if not properly and meticulously repaired. A misalignment by as little as 1 mm of the vermilion border, or "white line," can be easily noticed by the casual observer. It is a defect that cannot easily be revised after primary healing has taken place. Other important anatomic structures include the mucosal border (the portion of the lip that divides the intraoral and extraoral portion of the lip) and the underlying orbicularis oris muscle. Each of these structures requires careful and exact apposition to achieve the best structural and cosmetic result. Vertical through-and-through lacerations often violate all three of these structures.

Preparation for Closure

Although the mouth is replete with bacteria, and a lip laceration will not remain clean during the repair procedure, cleansing is only carried out to remove gross debris and

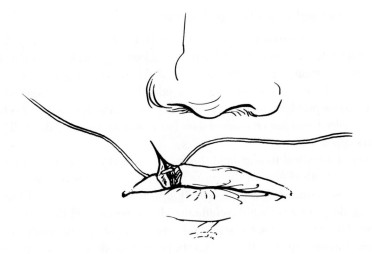

FIG. 11-14   The major goal when closing any lip laceration is to align the appropriate borders. Illustrated in this figure are the initial suture placement and alignment of the vermilion border. Once the vermilion border or "white line" is aligned, then the remainder of the laceration is closed.

dirt. If any teeth are broken, then a careful search is made in the wound for teeth fragments. Retained tooth particles can cause marked inflammation and infection leading to a complete breakdown of any attempted repair. Whenever a portion of a tooth cannot be accounted for, a lateral radiograph of the face using soft-tissue technique will reveal the missing fragment.

Anesthesia for lip repairs is best accomplished by either an infraorbital nerve block for the upper lip or a mental nerve block for the lower lip (see Chapter 5). Direct infiltration of the laceration can cause excessive distortion of the lip and create difficulties when attempting to properly align wound edges.

Uncomplicated Lacerations

Most lip lacerations usually do not require extensive revision or debridement. The key to closure is proper alignment of the anatomic structures listed previously. If the vermilion border is violated and the laceration is superficial, then the repair begins by placing the first suture, with careful precision, through that border on each side of the wound (Fig. 11-14). Once alignment is judged to be appropriate, then the remainder of the wound is closed with 6-0 nonabsorbable monofilament sutures. If the mucosal border is violated, it also is aligned meticulously. As a general rule, if the laceration extends beyond the mucosal border into the oral cavity, then 5-0 absorbable suture, such as chromic gut, is used to close that portion. Irradiated polyglactin 910 (Vicryl) is also recommended because it does not "stiffen" as much as gut and is rapidly absorbed.

Complicated and Through-and-Through Lacerations

Unlike many other structures of the face, the lip can be revised and significant portions of devitalized tissue, up to 25% of the upper or lower lip, can be excised without causing significant deformity except for the area of the upper lip just below the nose, the philtrum, and the oral commissures. Considerable judgment is required to deal with these cosmetic problems in image-conscious patients who have high expectations for excellent results. Consultation is advised for lacerations and injuries that will impact on the patient's appearance.

Repair of a vertical through-and-through laceration is illustrated in Fig. 11-15. The repair begins with closure of the vermilion border. Next, the orbicularis oris muscle is carefully reapproximated with deep 5-0 absorbable suture material like polyglycolic acid. The deep sutures should include the fibrous covering of the muscle to insure anchoring. The remainder of the repair proceeds with 6-0 nonabsorbable sutures for the skin and exposed lip. For the oral cavity portion inside the mucosal border, 5-0 absorbable sutures are used.

Aftercare

No dressing is placed on the lips. The patient is reminded not to bring excessive pressure to bear on the suture line while the sutures are in place. Rinsing the mouth after eating is recommended to prevent small particulate matter from penetrating the suture line. The extraoral sutures are removed after 4 to 5 days in adults and 3 to 5 days in children to prevent the formation of suture marks. A controlled study of intraoral lacerations suggests that there is some benefit to administering oral penicillin VK 4 times daily for 5 days as prophylaxis against infection.[14] Erythromycin or clindamycin may be considered as alternatives for the allergic patient.

ORAL CAVITY

The oral cavity consists of several structures, each of which requires separate considerations during management and repair. These are the buccal mucosa, gingiva, teeth, salivary glands and ducts, tongue, mandible, and the alveolar ridge of the maxillary bone. Injuries to the oral cavity can be a potential threat to airway patency.

Preparation for Repair

Other than airway considerations, the most important part of the evaluation of the oral cavity is the determination of the integrity of salivary structures, bone, and teeth. Visual inspection, as well as palpation, is necessary to complete the examination. Particularly troublesome are teeth, fragments of which must be accounted for if possible. They can easily lodge in the mucosa and the deep tissue of the lip where they can cause severe inflammation and infection if not removed before closure. If there is any question about the location of a tooth or fragment, radiographs of the soft tissues should be performed.

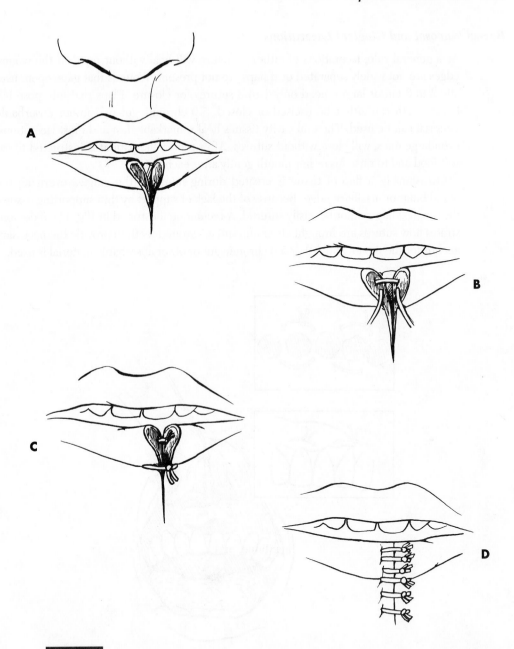

FIG. 11-15   **A,** Demonstration of a through-and-through laceration of the lip involving the orbicularis oris muscle. **B,** Closure of the orbicularis oris muscle is carried out by using absorbable deep sutures such as polyglycolic acid. **C,** Once the orbicularis oris muscle is approximated, the vermilion border or "white line" is approximated. **D,** The remainder of the laceration is closed with simple percutaneous monofilament nylon sutures.

Buccal Mucosal and Gingival Lacerations

As a general rule, lacerations of either structure will heal without repair if the wound edges are not widely separated or if flaps are not present. Wounds that gape open, usually 2 to 3 cm or larger, need only 1 to 3 sutures for closure. Flaps that interpose between teeth can either be excised or closed. 5-0 chromic gut or another absorbable material can be used. The oral cavity tissues heal remarkably fast and most lacerations, even large ones, will close without sutures. After repair, the patient is instructed to eat soft food and to rinse his or her mouth gently after each meal.

Occasionally, a flap of tissue is created during injury to the gingiva overlying the mandibular or maxillary ridge. Because of the lack of support by thin supporting tissues, the gingival flap cannot be easily sutured. A technique illustrated in Fig. 11-16 demonstrates how sutures are brought circumferentially around teeth to provide the necessary anchor for the repair, and 4-0 or 5-0 chromic gut or other absorbable material is used.

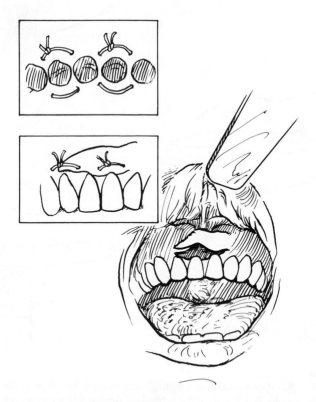

FIG. 11-16   Illustration of avulsion of gingival/mucosal tissue. The technique to close this injury is illustrated. The sutures are brought around the teeth and through the avulsed tissue flap. (Adapted from Zukin D, Simon R: *Emergency wound care: principles and practice*, Rockville, Md., 1987, Aspen Publishers.)

Tongue Lacerations

Repairing a lacerated tongue can be challenging. Small lacerations that do not gape widely when the tongue is extended will heal without intervention. Lacerations that gape widely, actively bleed, are flap shaped, or involve muscle probably need closure. The key to the repair of those lacerations is to gain the confidence of the patient. With frightened children this is often difficult, and the patient might be best served in a surgical setting where sedation and anesthesia can be delivered. An assistant is required to gain control of the tongue with dry gauze sponges, or a towel clip is placed in the previously anesthetized tip. A bite block can be fashioned to prevent injury to the assistant or the operator. The wound area is anesthetized by direct infiltration without epinephrine. The tongue heals rapidly and can be closed with an absorbable suture, such as 4-0 chromic, polyglycolic acid, or Vicryl. The sutures are placed in large bites to include both the mucosa and muscle.

Aftercare

For the first 2 or 3 days after repair of an intraoral laceration, soft foods and liquids are recommended. Rinsing the oral cavity after eating is also helpful.

Dental Trauma

Teeth are often loosened by trauma to the oral cavity. Minimal loosening, less than 2 mm, as determined by gentle "rocking" of the tooth between the examining fingers, usually reverses without intervention. Marked loosening or subluxation with an accompanying fracture of the alveolar ridge needs to be repaired with dental stabilization.

Intact teeth can also become avulsed. These teeth can be replaced in an anatomically intact socket, but the prognosis for salvage decreases with each minute that passes. On arrival in the emergency department, an attempt should be made to insert the avulsed tooth in the socket if possible.[1] If the socket contains debris, gentle removal is tried. Vigorous intervention is to be avoided. The tooth can be handled by the crown but not the root. To avoid damage to the periodontal ligament, cleaning of the tooth is not recommended. Even saline may be harmful to ligament cells.

If the tooth cannot be easily reinserted, it can be "stored" in one of three ways until a dentist or oral surgeon can be consulted. The three storage methods are: between the buccal mucosa and gum of the patient's mouth, in Hank's solution, or in milk.[16] Saline is avoided. After 30 minutes outside of the socket, the prognosis for salvage worsens rapidly. Even if the periodontal ligament survives and the tooth reattaches, later root canal intervention will be necessary to deal with the sequelae of the loss of neurovascular supply.

PERINEUM

Injuries to the perineum (i.e., penis, scrotum, and female introitus) can involve important structures that will need special attention. During the examination of wounds of the perineum, the urethra, corpora, testicles, and rectum must be assessed. Blood coming from the urethral meatus or difficulty urinating suggests urethral injury. The shaft of the penis is covered by very thin skin; violation of the corpora cavernosa or spongiosum often accompanies lacerations of the penis. The testicle is covered with a capsulelike fibrous covering called the tunica albuginea. Interruption of the corpora or tunica requires repair by a specialist. Most labial lacerations are uncomplicated but occasionally the female urethra or rectum is involved.

Preparation for Closure

Wounds to the perineum are prepared with a cleansing agent and are irrigated with saline as previously described. Uncomplicated lacerations can be anesthetized directly with lidocaine or bupivacaine. Care is taken not to use adrenaline-containing solutions for anesthetizing the penis because of potential ischemia and constriction of end-arteries.

Lacerations of the Penis and Scrotum

Because the skin of the penis is so thin, lacerations are closed with a single layer of non-absorbable suture like 5-0 nylon. Closure of the scrotal skin is carried out with chromic gut sutures that fall out within 10 days. If chromic is unavailable, another absorbable suture material can be substituted, but it may not fall out as soon. Healing takes place rapidly and removal of sutures from the rugated skin, which can be difficult, is unnecessary.

Lacerations of the Introitus

Lacerations of the labia can involve the deeper supporting muscles. If that is the case, closure has to take place in two layers to ensure reapproximation of the muscles. The skin over the labia majora can be closed with a nonabsorbable material such as nylon or polypropylene. The labia minora is covered with mucosa and can be closed with absorbable material. Uncomplicated lacerations of the vagina, unless they are extensive, will heal without sutures. Extensive or complex wounds are best referred to consultants.

Aftercare

Dressings for the genital area are hard to fashion. Gauze sponges supported by an athletic supporter are an option for men. Perineal pads are suggested for women. Hygiene of the genital area is important and daily gentle cleansing with soap and water is acceptable. Neosporin applied after bathing and before dressing application is recommended. Sutures of the penis are removed in 7 to 10 days for adults and 6 to 8 days for children.

KNEE

Careful examination of knee lacerations is important because of the structures that can be damaged. The peroneal nerve, patellar tendon, medial and lateral collateral ligaments, and patella all have to be tested for function and integrity before repair. Of particular importance is the joint space itself. If penetration is suspected, then 50 ml of normal saline with a few drops of methylene blue are injected into the joint, in a sterile fashion, at a site distant from the laceration. Arthrocentesis technique is used. If the capsule is violated, then the dye will leak out of the laceration. For more subtle injuries, fluorescein dye can be used with an ultraviolet light detection lamp.

Knee lacerations can be contaminated with grit and ground-in dirt. Although time consuming, meticulous cleansing, irrigation, and debridement are often necessary to render the wound ready to close. Uncomplicated, nonpenetrating lacerations are closed with monofilament nylon after local anesthetic infiltration. Occasionally deep (dermal) sutures are required using an absorbable material.

Aftercare

The key to good healing of knee lacerations is proper immobilization and elevation for several days. Crutches can be used for at least 48 to 72 hours if the extensor surface of the knee is involved or the wound is extensive. Knee flexion can be reduced by the application of a bulky dressing. Sutures are removed in 10 to 14 days in adults and 8 to 10 days for children.

LOWER LEG

The most vexing consideration with lower leg (shin) lacerations is the significant tension that occurs at the wound edge. Skin overlying the tibia is under a higher natural tension than most other regions of the body. Fig. 11-17 illustrates a technique for approximating the wound edges with as little tension as possible. 4-0 monofilament nylon is passed through sterile cotton-retaining pledgets obtained from the operating room. This technique allows for even distribution of tension along the wound edge without tearing. This pledget technique is particularly useful for older and thinner skin. Undermining and deep suture placement can assist in reducing tension.

Another technique for the closure of avulsion/flap wounds of the shin in older patients is the use of wound tapes.[10] Tapes avoid the problem of skin tearing with sutures and staples. Tapes can be left on until they naturally fall off. This technique allows for minimal potential disruption of the healing wound.

Aftercare

Elevation is an important element for lacerations and wounds of the lower leg. Dependent edema should not be allowed to develop. Sutures are removed after 8 to 12 days for adults and 6 to 10 days for children.

FOOT

The foot is anatomically complex and has similarities to the hand. Complete lacerations to the flexor tendons need to be repaired as they are in hands. Extensor tendons can be

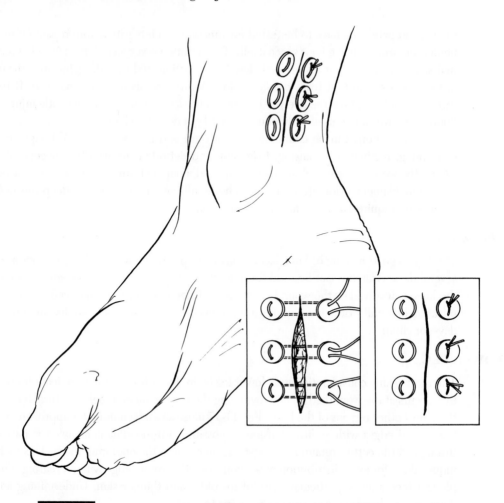

FIG. 11-17   Because of the high tension usually associated with lacerations in the lower leg (shin area), sterile cotton pledgets can be used as support for 3-0 or 4-0 monofilament nylon sutures. (Adapted from Zukin D, Simon R: *Emergency wound care: principles and practice*, Rockville, Md., 1987, Aspen Publishers.)

treated with primary skin closure and splinting. Consultation is recommended under these circumstances. Anesthesia for the plantar surface of the foot is best carried out by a posterior tibial nerve or sural nerve block, described in Chapter 5. Occasionally this method of administering anesthesia needs to be supplemented by local infiltration. Superficial dorsal lacerations are closed with 4-0 or 5-0 monofilament nylon. Lacerations of the plantar surface, or sole, can be closed with 3-0 monofilament. Lacerations of the web spaces between the toes have the same significance as lacerations of web spaces of the hand. There are no crucial structures passing through these areas and repair of the skin alone should suffice.

Aftercare

Like any lower-extremity injury, elevation is an important adjunct to care. Crutches are useful, particularly for wounds on the plantar surface. Sutures are removed in 10 to 12 days for adults and 8 to 10 days for children.

REFERENCES

1. Bringhurst L, Herr RD, Aldous JA: Oral trauma in the emergency department, *Am J Emerg Med* 11:486-490, 1993.

2. Burr WE: Auricular hematoma: treatment options, *Aust NZ J Surg* 57:391-392, 1987.

3. Cruse P, Foord R: A five year prospective of 23,649 surgical wounds, *Arch Surg* 107:206-209, 1973.

4. Duschoff IM: About face, *Emerg Med* Nov:25-77, 1974.

5. Edlich RF, et al: Principles of wound management, *Ann Emerg Med* 17:1284-1302, 1988.

6. Edlich R: Special considerations in wound management, *Am J Emerg Med* 19:1089, 1990.

7. Fullarton GM, MacEwen CJ, MacMillan R, et al: An evaluation of open scalp wounds, *Arch Emerg Med* 4:11-16, 1987.

8. George TK, Simpson DC: Skin wound closure with staples in the accident and emergency department, *J R Coll Surg Edinb* 30:54-56, 1985.

9. Howell JM, Morgan JA: Scalp laceration repair without prior hair removal, *Am J Emerg Med* 6:7-10, 1988.

10. King MT: Flap wounds of the skin, *Injury* 12:354-359, 1981.

11. Pecora D, Landis R, Martin E: Location of cutaneous microorganisms, *Surgery* 64:1114-1117, 1968.

12. Roth JH, Windle BH: Staple versus suture closure of skin incisions in a pig model, *Can J Surg* 31:19, 1988.

13. Seropian R, Reynolds B: Wound infections after preoperative depilatory versus razor preparation, *Am J Surg* 121:251-254, 1971.

14. Steele MT, Sainsbury CR, Robinson WA, et al: Prophylactic penicillin for intraoral wounds, *Ann Emerg Med* 18:847-852, 1989.

15. Tandon SC, Kelly J, Turtle M: Irradiated polyglactin-910: a new synthetic absorbable suture, *J R Coll Surg Edinb* 40:185-187, 1995.

16. Trope M: Clinical management of the avulsed tooth, *Dent Clin North Am* 39:92-112, 1995.

12 *The Hand*

· ·

A thorough understanding of the structure and function of the hand is essential to its care, even for seemingly minor injuries and problems. The complexity and relative density of important structures make the hand particularly vulnerable to injury with the added risk of serious, permanent impairment. With the use of conventional terminology, information concerning the examination can be properly recorded in the medical record and communicated to others. Problems that are appropriately managed by emergency wound-care personnel are discussed in the following section. When there is any doubt concerning the proper course of management, every attempt is made to initiate an appropriate consultation.

INITIAL TREATMENT

Before a thorough and careful examination of a patient with an injured hand can take place, certain preparatory steps have to be taken. Except for the most trivial injuries, the patient is best managed by placing him or her on a stretcher on arrival at the medical care facility. Hand injuries are often painful and provoke anxiety. Placing the patient in a supine position prevents unexpected vasovagal syncope. The recumbent position allows for easy placement of the hand in an elevated position to decrease the swelling that occurs following injury.

Any rings or constricting jewelry are removed to prevent ischemia of a digit. Most rings can be removed by using a lubricant and applying gentle, persistent traction. Ring removal from swollen fingers can be carried out by using a specially designed ring cutter and spreading the ring open with two Kelly clamps applied to the edges of the cut portion (see Fig. 1-2). Reassure patients who are concerned about damaged rings that jewelers can restore rings to their original condition. Another method for the removal of rings is illustrated in Fig. 12-1. Umbilical tape or O-silk suture can be firmly wrapped around the finger and passed under the ring with a small forceps. The ring is extracted as the tape or suture is unwound proximally to the ring.

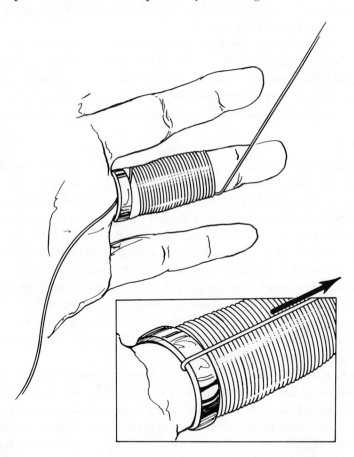

FIG. 12-1   The technique to remove a ring by finger-wrapping with large silk suture or umbilical tape. Note that the suture is begun distally over the distal interphalangeal (DIP) joint and brought back to the ring. The tail end portion of the wrap is brought under the ring, usually with a small hemostat. The removal of the ring is begun by unraveling the wrap and tugging on the string that is proximal to the ring portion. As it unravels, the ring will gently travel forward distally over the finger.

Most patients attempt to bandage the injured hand before proceeding to a medical care facility. These hastily fashioned, unsterile dressings should be carefully removed. Until treatment can be administered, sterile sponges moistened with normal saline should be applied, followed by a 2-inch or 3-inch gauze wrap. Any active bleeding requires manual pressure with gauze sponges. Rarely is an extremity tourniquet needed to stop excessive hemorrhage.

If the wound is grossly contaminated with soil or other debris and if there will be a delay before treatment is administered, the hand is gently cleaned with a wound-cleansing agent followed by irrigation with normal saline.[4] The chance of infection increases with each passing hour from the time of injury to repair. Early cleansing and irrigation can extend this safe period.

It is a common but unsupported practice to soak hand injuries in a wound-cleansing solution before repair. Although soaking is believed to loosen debris and help kill contaminating bacteria, there is no scientific evidence to support these beliefs.[16,21] Brief extremity immersion is recommended only to help remove gross soil and debris from the area surrounding the wound before proper skin cleansing and wound irrigation.

TERMINOLOGY

Knowledge of the conventional terminology is required to properly document and communicate information about injuries of the hand and fingers. All lacerations and wounds can be accurately located by the use of appropriate terms. For example, a ½-inch laceration on the back of the index finger at the first knuckle is described accurately as "a 1 cm superficial laceration of the index finger on the dorsal surface at the proximal interphalangeal joint (PIP)." Figs. 12-2 and 12-3 illustrate the various descriptive landmarks and joints. The back of the hand is the dorsal surface, whereas the palm side is the palmar or volar surface. Common landmarks of the palm are the thenar and hypothenar eminence. The digits are best remembered and recorded, when necessary, as the thumb, index, middle, ring, and little finger. Each segment of the finger is named for the underlying bony phalanx. Although the joints are descriptive of their location, it is the convention to use the abbreviations noted in Fig. 12-2.

Instead of using terms such as inside and outside or medial or lateral, the sides of the hands and fingers are referred to as radial or ulnar. This convention eliminates the confusion elicited by the other terms. Any injury to any surface on the side of the hand or finger corresponding to the radius is so described. For example, a laceration of the side of the little finger is either radial or ulnar depending on whether it is on the side of the ulna or the radius (Fig. 12-3).

PATIENT HISTORY

Certain key historical facts help determine the timing and choice of repair, as well as other supportive treatment. As previously discussed, how much time has elapsed from the time that the injury was sustained influences the decision of when to repair the

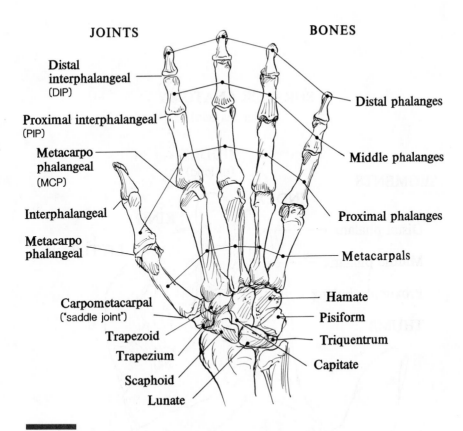

JOINTS   **BONES**

Distal interphalangeal (DIP)

Distal phalanges

Proximal interphalangeal (PIP)

Metacarpo phalangeal (MCP)

Middle phalanges

Interphalangeal

Metacarpo phalangeal

Proximal phalanges

Metacarpals

Carpometacarpal ("saddle joint")

Hamate

Pisiform

Trapezoid

Trapezium

Triquentrum

Scaphoid

Capitate

Lunate

FIG. 12-2   Descriptive anatomy of the joints and bones of the hand.

wound. Clean wounds that are caused by shearing forces can probably be safely repaired up to 6 to 8 hours after the injury. Wounds caused by tension and compression mechanisms are more vulnerable and should be considered for closure sooner. Severely contaminated wounds or those caused by mutilating forces are best left for consultation and possible delayed closure. This decision is made on a case by case basis.

A seemingly innocuous mechanism of injury is the puncture wound of the hand. Although the entry point is quite small and innocent appearing, special care has to be taken not to miss a transected nerve or tendon. In addition, the possibility of a foreign body being retained in a puncture wound has to be considered, and a radiographic examination should be carried out when the suspicion is raised.

Other historical points of importance are the patient's hand dominance, history of prior hand deformities, profession, and hobbies. Although these considerations are seemingly not as important for patients with emergency lacerations and wounds, a simple matter of a mismanaged fingertip injury can significantly affect an activity like

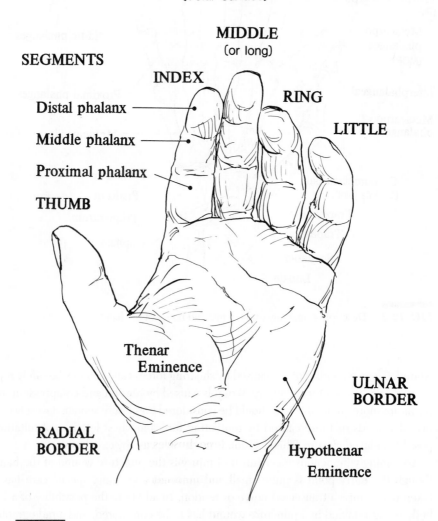

SURFACE ANATOMY
(Volar Surface)

MIDDLE
(or long)

SEGMENTS

INDEX

RING

LITTLE

Distal phalanx

Middle phalanx

Proximal phalanx

THUMB

Thenar
Eminence

ULNAR
BORDER

RADIAL
BORDER

Hypothenar
Eminence

FIG. 12-3   Descriptive anatomy of the surface of the hand. Note the ulnar and radial borders.

playing the guitar. For the guitar player, every step is taken to preserve the nail matrix. Preservation attempts might not be so necessary for an individual who does not require this anatomic part for either a job function or hobby.

Finally, any allergies the patient may have should be verified from a patient's history. Many drugs are given to patients with hand injuries. These drugs include tetanus toxoid, local anesthetics, pain medications, and a variety of antibiotics.

EXAMINATION OF THE HAND

The actual examination of the injured hand consists both of careful inspection of the wound and thorough functional testing. Nerve function is evaluated by assessing both motor and sensory components. The integrity of tendons can most often be determined by specific functional maneuvers. However, because tendons are often only partially severed and function is preserved, direct visualization by exploration is frequently necessary. In emergency wounds, circulation is so profuse that severed, bleeding vessels that travel in neurovascular bundles are often better indicators of nerve injury than actual threats to perfusion of the hand or finger. When necessary, radiographs are obtained to assist in the examination to rule out either fractures or foreign bodies. Finally, there is no substitute for exploration and direct visualization to discover structural damage of any type.

Nerve Testing
Motor Function

Three major nerves are responsible for both motor and sensory function of the hand. The radial nerve innervates the extrinsic muscles of the forearm that are responsible for extension of the wrist and fingers. This nerve does not innervate any muscle within the confines of the hand itself. The motor function of this nerve is tested by having the patient dorsiflex his or her wrist and fingers against a resisting force, such as the examiner's hand (Fig. 12-4). Intact motor strength, as provided for by an intact radial nerve, should prevent the examiner from overcoming the dorsiflexed wrist when a good deal of counterforce is applied.

In addition to the flexor carpi ulnaris and part of the flexor digitorum profundus, the ulnar nerve innervates most of the intrinsic muscles of the hand itself, including all of the interossei muscles and the little and ring fingers lumbricals. The motor portion of this nerve is responsible for the ability of the fingers to spread and close in a fanlike manner. A specific test for ulnar motor function is to have the patient adduct his fingers (close) against an object, such as a pen (Fig. 12-5). With an intact nerve, the examiner cannot easily remove the object. Each finger can be tested in this manner.

The median nerve provides motor innervation to wrist flexors, the flexor digitorum superficialis, part of the flexor digitorum profundus (shared with the ulnar nerve), and the remaining intrinsic muscles of the hand, most notably those of the thumb that are

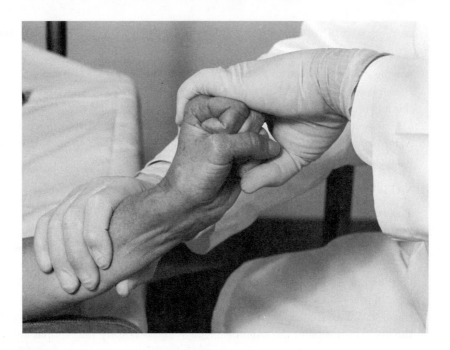

FIG. 12-4   Testing for radial nerve function. With the patient's fist dorsiflexed, the examiner tries to "break" the resistance created by the dorsiflexion.

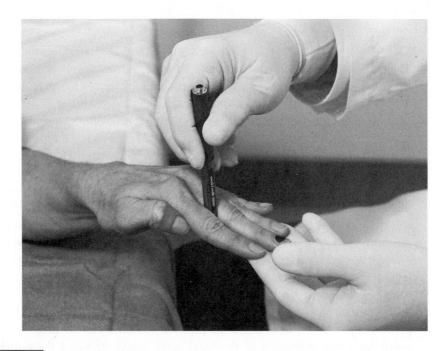

FIG. 12-5   Testing for ulnar nerve function. The patient is asked to resist the examiner's attempt to pull an object, such as a pen, from between the adducted fingers.

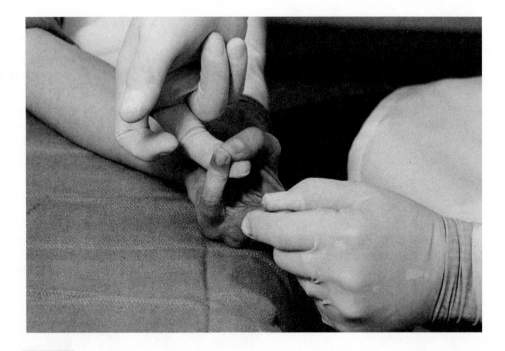

FIG. 12-6 Testing for median nerve function. The thumb is apposed to the little finger to form a tight ring. This ring should not be easily broken by the examiner.

responsible for opposition. Opposition to some degree is also mediated by the adduction component of the interossei as supplied to the ulnar nerve. The testing maneuver is completed by having the patient oppose his or her thumb with the tip of the little finger. A properly made "ring" consisting of the thumb and little finger should be hard to break by the examiner if the median nerve is intact (Fig. 12-6).

Sensory Function

A variety of stimuli can be delivered to the skin of the hand to test sensory function. Gross touch with a blunt object is the easiest but least specific. It can be useful, however, for rapid screening to assess the possibility of nerve damage especially when comparison testing is done between the injured and noninjured hands. If there is a nerve injury, the patient will often be able to report a difference in feeling. Pinprick stimulus is the most commonly used modality for testing. Pinprick is useful when alternated with blunt stimulus. In a complete nerve transection, the patient cannot tell the difference between a blunt and a sharp stimulus. Pinprick testing, nevertheless, is difficult to assess on the fingertips, especially in a manual laborer whose finger pads are covered with thick calluses.

A more accurate method of assessing sensory function is two-point discrimination.[10] A paper clip can be fashioned so that two ends can be opened or closed to varying distances from each other (Fig. 12-7). A patient with a normally innervated fingertip should be able to distinguish two simultaneously delivered stimuli 6 mm or more apart from each other. Most patients can tell a difference down to 3 mm. When identification of separate stimuli is reported by the patient at 8 mm apart or more, the examination is clearly abnormal.

Of the major nerves, the radial nerve provides the least important sensory innervation to the hand. This nerve supplies sensation to the radial portion of the dorsum of the hand, the dorsum of the thumb, and the proximal portion of the dorsal side of the second and third digits and half of the ring finger (Fig. 12-8). To rapidly test gross radial sensory function, a stimulus is supplied to the first web space, an area of pure radial distribution.

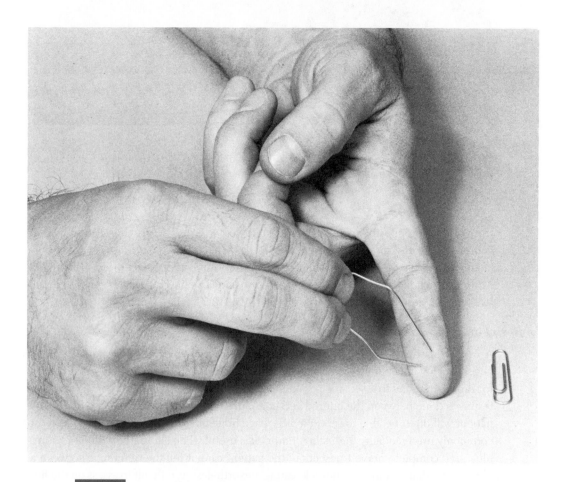

FIG. 12-7   Technique for testing sensory nerve function by two-point discrimination. A paper clip is bent in a manner to provide variable distance stimuli. See text for a complete description.

Sensory distribution of the ulnar nerve includes the dorsal and volar surfaces of the ulnar side of the hand, the entire fifth digit, and the ulnar half of the fourth digit. To test an intact sensory component of the ulnar nerve, an appropriate stimulus is delivered to the area of purest ulnar distribution, the tip of the fifth digit.

The remainder of the hand is innervated by the median nerve. The radial side of the palm and volar surfaces of the thumb, index, middle, and radial half of the ring fingers comprise the area of sensory distribution. As depicted in Fig. 12-8, it is important to note that median nerve innervation extends to all of the fingertips of the thumb, index, and middle fingers, including the dorsal portion of the distal phalanges. Pure median sensation can be found at the tip of the index finger.

More common than injuries to the major nerves are injuries and lacerations to the digital nerves that lie within the hand itself. There are four digital nerves for each digit. The two palmar nerves (Fig. 12-9) are the largest and most important. Sensation to the palmar surface, as well as the nailbed area of the fingertip, is carried through these two

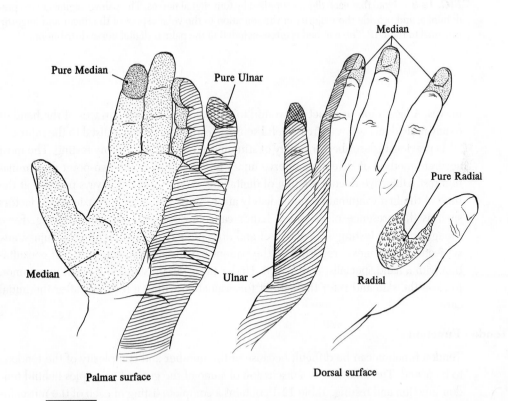

Palmar surface   Dorsal surface

FIG. 12-8   The distribution of the three major nerves providing sensory innervation of the hand. Note the areas of pure median, ulnar, and radial sensation.

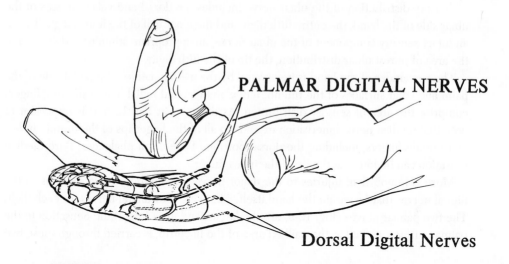

PALMAR DIGITAL NERVES

Dorsal Digital Nerves

FIG. 12-9   Note that each digit is supplied by four digital nerves. The palmar digital nerves predominate and provide the majority of the sensation to the volar aspect of the finger and fingertip proximal to the DIP. The nail bed is often included in the palmar digital nerve distribution.

nerves. A laceration or puncture wound to the palmar or dorsal surfaces of the hand or to any individual digit requires careful sensory testing of the digits distal to the injury.

As previously described, a variety of stimuli can be used for sensory testing. The most accurate method of detecting a nerve injury in this setting is the two-point discrimination test. Objective documentation of digital nerve injuries is not always possible at the time of the first examination immediately after injury. Patient pain, anxiety, and factors such as the presence of calloused hands can interfere with two-point testing. Even though stimulus testing is inconsistent and does not clearly document nerve injury, any subjective "numbness" reported by the patient has to be taken seriously and consultation with a hand specialist considered. Under these circumstances, it is not uncommon to close the skin and refer the patient for evaluation within a few days after the initial care.

Tendon Function

Tendon function can be difficult because of the number and complexity of the tendons to be tested. The following is a discussion of some of the general principles behind tendon function and testing. Table 12-1 contains a complete listing of each of the musculotendinous units in the hand and of their related nerve control.

Table 12-1 *Components of Hand Function*

Joint/Action	Musculotendinous Unit	Nerve Control
WRIST		
Flexion	Flexor carpi radialis	Median
	Palmaris longus	Median
	Flexor carpi ulnaris	Ulnar
Extension	Extensor carpi radialis	Radial
	Extensor carpi ulnaris	Radial
Radial deviation	Extensor carpi radialis	Radial
	Flexor carpi radialis	Median
Ulnar deviation	Extensor carpi ulnaris	Radial
	Flexor carpi ulnaris	Ulnar
METACARPOPHALANGEAL		
Flexion	Interosseous	Ulnar
	Lumbrical	Median/Ulnar
Extension	Extensor digitorum communis	Radial
	Extensor indicis proprius	Radial
	Extensor digiti minimi	Radial
Abduction	Dorsal interossei	Ulnar
Adduction	Volar interossei	Ulnar
PROXIMAL INTERPHALANGEAL		
Flexion	Flexor digitorum sublimis	Median
Extension	Interossei	Ulnar
	Lumbricals	Ulnar/Median
	Extensor digitorum communis	Radial
	Extensor indicis proprius	Radial
	Extensor digiti minimi	Radial
DISTAL INTERPHALANGEAL		
Flexion	Flexor digitorum profundus	Median/Ulnar
Extension	Same for proximal interphalangeal joint	
THUMB-CARPOMETACARPAL		
Flexion/Adduction	Adductor pollicis	Ulnar
	Flexor pollicis brevis	Ulnar
	Dorsal interosseous	Ulnar
	Flexor pollicis longus	Median
Extension/Abduction	Extensor pollicis longus	Radial
	Extensor pollicis brevis	Radial
	Abductor pollicis longus	Radial
	Abductor pollicis brevis	Median
Opposition	Abductor pollicis brevis	Median
	Flexor pollicis brevis	Median
	Opponens pollicis	Median

Continued

Table 12-1   *Components of Hand Function—cont'd*

Joint/Action	Musculotendinous Unit	Nerve Control
THUMB METACARPOPHALANGEAL		
Flexion	Flexor pollicis longus	Median
	Thenar intrinsics	Median/Ulnar
Extension	Extensor pollicis brevis	Radial
THUMB INTERPHALANGEAL		
Flexion	Flexor pollicis longus	Median
Extension	Extensor pollicis longus	Radial

Extensor Function

Extensor tendon function can be simply tested by having the patient extend his or her fingers against the force of the examiner (Fig. 12-10). Although this maneuver appears to be easy enough, there are complexities of the tendon anatomy than can cause confusion when interpreting the results of the examination. The wrist itself has three main extensor tendons that are responsible for proper extension at the wrist. If these tendons are cut, the wrist can be extended by the finger extensors but with far less force and can be easily overcome by the examiner. The thumb is served by an abductor and two extensor tendons. If one is cut, the second can still function. Each finger has one main extensor tendon responsible for extension with power. The second and fifth digits, however, have small accessory tendons that can weakly extend these fingers if the main extensors are knocked out of action.

Another anatomic point that can possibly cause misinterpretation in the examination for extension of the digits is that, as extensor tendons cross the wrist, they flatten out and interconnect with other extensors over the dorsum of the hand (Fig. 12-11). Weak extension of a severed tendon can occur by the action of the adjacent interconnecting tendon. These interconnections also can prevent severed extensor tendons from slipping back into the forearm after they are cut. This anatomic property of extensors makes anastomosis easier for extensors than for flexor tendons because the two severed ends can be readily retrieved during repair.

Whenever there is doubt about extensor tendon function, careful exploration has to be carried out through the laceration itself. Extensor tendons are quite superficial and can be easily identified with proper and gentle exposure. A key factor to remember is that the position of the hand at the time of examination and exploration may be different from the position of the hand during injury. If that should be the case, then the actual laceration to the tendon may be at a location away from the laceration on the skin (Fig. 12-12). Therefore active flexion/extension of the finger to cause the tendon to slide back and forth is encouraged during the exploration.

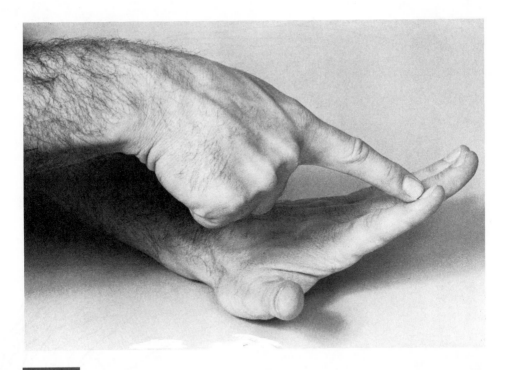

FIG. 12-10 Testing the extensor tendon function. Each finger is extended against a resisting force. This force should not be easily overcome.

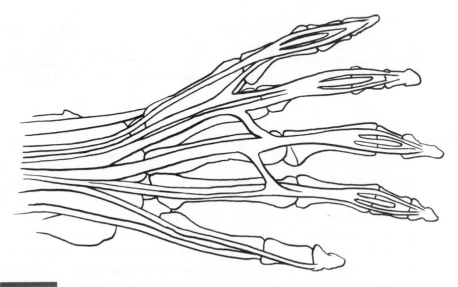

FIG. 12-11 The extensor tendon anatomy of the hand. Note in particular the cross-linkages of extensor tendons at the distal metacarpal level. Severance of a extensor tendon proximal to these cross-linkages can give the examiner the false sense that the affected digit can be extended because of the help that cross-linkage provides through the adjacent tendon.

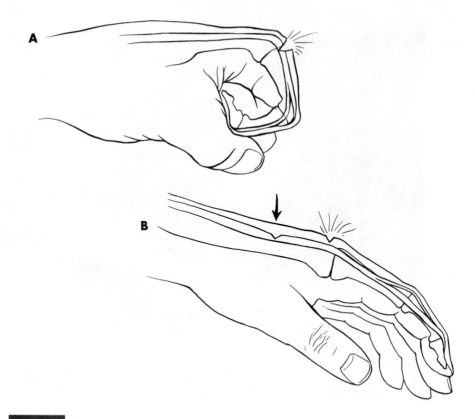

FIG. 12-12   Tendon-skin wound mismatch. **A,** A tendon can be partially lacerated in one position, such as a closed fist. **B,** However, when the wound is explored, the tendon injury might be missed because the site of the tendon injury has retracted when the hand is extended for care. The examiner must carry out the exploration by trying to recreate the position of injury.

Flexor Function

The thumb has only one flexor tendon, but the index, middle, ring, and little fingers have two main flexor tendons. The volar surface of the wrist is a complex and vulnerable area, replete with important structures. As illustrated in Fig. 12-13, the median nerve lies just deep and radial to the palmaris longus, the most superficial tendon. Even trivial-appearing lacerations to the wrist can cause serious tendon and nerve damage.

The flexor tendons to each finger are paired. The flexor digitorum profundus tendons are responsible for power and mass action such as is needed for gripping. These tendons run deep to the flexor digitorum sublimis tendons, but at the level of the middle phalanx, the profundus splits through the sublimis and goes on to attach to the distal phalanx (Fig. 12-14). To test profundus function, the action of the sublimis tendon has to be

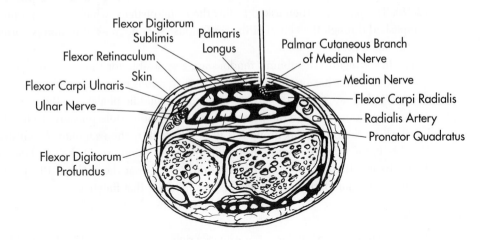

FIG. 12-13 Cross-sectional anatomy of the wrist. Note in particular the superficial location of the median nerve. Any visible tendon laceration, such as to the palmaris longus, has to raise the suspicion of an injury to the median nerve.

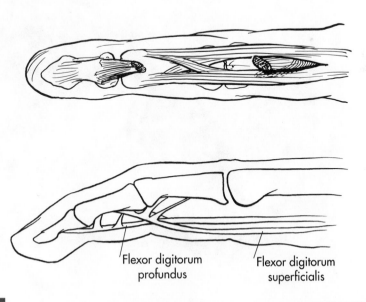

FIG. 12-14 Note the relationship of the flexor digitorum profundus to the flexor digitorum superficialis. The profundus splits through the superficialis, which is attached on the middle phalanx. The profundus attaches to the distal phalanx.

blocked by holding each digit, one at a time, in extension at the middle phalanx (Fig. 12-15). The patient is then asked to flex the distal phalanx, which now can only be accomplished through the action of the profundus. Sixty degrees of flexion is normal during this maneuver.

The flexor digitorum sublimis tendons are responsible for the positioning of the fingers so that power flexion can take place. These tendons run superficial to the deep tendons until they are split at the distal portion of the middle phalanx by the profundi. The sublimis tendons attach to the proximal portion of the middle phalanx. To test for sublimis action, the profundus group has to be blocked by the examiner. As illustrated in Fig. 12-16, the examiner holds all the fingers in extension except the one being tested. The patient is then asked to fully flex his or her finger at the MP and PIP joint. If the sublimis is lacerated, the patient will be unable to flex that finger.

CIRCULATION

The circulation of the hand is extraordinarily rich and redundant (Fig. 12-17). Most people can suffer complete loss of either the radial or ulnar arteries and maintain adequate

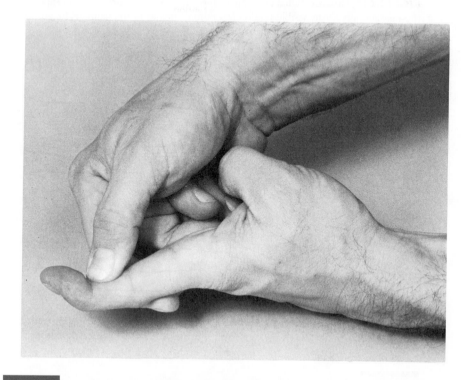

FIG. 12-15   Testing for function of the flexor digitorum profundus. The distal phalanx of the finger is forcibly flexed, while the action of the superficialis tendon is blocked. Only the profundus can flex the distal phalanx.

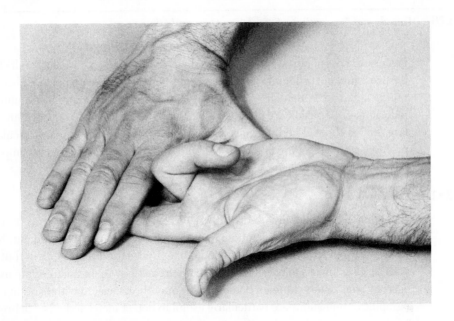

FIG. 12-16 Testing for function of the flexor digitorum superficialis. The mass action of the profundus can be blocked by holding the nontested fingers in extension. The tested finger can only be flexed at the PIP by the superficialis tendon.

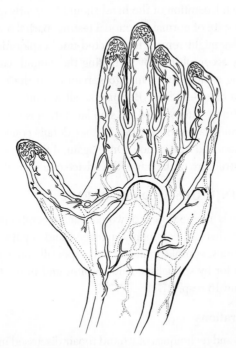

FIG. 12-17 The profuse and redundant vascularity of the hand. It is not uncommon to be able to sacrifice either the radial or ulnar artery and still have complete perfusion of the hand. Lacerations of the digital arteries arouse suspicion of a lacerated digital nerve.

perfusion. Loss of perfusion because of damage to the vessels usually results from an extensive injury not ordinarily repaired by emergency wound-care personnel and consultation is obtained. Although pulses are always documented in any hand injury, the best indicators of perfusion are color, skin blanching with pressure, temperature, and capillary refill at the nail bed. Because arteries travel with nerves in neurovascular bundles, profuse arterial bleeding of the digit should raise the suspicion of an accompanying digital nerve injury.

RADIOGRAPHY

Radiographs are liberally used to assist in the evaluation of the hand. For any blunt trauma associated with a laceration, underlying fractures must be ruled out. Not only do hand fractures require careful and sometimes specialized management, but a fracture with a laceration has to be considered an open fracture. Open fractures are usually managed by consultants. Foreign bodies are frequently associated with hand injuries. Radiographic examinations are particularly useful to detect metal and other debris. Contrary to a common misconception of many clinicians, almost all types of glass, in up to 90% of cases, are easily detectable by radiographs[27] (see Chapter 15).

WOUND EXPLORATION

Ultimately, each laceration of the hand should be gently and carefully explored just before repair. In spite of normal functional testing, partial tendon lacerations and violation of joint capsules might remain undetected until exploration is carried out. This procedure is usually accomplished by retracting the wound with an Adson forceps or a skin hook and using a mosquito clamp to spread open the deeper tissue for a good look, preferably in a bloodless field. Because small wounds can harbor serious injury to underlying structures, extension of the skin laceration is sometimes necessary to gain adequate exposure. Chapter 8 provides further details concerning tourniquet application, wound extension, and exploration. Once again, if there is ever a doubt about an injury to an important structure of the hand, the advice of a specialist should be sought.

SELECTED HAND INJURIES AND PROBLEMS

Although there is a large variety of wounds and lacerations to the hand, those described here are those that are commonly managed and repaired by emergency wound-care personnel. Serious, complex injuries, and especially ones that cause functional deficits, are best cared for by specialists. Animal bites and burns to the hands are discussed in Chapters 14 and 16 respectively.

Uncomplicated Lacerations

The principles and techniques of wound repair discussed in Chapter 9 also apply to closing hand lacerations. Most lacerations of the dorsal and volar surfaces of the hand can be anesthetized by direct wound infiltration (see Chapter 5). Large lacerations can be managed by wrist blocks. Wounds beyond the proximal phalanx are best anesthetized with digital blocks.

Debridement of the hand, when indicated, is carried out with great caution. Excessive removal of skin can lead to failure of adequate coverage, eventual wound contraction, and a resulting functional deficit. Fat is a good substrate for bacterial growth, and less care has to be taken when debriding away contaminated and devitalized tissue. On the other hand, injured fat does not regenerate. The padding role that fat provides the volar surface of the hand can be endangered. In cases where large amounts of fat must be sacrificed, the opinion of a consultant is recommended.

Because of the number of important structures that lie within the small confines of the hand, deep closures with any suture material are discouraged. Any "foreign" material can provoke inflammation and tissue scarring that might interfere with such important and vulnerable functions as tendon gliding. By closing the skin alone, very little dead space is left behind in hand injuries. In addition, natural tension across the wound is usually minimal in hand lacerations and deep closures are not needed to reduce that tension.

The recommended suture material for skin closure is 5-0 nonabsorbable monofilament nylon. Only as many sutures as are necessary to achieve appropriate wound edge approximation are placed. Hand lacerations heal with little scarring, and no purpose is served by excessive sutures in search of the perfect repair. Simple interrupted technique suffices for most wounds. However, skin on the hand tends to invert with closure, particularly on the dorsal surface. In this case, the horizontal mattress technique is quite useful.

Fingertip Injuries

The management of fingertip injuries is quite controversial. There are very few actual controlled studies of fingertip and fingernail problems. Therefore the strategies and choices of repair techniques vary considerably between personnel who take care of these problems. Just the issue of whether to remove the nail following an injury evokes widely varying opinions. Certain principles, however, guide the repair process. These are preservation of finger length, nail growth capacity, fingertip padding, and sensation.[18]

The fingertip and fingernail apparatus comprise a complex anatomic and functional unit (Fig. 12-18). The fleshy volar pad is replete with nerve endings and capillaries. There is sufficient soft tissue to effectively pad the fingertip and distal phalanx against undue trauma. Preservation of sensation of the fingertip is crucial to all manual activities. Even with full-thickness loss of the finger pad, healing and regeneration of tissue can usually be relied on to restore a functional pad. Numerous fibrous bands called *septa* anchor the skin to the underlying bony structure (Fig. 12-19). These structures prevent sliding or slipping of the skin during use of the fingers. Septa should be kept anatomically intact whenever possible.

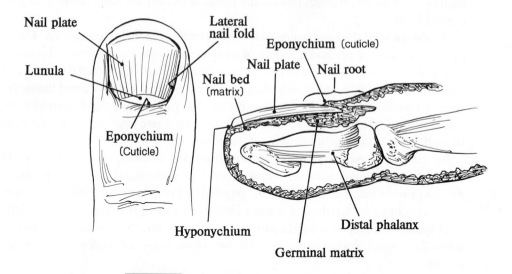

FIG. 12-18   Anatomy of the distal finger and nail components.

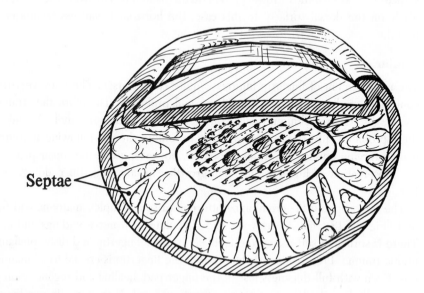

FIG. 12-19   The fibrous septa that connect the skin to the underlying phalanges. The septa provides stability to the soft tissue of the finger.

The nail apparatus has several components. The nail itself is divided into the nail root, which is the portion that lies under the eponychium, and the nail plate, which adheres to the sterile matrix. The matrix also has two parts, the germinal matrix from which new nail is generated, and the sterile matrix, or nail bed, over which the nail passes during normal growth. The eponychium, commonly referred to as the cuticle, is the fold of skin that overlies the nail root. One of the main principles of nail management is to prevent the eponychium from adhering and scarring down onto the germinal matrix. Should this unfortunate event take place, nail regeneration can be significantly impaired. Techniques to prevent this occurrence are discussed in the following sections.

Fingertip injuries can be divided into three groups: (1) blunt injuries—subsequent hematoma, (2) nail and nail bed lacerations, and (3) avulsion injuries with tissue loss. Foreign bodies lodged under a fingernail are discussed in Chapter 15.

Blunt Injuries: Subungual Hematoma

The treatment of subungual hematoma is controversial and dependent on the clinical training and personal experience of the physician. Until recently, there have not been many studies to clarify the issues surrounding this problem and provide guidance.

It has been thought and taught that the presence of a large hematoma (> 50% of the nail surface) signifies a probable laceration of the nail bed; therefore the need for nail removal and repair. In a study of 47 patients, 60% with a large hematoma had a nail bed laceration.[24] If a distal phalanx fracture was also present, the likelihood of a laceration rose to 97%. The authors concluded that nail removal, with bed repair, should be carried out in patients with large hematomas (at least 50% of the nail). Smaller hematomas could be treated with trephination alone.

The argument for limited nail removal and bed repair is supported by a study of 45 patients with subungual hematoma who were followed for at least 6 months post-treatment.[23] All patients, including 16 patients with a 50% hematoma and 14 with distal phalanx fracture, were trephinated as their *only* treatment. They were splinted for protection for 1 week. The outcome was uniformly good with no wound infections, osteomyelitis, or significant later nail deformities. Excluded from the study were patients with nail disruption and prior existing nail deformities. While this is a solitary study favoring limited intervention, it is consistent with this author's experience.

Nail trephination can be carried out by a variety of methods. The heated paper clip creates an appropriate diameter drainage hole, but this technique requires considerable practice and skill. The clip has to be heated until it is red hot and transferred quickly to the nail. Heat is quickly lost, and it is not uncommon to have to repeat the procedure to gain full nail penetration. Eighteen-gauge needles and #11 scalpel blades can be used to create a drainage site using a rotating or drilling motion. The drainage holes are often small and close prematurely with a blood clot. There is considerable pressure brought to bear on the fingertip when applying this technique. More effective and less painful is the battery-powered drill.

The most efficacious and least painful device is the disposable electric cautery that can be handled like a pencil and placed with ease and precision over the hematoma (Fig. 12-20). The drainage hole is adequate, and the patients tolerate the procedure very well once they understand that the heat tip will not burn them. With appropriate technique, once the heat tip passes through the nail, heat will be rapidly dissipated by the underlying hematoma.

In summary, the following guidelines are offered for the evaluation and management of subungual hematoma:

- Trephination alone is appropriate for subungual hematomas of any size in which the nail remains attached and there is not deformity of the fingertip suggestive of a displaced fracture. Even if a nail bed laceration or nondisplaced tuft fracture is present, healing will proceed without event and full function will be restored to the finger with splinting.

- Nail removal is reserved for patients in whom the nail is already partially avulsed, torn, or deformed from this injury. Under these circumstances, once the nail is removed, as described in the following, the bed is inspected and lacerations repaired.

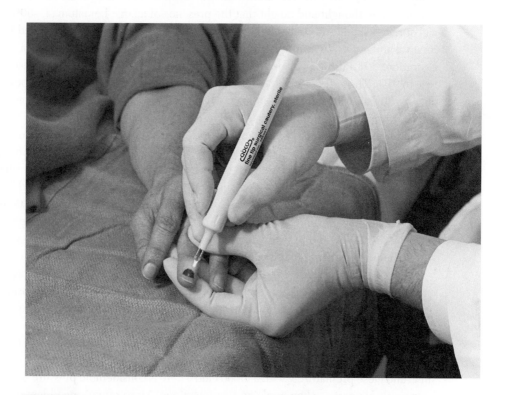

FIG. 12-20   Electric cautery to penetrate a nail to drain a subungual hematoma.

- Although subungual hematomas with associated fractures can technically be considered open fractures, in reality they do not need to be treated as such. Antibiotics are not indicated if the nail is left in place.

Nail Bed Lacerations

Exposed bed lacerations of the matrix, caused by blunt trauma, are repaired by careful reapposition of the wound edges and suturing with 5-0 or 6-0 absorbable suture material. If intact, an avulsed or removed nail can be replaced, for temporary splinting purposes, under the eponychium (Fig. 12-21). The main reason for using the nail as a splint is to prevent adhesions and granulation tissue buildup between the eponychium and germinal matrix of the bed. It also serves to splint any accompanying fracture and mold the healing wound site. To maintain the nail in place, two 5-0 nonabsorbable sutures can be placed through trephined holes (Fig. 12-21). If the nail cannot be used, a small piece of nonadherent dressing such as Adaptic or Penrose drain can be tucked under the eponychium (Fig. 12-22). The nail, or packing, is usually left in place for 7 to 10 days.

In children it is not uncommon for the nail root to partially avulse from the bed under the cuticle (eponychium). If the remainder of the nail appears intact and is firmly attached to the nail matrix, then the nail root can be replaced by the nail root retrieval technique (Fig. 12-23). If this procedure is too difficult to accomplish, then the nail root is excised and the eponychium is packed with a nonadherent dressing material for 10 to 14 days for the same reasons described earlier (Fig. 12-24). A new nail eventually grows out and extrudes the remaining portion of the old nail.

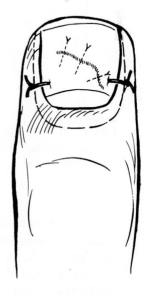

FIG. 12-21 Nail bed injury. If the decision has been made to remove the nail, and a laceration of the bed is discovered, this laceration is repaired with 6-0 absorbable suture such as polyglycolic acid. The nail, if removed intact, can be replaced as a splint for 7 to 10 days. The nail will prevent adherence of the germinal matrix to the eponychium. The nail is anchored by placing sutures as shown in the lateral aspect of the plate.

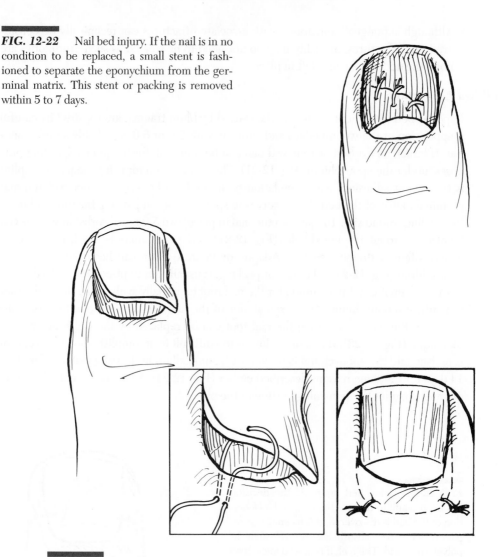

FIG. 12-22   Nail bed injury. If the nail is in no condition to be replaced, a small stent is fashioned to separate the eponychium from the germinal matrix. This stent or packing is removed within 5 to 7 days.

FIG. 12-23   Nail-root avulsion. Occasionally, the proximal aspect of a nail root is avulsed. The technique illustrated demonstrates how this nail root can be replaced under the cuticle. This is an injury more commonly seen in children.

Lacerations of the fingertip and nail apparatus caused by sharp or shearing forces can usually be managed by simple suturing. Transverse lacerations through the nail plate and matrix can be repaired by removing the distal portion of the nail plate to expose the lacerated nail bed. Repair of the matrix is carried out with 6-0 absorbable suture (Fig. 12-25). Maintaining the integrity of the nail root prevents nail growth problems with the germinal matrix.

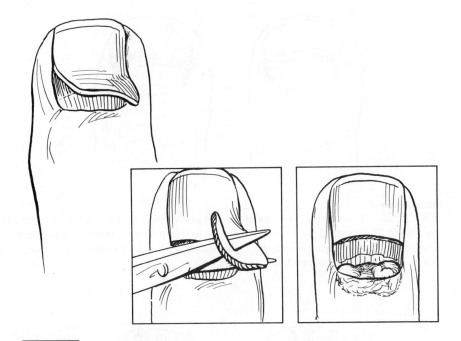

FIG. 12-24   Nail-root avulsion. If the nail root cannot be replaced, the nail root can be excised and a small Penrose or Adaptic packing is placed under the eponychium for 5 to 7 days. A new nail germinates and extrudes the remainder of the old portion.

Longitudinal lacerations through the matrix and eponychium require careful repair of both structures. The nail bed is repaired with 6-0 absorbable suture (Fig. 12-26). The eponychium and surrounding skin is closed with nonabsorbable material like nylon. If the nail plate is removed in its entirety, then a nail replacement or packing for 10 to 14 days, as previously described, is necessary to prevent eponychial adherence to the germinal matrix. Only the nonabsorbable sutures are removed after 10 to 12 days.

Nail Removal Technique

When the decision is made to remove the nail, the techniques illustrated in Fig. 12-27 are suggested. A small hemostat or iris scissors is inserted under the nail plate along the nail bed. The instrument is slowly advanced as it is spread open to lift the nail plate off the matrix. This process is carried back through to the nail root and germinal matrix area. Care is taken to avoid undue injury to the nail bed and germinal matrix. The eponychium is also gently pushed away from the nail plate. Once the nail plate has been loosened, a hemostat is used to grasp the nail plate firmly and pull it out from under the eponychium. The nail does not always come off easily and some measure of force must be applied.

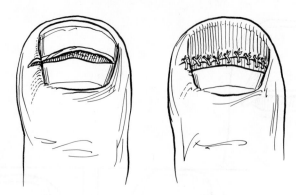

FIG. 12-25 Transverse lacerations of the nail bed can often be managed by leaving the nail root intact. The proximal portion of the nail is excised with tissue scissors proximally to the injury. The nail bed is then repaired with absorbable suture. The nail continues to grow over the suture line well after the sutures have been absorbed.

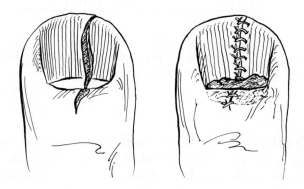

FIG. 12-26 Longitudinal lacerations of the nail bed are often best closed by removal of the nail entirely. Once the nail bed is repaired, packing of Penrose drain or Adaptic is used to separate the eponychium from the germinal matrix for at least 5 to 7 days.

Avulsion Injuries

Another area of controversy in fingertip management surrounds avulsion injuries with loss of tissue (Fig. 12-28). At issue is whether to close these avulsions by grafting or whether to leave them to heal spontaneously. There is consensus that any fingertip avulsion with less than 1 cm square area of tissue loss and no accompanying bony or nail bed injury can be managed by allowing spontaneous healing to take place.[17] At issue are avulsion injuries of larger areas or bone exposure. Losses up to 1.8 × 2.6 cm, even with

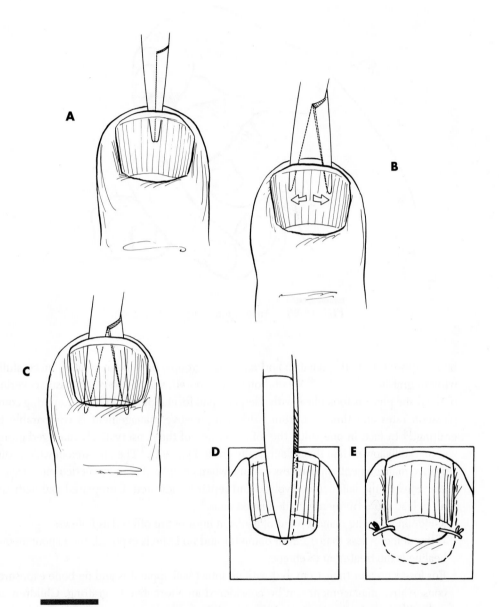

FIG. 12-27 Technique for removal of a nail. **A,** Introduce a small hemostat or iris scissors between the nail and the nail bed. **B,** Gently dissect the nail from the nail bed. **C,** Extend the dissection all the way back to the germinal matrix. **D,** Grasp the nail firmly and remove it from the nail bed. **E,** If the nail plate remains intact, it can be replaced as a splint or stent and anchored as shown with two 5-0 nonabsorbable sutures.

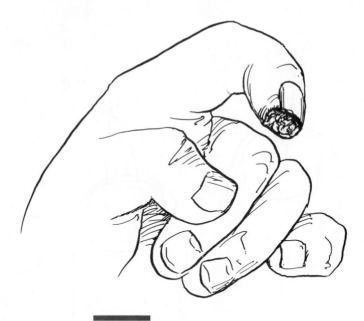

FIG. 12-28   An avulsion injury of the fingertip.

bone exposed, in both pediatric and adult age groups, have been treated successfully without grafting.[5, 9, 13, 15, 32] When bone was exposed, spontaneous soft tissue covering of the distal phalanx took place with adequate pad formation.[8, 32] When comparing complication rates and time lost from work, conservative management is comparable to grafting.[12] In fact, in one study the infection rate of the conservatively managed group was markedly lower than that of surgically grafted patients.[3] The one area in which conservative management appears less optimal when compared to more meticulous surgical repair is when the nail bed is involved and repair is indicated. Unrepaired nail matrixes tend to lead more frequently to deformed nails.[3]

Guidelines for the management of avulsion injuries are offered as follows:

- If the defect is less than 1 cm in diameter and no bone is exposed, then spontaneous healing is the treatment of choice.
- For losses greater than 1 cm, but with an intact nail apparatus and no bone exposure, conservative management can be considered an alternative to grafting. Children do well with conservative treatment. Local practice, which may necessitate consultation, often dictates the management of these injuries.
- For avulsions with nail apparatus involvement, repair or revision of the matrix is necessary. Consultation may be required.
- For injuries with exposed bone, consultation is recommended to assist in the decision regarding the treatment choice.

Proper dressings for fingertip avulsions include a nonadherent base, such as Xeroform or Adaptic, with a sponge covering and gauze wrapping as described in Chapter 17. As discussed in the later section on antibiotics for hand wounds, antibiotics are suggested for injuries with exposed bone.

Tendon Lacerations

All lacerations of flexor tendons (in the upper or lower extremity) are referred to specialists for care. An emergency wound-care setting is no place to repair flexor tendon injuries. Besides requiring a controlled surgical environment, these tendons are most effectively managed by trained surgeons using the proper instruments and magnification. Under the best of circumstances, flexor tendon injuries present considerable technical challenges, and repair can be fraught with complications. As illustrated in Fig. 12-29, injuries in zone II, known as No Man's Land, present the greatest challenge to the caregiver.

In many cases, flexor tendon lacerations can be repaired primarily up to 3 weeks post injury.[26] Anastomoses carried out within 7 to 10 days may have a better outcome.[28] After 3 weeks, reconstructive procedures have to be used. With agreement from the consultant, the skin can be closed and arrangements made for follow-up evaluation and decision regarding formal tendon repair. The skin closure is carried out after standard skin cleansing and irrigation. A splint is placed. An intravenous dose of a first general cephalosporin is administered in the emergency department followed by oral cephalosporin or dicloxacillin. Clindamycin can be given in the allergic patient. For injuries with excessive contamination, skin loss, unstable bony skeleton, or missing tissue, then immediate operative intervention may be necessary.

Simple, single lacerations of an extensor tendon on the dorsum of the hand, between the distal wrist and metacarpophalangeal joints (zone VI), can be repaired in the emergency wound care area by appropriately trained wound-care personnel.[2] It is recommended that training for extensor tendon repair include several supervised repairs under the guidance of a specialist. It is important to master appropriate techniques and understand proper splinting and the necessary follow-up care. The specialist should agree with the plan of care because he or she will pick up the aftercare.

Single extensor tendons can be repaired in the emergency department under the following circumstances: (1) if the injury is between the distal wrist and the metacarpophalangeal joints (zone VI); (2) if the skin and tendon wounds are sharp and not heavily macerated or contaminated; (3) if the injury is less than 8 hours old; (4) if the two ends of the tendon are easily visualized; (5) if appropriate instruments are available to minimize trauma to the tissues; and (6) if the patient is cooperative and will comply with follow-up care.

The technique for repairing an extensor tendon is shown in Fig. 12-30. A 4-0 nonabsorbable suture such as nylon or polypropylene on a straight needle is passed through the tendon in the figure-eight pattern until it is secure. The skin is closed with 5-0

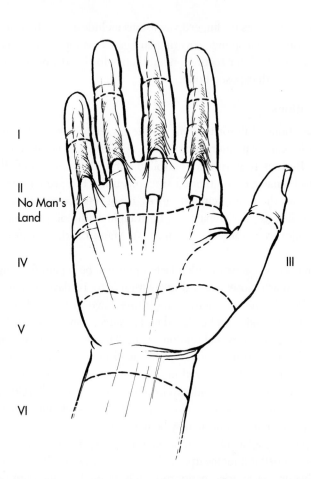

FIG. 12-29   Zones of tendon repair. The hand can be divided into zones that have different implications when considering tendon repair strategy and technique. Injuries in zone II, also referred to as No Man's land, are difficult to repair because of the complex and close relationship of the tendons and surrounding structures.

nonabsorbable suture material. A plaster splint is placed on the palmar surfaces of the forearm-wrist-hand-digit, over the appropriate nonadherent base and the gauze sponge/wrap surface dressing. The wrist is placed at a 30-degree angle of extension and the metacarpophalangeal joints are placed at a 20-degree angle of flexion. The fingers are only slightly flexed. The splint remains in place for 3 weeks; however, the patient is referred much sooner to the consultant for follow-up care.

On careful exploration of a laceration of the hand, it is not uncommon to discover partially lacerated extensor or flexor tendons. The management of these injuries is controversial. Unrepaired, these injuries have been reported to rupture, cause "triggering," or

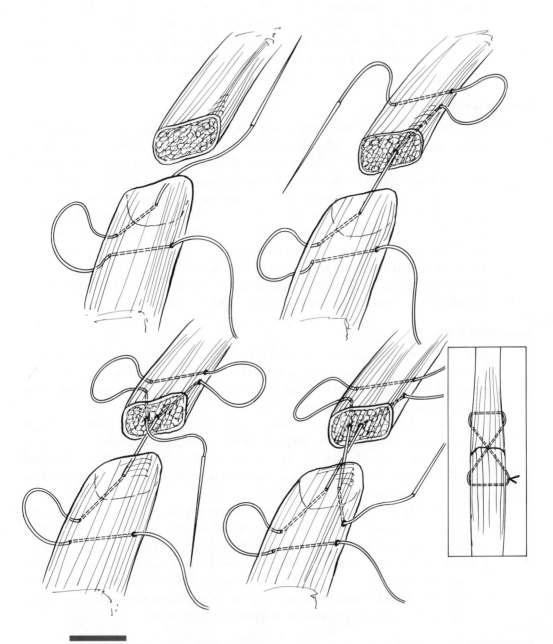

FIG. 12-30 The figure-eight technique to reappose sharply divided lacerated extensor tendons. See text for further explanation.

become entrapped.[26] On the other hand, successful treatment of these injuries has been reported with skin closure alone followed by splinting.[19,30] Treatment can be guided by cross-sectional size of the laceration. As a general rule, if the tendon is more than 50% transected, it should be repaired as if fully severed. Lesser injuries can be trimmed to prevent triggering or entrapment. Appropriate splinting, rehabilitation, and follow-up care are carried out under the direction of the specialist.

Nerve Injuries

Lacerations associated with sensory or motor deficits of one of the major nerves of the upper extremity require immediate referral to a consultant. Injuries to the digital nerves, however, can be handled somewhat differently. For uncomplicated severed nerves, delayed repair can have significant advantages over early repair.[20, 31] The repair setting and time are better controlled, the cut nerve ends and epineurium are better delineated, and early skin closure is an effective barrier against infection. The delayed repair is done through a sterile field and incision. In the emergency department, with consultative support, simple skin suturing is carried out, a dressing is placed, and the patient is referred to the specialist within 1 to 2 days. Nerve repair can be carried out on an elective basis within 2 weeks. When the injury is complicated by contamination, tissue devitalization, or associated injuries, early consultation is recommended.

Amputated Parts

Emergency physicians are often involved in the early management of patients with amputated parts. Although the injury is not within the realm of emergency wound-care personnel to manage, proper handling of the injured extremity and severed part is important, especially if there is a chance of reimplantation by a specialist.

The injured extremity is gently cleansed and wrapped in lightly saline-moistened gauze sponges followed by gauze wrapping. Rarely is a tourniquet needed to stop hemorrhage because natural vasospasm and platelet plugging of the severed vessels occurs rapidly after injury. It is common to administer a dose of intravenous first generation cephalosporins to the patient as prophylaxis.

The severed part is placed in a dry sterile sponge wrapping. Saline soaking causes unnecessary and unwanted edema and makes reimplantation much more difficult. The wrapped severed part is then placed in a small plastic wrap or bag. The bag and its contents can then be put in a container with ice to cool the tissue. Great care has to be taken to make sure that ice does not come into direct contact with the severed part so as not to cause necrosis from freezing. Once these steps have been taken, the patient can wait for the specialist or can be transported to an appropriate care facility.

Paronychia

The most common hand infection is a paronychia.[1] A paronychia is an infection of the eponychium and it is usually associated with a collection of pus between the eponychium and the nail root. The infection is most often localized to one side of the epony-chium, the lateral nail fold. However, it can include the eponychium in the midline or proceed in "horseshoe" fashion to involve the entire eponychium. Pus can also invade the space under the nail plate. The most common bacteria found in a paronychia are gram-positive cocci, either *Streptococcus pyogenes* or penicillin-resistant *Staphylococcus aureus.*[1, 6]

The simplest and most effective manner to drain a paronychia is to insert a #11 blade between the eponychium and the nail plate and gently sweep the blade to elevate the eponychium (Fig. 12-31). With deft technique in a calm patient, this procedure can be carried out with anesthesia. Otherwise, a digital block is performed before drainage. Following drainage, a simple Band-Aid dressing is applied. The patient is instructed to remove the Band-Aid and soak the finger in warm, soapy water twice a day. Band-Aids can be reapplied between soakings. Some authorities recommend placing drains under the eponychium. Uncomplicated paronychia in patients without risk factors such as diabetes do not need these measures. Antibiotics are often prescribed but are unnecessary if the pus is completely drained and there is no surrounding digital cellulitis. If there is, a first generation cephalosporin, or clindamycin (for allergic patients) can be prescribed for 7 days.

Occasionally, a paronychia extends below the nail plate between the nail and matrix. Pus can be seen through the semitranslucent nail. If pus is suspected to be in this space, partial or complete nail removal is recommended. Merely sweeping a #11 blade under the eponychium does not suffice. Fig. 12-32 demonstrates a method of partial nail removal to accomplish the drainage of both the paronychia and the pus under the nail plate. A paronychia that involves the entire eponychium and nail root area can be managed as illustrated in Fig. 12-33. An incision of the eponychium is made to free the nail root for removal. Occasionally, the entire nail must be removed to effect complete

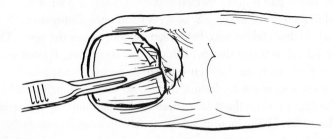

FIG. 12-31 Technique for draining simple paronychia. Note that the #11 blade is brought between the nail and the eponychium parallel to the nail plate. This simple maneuver drains the vast majority of paronychias.

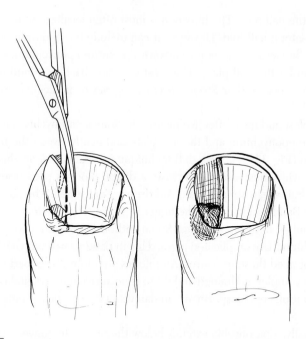

FIG. 12-32   When a paronychia extends below the nail and insinuates between the nail bed and nail plate, partial nail removal must take place. Once the nail removal is accomplished, a small packing or drain is left in place for 5 to 7 days.

drainage. Antibiotics are often recommended for complex paronychia. See the following discussion on antibiotics for hand wounds.

Felon

A felon is an infection with a collection of pus in the pulp space of the fingertip (Fig. 12-34). The finger pad is quite swollen and exceedingly tender. The most common bacteria found in these infections are *S. pyogenes* and penicillin-resistant *S. aureus*.[1, 6] Several methods to drain felons have been recommended over the years. The so-called fish mouth and lateral incisions that cut through the supporting fibrous septa of the finger pad are thought to increase the occurrence of unnecessary sequelae.[14]

The simplest technique to drain a felon is to make a longitudinal incision directly through the finger pad on the volar surface of the digit into the pulp space and pus collection (Fig. 12-35).[14] The incision is kept open with a small loose-fitting wick made of a nonadherent dressing material or a small sliver of rubber such as part of a Penrose drain or a rubber band. The drain is removed at follow-up at 48 hours, after which a soaking routine similar to the one used for paronychia is encouraged. These patients are then started on antibiotics. See the discussion on antibiotics for hand wounds later in this chapter.

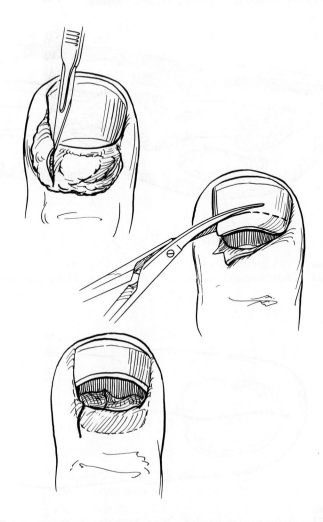

FIG. 12-33 A complex "horseshoe" paronychia usually needs to be drained both by incising the paronychia directly and removing either a portion or all of the nail. Note that a packing is left in place for 5 to 7 days to prevent adherence of the eponychium to the germinal matrix.

Pressure Injection Injuries

An injury to the hand that initially seems benign is caused by a high-pressure injection device such as a paint sprayer or grease gun. Through a pinhole, such a device can create a needle-thin stream that can have a pressure of up to 15,000 lbs/in.[2] A variety of paints, petroleums, and other chemicals can easily pierce the skin and, under the pressure created, spread throughout the hand along natural tissue planes and tendon sheaths. Grease and paint are the two most common substances.[22]

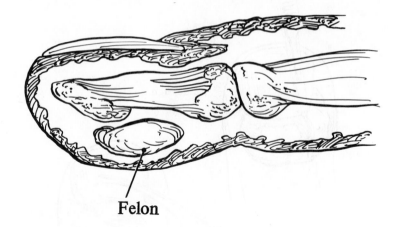

FIG. 12-34   Illustration and location of a felon in the pulp of the finger space.

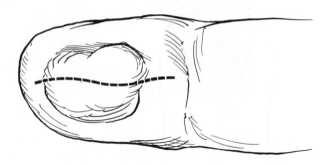

FIG. 12-35   Technique for draining a felon. Note that the incision is made directly over the area of maximal tenderness and fluctuance.

The entry wound is often no more than a small puncture. The most common site of entry is the tip of the index finger, a result of "testing" to see if the device works. Some of the injectable chemicals, such as the petroleums, do not cause an immediate reaction or pain. The patient often has minimal complaints. The combination of the small wound and relative lack of symptoms is deceptive. These injuries can progress over hours to marked pain, swelling, and inflammation of the entire hand. They require immediate consultation. Some authorities recommend fasciotomies of the hand before significant swelling develops to forestall ischemia created by an increase in tissue pressure from the intense reaction, to remove the chemical, and to debride necrotic tissue. The overall incidence of amputation has been reported to be 48%.[22]

ANTIBIOTICS FOR HAND WOUNDS

The use of antibiotics in patients with hand injuries is largely empirical because there are few definitive, well-designed studies examining their use. Several studies have shown that prophylactic antibiotics are of no value in uncomplicated lacerations of the hand.[11, 21, 29] In more complicated injuries such as avulsions of the fingertip, antibiotics are often prescribed, but again, there are no definitive studies to support this practice. In fact, some studies have found that antibiotics are of no value.[9, 15]

It is common to treat fingertip injuries with prophylactic antibiotics. However, in a large study of 299 patients treated without antibiotics for injuries ranging from simple lacerations to avulsions, only 2 infections developed.[33] Only when bone is exposed under severe crushing forces has one group found a decrease in the infection rate with the use of antibiotics.[25] It is not even clear in the face of a paronychia that antibiotics improve outcome. In spite of this controversy, some recommendations that rely more on traditional practice and clinical judgment can be made. Use antibiotics for:

- Wounds greater than 8 hours old
- Wounds caused by a crushing mechanism in which some tissue compromise is suspected
- Contaminated or soiled wounds in which extensive cleansing and debridement have been necessary
- Fingertip avulsions with exposed bone
- Open fractures
- Tendon or joint involvement
- Mammalian bites (see Chapter 14 for further discussion and special circumstances)
- Complex paronychia with pus under the nail
- Felons
- Immunocompromised patients or those who have diabetes

The choice of antibiotics for hand injuries also generates debate. A good first choice are the first generation cephalosporins that are effective against most of the common gram-positive and gram-negative organisms that are implicated in wound care. These antibiotics include cephalexin (Keflex), cephradine (Velosef), and cefadroxil (Duricef). For penicillin-allergic patients, clindamycin (Cleocin) is appropriate. For antibiotics to have any value, they must be administered as soon as possible in the emergency department, preferably within 3 to 4 hours from the time of injury.[7] For maximal effectiveness, the initial dose should be given intravenously. An intravenous first generation cephalosporin preparation that is recommended is cefazolin (Ancef) or Clindamycin can be used for penicillin-allergic patients. For prophylaxis, the duration of administration is no longer than 4 to 5 days.

DRESSINGS AND AFTERCARE

The basic finger dressing is described in Chapter 17. Xeroform is a popular nonadherent base, as is Adaptic. The latter is probably somewhat less adherent in wounds where there is more exudate and crusting. All fingertips are well padded with gauze sponges. A metal protective splint is recommended for patients who are going to return to work or resume manual activities.

Most hand wounds are best followed up within 48 hours with dressing removal for inspection. If a suture line becomes infected, suture removal and wound cleansing with thorough irrigation are carried out as soon as possible. Infections of the hand can be disastrous and often spread rapidly to important structures from a small nidus. Most sutures of the hand are removed in 8 to 10 days.

REFERENCES

1. Bell M: The changing pattern of pyogenic infections of the hand, *Hand* 8:298-302, 1976.
2. Blair WF, Steyers CM: Extensor tendon injuries, *Orthop Clin North Am* 23:141-149, 1992.
3. Chow S, Ho E: Open treatment of fingertip injuries in adults, *J Hand Surg* 7:470-476, 1982.
4. Custer J, Edlich RF, Prusak M, et al: Studies in the management of the contaminated wound, *Am J Surg* 121:572-575, 1971.
5. Douglas BS: Conservative management of guillotine amputation of the finger in children, *Aust Ped J* 8:86-89, 1972.
6. Eaton R, Butsch D: Antibiotic guidelines for hand infections, *Surg Gynecol Obstet* 130:119-121, 1970.
7. Edlich RF, Smith OT, Edgerton MT: Resistance of the surgical wound to antimicrobial prophylaxis and its mechanism of development, *Am J Surg* 126:583-586, 1973.
8. Farrell RG, Disher WA, Nesland RS, et al: Conservative management of fingertip amputations, *J Am Coll Emerg Phys* 6:243-246, 1977.
9. Fox JW, Golden GT, Rodeheaver G, et al: Nonoperative management of pulp amputation by occlusive dressings, *Am J Surg* 133:255-256, 1977.
10. Gellis M, Pool R: Two-point discrimination distances in the normal hand and forearm, *Plast Reconstr Surg* 59:57-63, 1977.
11. Grossman JAI, Adams JP, Kunec J: Prophylactic antibiotics in simple hand lacerations, *JAMA* 245:1055-1056, 1981.
12. Holm A, Zachariae L: Fingertip lesions: an evaluation of conservative treatment versus free skin grafting, *Acta Orthop Scand* 45:382-392, 1974.
13. Ipsen T, Frandsen PA, Barfred T: Conservative treatment of fingertip injuries, *Injury* 18:203-205, 1987.
14. Kilgore ES, Brown LG, Newmeyer WL, et al: Treatment of felons, *Am J Surg* 130:194-197, 1975.
15. Lamon RP, Cicero JJ, Frascone RJ, et al: Open treatment of fingertip amputations, *Ann Emerg Med* 12:358-360, 1983.
16. Lammers RL, et al: Effect of povidone-iodine and saline soaking on bacterial counts in acute, traumatic, contaminated wounds (abstract), *Ann Emerg Med* 19:709, 1990.
17. Louis D, Palmer A, Burney R: Open treatment of digital tip injuries, *JAMA* 244:697-698, 1980.
18. Margles S: Principles of management of acute hand injuries, *Surg Clin North Am* 60:665-685, 1980.
19. McGeorge DD, et al: Partial flexor tendon injuries: to repair or not (abstract), *J Hand Surg Br* 17B:176, 1992.
20. Millesi H: Reappraisal of nerve repair, *Surg Clin North Am* 61:321-340, 1981.
21. Roberts AHN, Teddy PJ: A prospective trial of prophylactic antibiotics in hand lacerations, *Br J Surg* 64:394-396, 1977.

22. Schoo MJ, Scott FA, Boswick JA: High-pressure injection injuries to the hand, *J Trauma* 20:229-238, 1980.

23. Seaberg DC, Angelos WJ, Paris PM: Treatment of subungual hematomas with nail trephination, *Am J Emerg Med* 9:209-210, 1991.

24. Simon RR, Wolgin M: Subungual hematoma: association with occult laceration repair, *Am J Emerg Med* 5:302-304, 1987.

25. Sloan JP, Dove AF, Maheson AN, et al: Antibiotics in open fractures of the distal phalanx, *J Hand Surg* 12B:123-124, 1987.

26. Steinberg DR: Acute flexor tendon injuries, *Orthop Clin North Am* 23:125-141, 1992.

27. Tanberg D: Glass in the hand and foot, *JAMA* 248:1872-1874, 1982.

28. Tottenham VM: Effects of delayed therapeutic intervention following zone II flexor tendon repair, *J Hand Ther* 8:23-26, 1995.

29. Worlock P, Boland P, Darrell J, et al: The role of prophylactic antibiotics following hand injuries, *Br J Clin Pract* 34:290-292, 1980.

30. Wray R, Weeks P: Treatment of partial tendon lacerations, *Hand* 12:163-166, 1980.

31. Wyrick JD, Stern PJ: Secondary nerve reconstruction, *Hand Clin* 8:587-597, 1992.

32. Young WA, Andrassy RJ: Conservative management of fingertip amputations in children, *Texas Medicine* 79:58-60, 1983.

33. Zook EG, Guy R, Russell RC: A study of nail bed injuries, *J Hand Surg* 9(A):247-252, 1984.

13 *Alternative Closures: Tape, Staples, and Adhesives*

Wound Taping
Wound Stapling
Wound Adhesives

Over the last decade, the use of alternative wound closure techniques, wound taping and stapling, has increased dramatically. Although the ease of application of tapes and the speed with which staples can be inserted has focused attention on these techniques, clinical experience and scientific studies have supported the validity of their use under specified conditions. Tapes are not only used for primary wound closure but are also an important support for lacerations after suture removal.

Once thought to be limited to surgical settings for the closure of cosmetically unimportant incisions, staples have been found to compare favorably with standard suture techniques for closure of a variety of traumatically induced wounds. In recent years, many studies of wound adhesives have been published providing a growing body of evidence that this wound closure method has excellent potential and is a viable technique. As of the date of this publication, however, wound adhesives have not been approved for use by the Food and Drug Administration (FDA) in the United States.

WOUND TAPING

When compared with suturing, there are several advantages to wound taping. These include a reduced need for anesthesia, ease of application, even distribution of tension across the wound, no residual suture marks, application by nonphysician personnel, and the elimination of need for suture removal.[16] They also have advantages in closing flap lacerations and have a greater resistance to wound infection than sutures.[2,4] On the other hand, tapes do not work well on surfaces that are oily or hair-bearing, joint surfaces, lax skin, gaping wounds under tension, or in very young or uncooperative children.

A bewildering variety of wound tapes are currently on the market. Steri-Strips by 3M are the best known but other brands include Shur-Strip, Cover-Strips, Suture-Strip,

Clearon, Nichi-Strip, and Curi-Strip. They have differing porosity, adhesion, flexibility, breaking strength, and elongation capability. An early study that compared Clearon and Steri-Strip demonstrated a better overall performance by Steri-Strip than the others.[9] In another comparison study of six tapes (Curi-Strip, Steri-Strip, Nichi-Strip, Cicagraf, Suture-Strip, and Suture-Strip Plus), an overall scoring method was devised to rank their performance under laboratory conditions.[12] The three highest ranking tapes were the Nichi-Strip, Curi-Strip, and Steri-Strip. Under experimental conditions, tape closures resisted wound infection better than nylon sutures. Tapes are also well suited for supporting grafts and flaps.

Indications for Taping

Wound taping can be considered under the following conditions:
- Superficial, straight lacerations under little tension. Areas suitable for taping include the forehead, chin, malar eminence, thorax, and nonjoint areas of the extremities.
- Flaps in which sutures might compromise vascular perfusion at the wound edges.
- Lacerations with a greater-than-usual potential for infection.
- Lacerations in the elderly or steroid-dependent patient who has thin, fragile skin.
- Support for lacerations after suture removal.

Tapes do not work well on irregular wounds, those that cannot be made free of blood or secretions, intertriginous areas, scalp, and joint surfaces.

Taping Technique

Most taping of emergency wounds can be done with ¼-inch wide tape of varying lengths. For wounds that are greater than 4 to 5 centimeters in length, ½-inch width is preferable.

The following steps are carried out:
- The wound is cleansed, irrigated, and debrided if necessary. Hemostasis has to be complete and the skin surface completely dried.
- Benzoin is applied to the surrounding skin to increase adhesion. Care is taken not to spill this agent into the wound. It is left to dry until it becomes tacky.
- Tapes are cut to the length desired while they are still on the backing sheet. Usually 2 to 3 cm of overlap is allowed for each side of the wound (Fig. 13-1).
- One of the perforated end tabs is gently removed to prevent deforming of the tape ends (Fig. 13-2).
- Individual tapes are removed from the backing with forceps by pulling directly away from the backing (Fig. 13-3).
- One half of the tape is securely placed on one side of the midportion of the wound and held securely. The opposite wound edge is apposed with a finger of the opposite hand (Fig. 13-4). After edge apposition, the tape is completely secured (Fig. 13-5).
- Further tapes are evenly placed adjacent to the original midwound tape (Fig. 13-6). Repeat this process with further tapes until the wound edges are completely

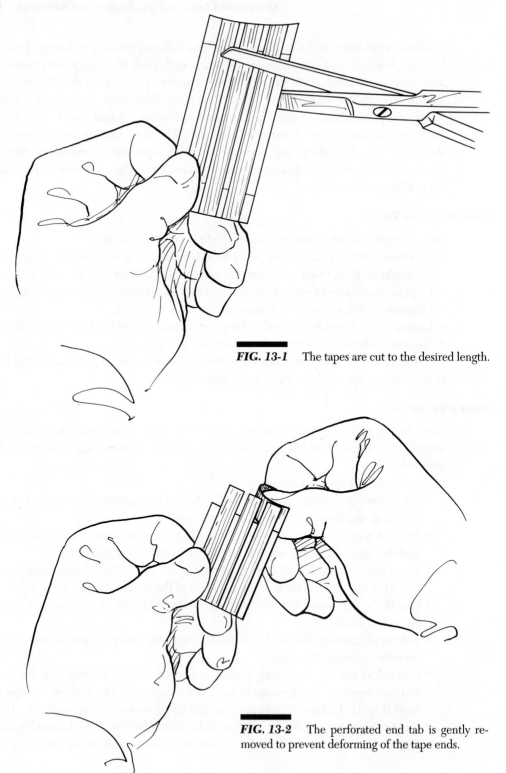

FIG. 13-1 The tapes are cut to the desired length.

FIG. 13-2 The perforated end tab is gently removed to prevent deforming of the tape ends.

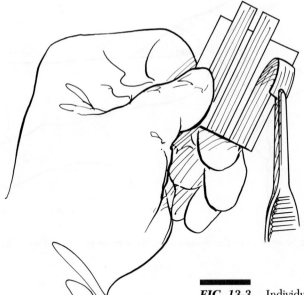

FIG. 13-3   Individual tapes are removed with forceps.

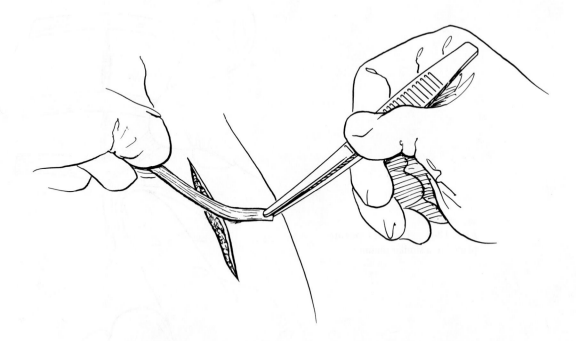

FIG. 13-4   The tape is firmly secured on one side of the wound.

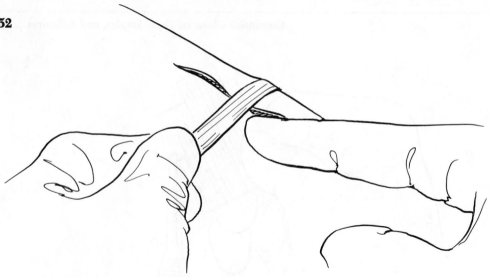

FIG. 13-5   The tape is brought over the wound after the wound is apposed with the finger of the opposite hand.

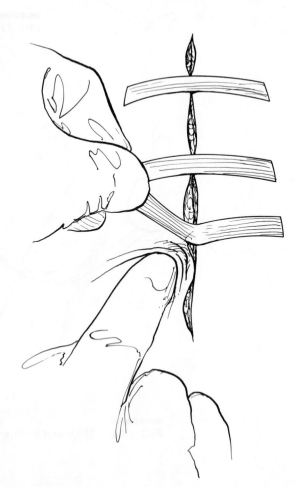

FIG. 13-6   Further tapes are placed in a similar manner.

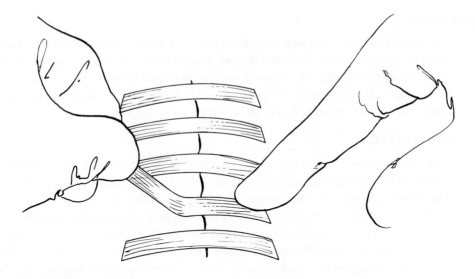

FIG. 13-7 Enough tapes are placed so that wound gapping does not occur. Usually there are 2 to 3 mm between tapes.

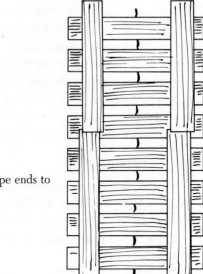

FIG. 13-8 Cross stays are placed over the tape ends to prevent skin blistering and premature removal.

apposed (Fig. 13-7). Wound tapes should have a gap between them that is at least 2 to 3 mm wide. Complete occlusion of the wound by tapes can cause normal wound seepage to dissect under the tapes and lead to premature removal.
- The final step is to place cross stays to prevent elevation of the tape ends and minor skin blistering caused by tension of the tape ends (Fig. 13-8).

Tape Aftercare

Tapes are maintained in place for at least as long as sutures would be for the anatomic area in question. Unlike a sutured wound, a taped wound cannot be washed or moistened because premature tape removal can lead to wound dehiscence.

Note: Tapes should never be wrapped around a digit in a circumferential manner because they are not expandable and can act as a constricting band.

WOUND STAPLING

Since the introduction of automatic skin-stapling devices, there has been a reluctance to use them beyond their intended purpose of closing surgically-made incisions. In spite of the remarkable amount of time saved by placing staples instead of sutures, early animal and clinical investigations questioned whether staples could accurately appose wound edges or promote wound tensile strength as effectively as sutures.[7] Studies in animals, however, have suggested that wound tensile strength is actually greater for staples when compared to sutures.[13, 18] Additionally, less wound inflammatory response has been noted with staples, and they resist infection more effectively than sutures.

Clinical studies of staple use in traumatic lacerations demonstrate that, when compared to standard suturing methods, the ultimate cosmetic result as judged by blinded observers is no different.[3, 6] In these studies, body regions that were chosen for the comparisons included the scalp, neck, arm/forearm, trunk, buttocks, and legs. Both adult and pediatric groups were studied. The time required for staple closure was approximately four to five times less than that required for suture placement. Cost has been cited as a drawback to the use of staples; however, the time saved by a busy physician and the reduced need for wound closure instruments balances that factor.[8] Patients appear to tolerate staples well while they are in place; however, there does appear to be increased discomfort on removal when compared to sutures.[13]

Indications for Stapling

Wound stapling can be recommended under the following circumstances:

• Linear, sharp (shearing mechanism) lacerations of the scalp, trunk, and extremities. Although they have been used in hand lacerations, experience is not extensive enough to confidently recommend them for that area. Stapling is similarly avoided for facial wounds.

• Temporary, rapid closure of extensive superficial lacerations in patients requiring immediate surgery for life-threatening trauma.

Staples are avoided in anatomic areas to be studied by computed tomography (CT) scan or magnetic resonance imaging (MRI). They can produce streak artifact on a CT scan, but in critical circumstances, clinically useful scans can be obtained in spite of their presence. Staples can move with MRI and should not be placed if that study is anticipated.

Stapling Technique

Stapling devices have evolved significantly in the last several years, and a number of products are available. The Reflex One is representive of a multiple-staple device (35 staples per cartridge) with a wide staple that closes into a rectangular configuration (Fig. 13-9). This stapler is commonly used for surgical incisions or long lacerations of the trunk or extremity. The Precise Ten Shot stapler holds 10 staples that close into a smaller arcuate configuration. This device is useful for shorter, traumatically induced lacerations that might require greater precision and control. In addition to the stapler, the equipment required includes basic wound-care instruments and standard anesthetic agents.

The following steps are followed to insert staples:

- Forceps are used to evert the wound edges before placement of each staple (Fig. 13-10). When possible, a second operator can be very helpful in everting the edges while the primary operator uses the stapler.
- Before triggering, the stapler should be placed gently on the skin over the wound without indenting the skin (Fig. 13-11).

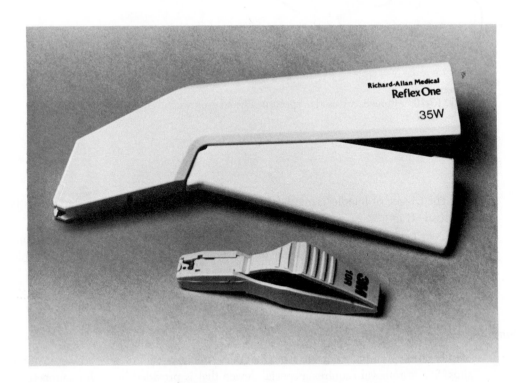

FIG. 13-9   Examples of wound stapling devices.

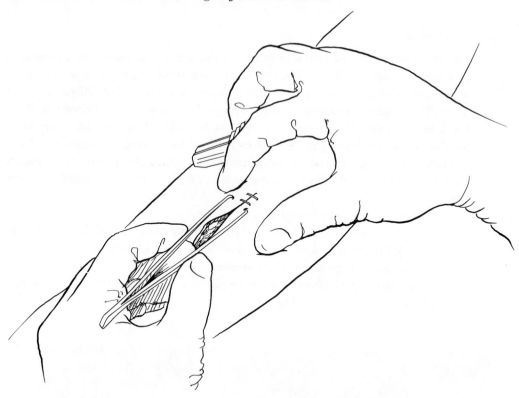

FIG. 13-10   Forceps are used to approximate and evert wound edges during stapling.

- The trigger, or handle, is gently and evenly squeezed to advance the staple into the tissue (Fig. 13-12).
- Once placed, a space should be visible between the staple and skin. A common mistake in placing staples is to apply excessive downward pressure causing the staples to seat deep in the wound.
- Because of the configuration of the bending mechanism of the stapler, once the staple is seated, the stapler has to be "backed out" of the staple loop to disengage it.

Staple Aftercare

Staples are kept in place for the same length of time as are sutures in similar anatomic sites. Staple removal requires a special device that is provided by each manufacturer. The lower jaw is placed under the crossbar of the staple and the upper jaw is closed to open the loop of the staple as seen in Fig. 13-13.

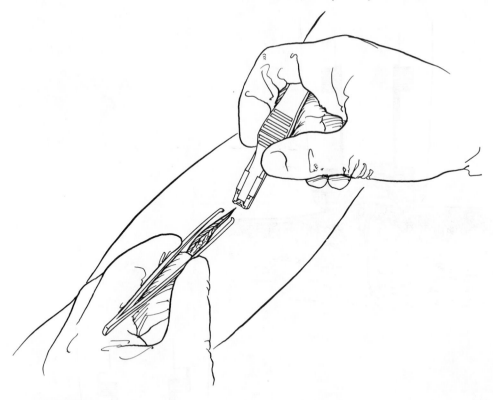

FIG. 13-11 During stapling the stapler is placed gently on the skin before triggering. Indenting the skin with too much pressure causes staples to be placed too deep.

WOUND ADHESIVES

Currently, there is one practical tissue adhesive for emergency wound care, N-butyl-2-cyanoacrylate.[5, 19] Others are under investigation or development. The cyanoacrylate adhesives have been approved for use in Canada, Great Britain, Israel, and other countries, but, as of this publication, have not been approved for use by the Food and Drug Administration of the United States.[19] Another tissue adhesive option, fibrin glue, is in use for skin grafting and bonding of tissue flaps.[5] Fibrin glue has several technical drawbacks, including expense, which make it impractical for emergency wound-care use.

The most attractive features of wound adhesives are short wound closure time and no requirement for anesthesia. Wound closure time is approximately 20% to 50% of the time necessary for standard suturing.[11, 17, 19] Adhesives polymerize 1 second after application, and the wound needs manual support for only 30 to 60 seconds after application of the final spot or line weld. Wounds closed with adhesives are at greater risk for breaking

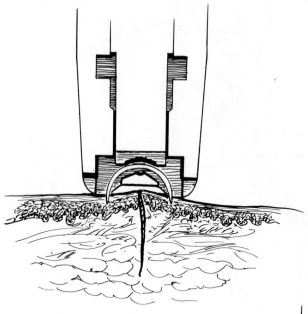

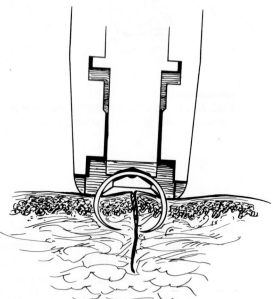

FIG. 13-12 During triggering the staple is reconfigured to approximate wound edges.

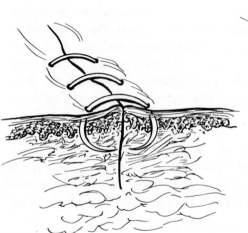

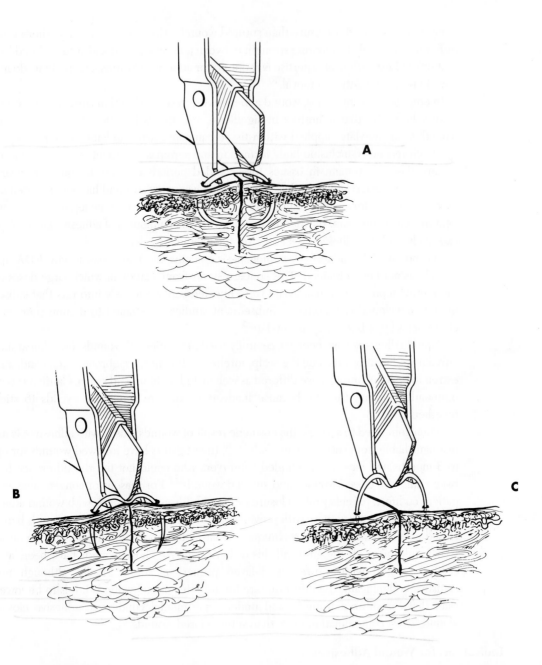

FIG. 13-13   The following procedure is used to remove staples. **A,** The lower jaws of the staple removing device are positioned under the staple cross-bar. **B,** The upper jaw is used to gently compress the staple. **C,** Once complete compression has taken place, the staple has been reconfigured for easy and gentle withdrawal.

open immediately after closure than sutured wounds. However, after 7 days there is no difference in tensile or bursting strength between adhesive closed and suture closed lacerations.[10] Less technical expertise is required for adhesive closures, and patients do not have to return for suture removal.[10]

In emergency wound care, wound adhesives are restricted to skin surfaces, and there is very little risk that adhesives in significant amounts will penetrate deep into the wound. Cyanoacrylates applied within tissue can cause acute inflammatory responses, giant cell reactions, inclusion body formation and seromas.[15] Subcutaneously or within organs, they can remain in tissues for extended periods of time, beyond one year.[5] N-butyl-2-cyanoacrylate is the least toxic of the cyanoacrylates and has accumulated an excellent record for use in wound care.[14] In large amounts, they generate exothermic heat that can cause pain. In wound care, only very small amounts of adhesive are applied externally, and the adhesives peel off after the wound is healed.

The potential for adhesive carcinogenesis remains the main reason why FDA approval has not been obtained. This concern stems from a study in which large doses of the methyl monomer cyanoacrylate were injected subcutaneously into rats that subsequently developed carcinomas.[15] Subsequent studies have failed to demonstrate carcinogenesis by N-butyl-2-cyanoacrylate.[5]

Wound adhesives have been successfully used in a variety of wounds, both linear and curvilinear. Locations include the scalp, forehead, chin, nose, eyebrows, ears, hand, and extremities. Mechanisms have differed as well including blunt and sharp. Caution is recommended around the eye because inadvertent spillage can cause eyelids to stick together.

When compared to sutures, the cosmetic result of wounds closed with adhesives is indistinguishable from sutured wounds.[1, 11, 19] Investigators have followed wounds for up to 3 months and have used "blinded" observers who could not tell the difference between adhesive closed wounds and sutured wounds.[11] For reasons of convenience and patient comfort, parents prefer closure of their children's lacerations with wound adhesives when asked to compare with previous experiences of their children's wounds being closed with standard suturing techniques. It has been reported, however, that an occasional child picks off the glue with his or her fingers.[17] These wounds have been successfully closed with sutures as delayed primary closures. Finally, although not statistically significant, the infection rate for adhesive closed wounds tends to be lower than that for sutured wounds, and under experimental conditions, adhesive closed wounds resist contamination more than suture closed wounds.[10]

Indications for Wound Adhesives

Wound adhesives can be recommended for the following circumstances:
- Linear and curvilinear lacerations under little tension (< 0.5 cm wide) where no deep sutures are required.
- Lacerations with "tidy" or sharp wound edges before or after debridement.

- Lacerations 5 cm or less. Tissue bulk and shear forces of long lacerations can disrupt adhesive closure.

  Adhesives are not effective for lacerations over joints, with excessive bleeding, or with high static tension as evidenced by edge gaping. Caution is used for lacerations near the eye. Hair-bearing areas are not a contraindication for adhesive closure.

Adhesive Wound Closure Technique

Histoacryl Blue is a combination of an adhesive and blue dye that facilitates its use. It is supplied in 0.5 ml plastic containers for single use. However, it can be configured for multiple patient use by cutting off the plastic applicator tip and attaching a 25-gauge needle.[5] This needle allows for very fine control and can be discarded after use. Each vial costs approximately $28 to $30, but contains sufficient adhesive to close approximately 8 lacerations of 2 cm in length. Guidelines and restrictions for handling of adhesives in the United States have yet to be developed by the FDA.

- After wound cleansing and any necessary debridement, any significant bleeding should be controlled. However, the wound does not have to be strictly dry because polymerization occurs in the presence of a liquid, either water or blood.
- The adhesive material can be applied with three different techniques: spot weld, line weld (like a wound tape), or contiguous with the wound (Fig. 13-14). The applicator

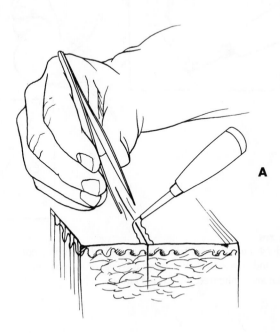

FIG. 13-14   Wound adhesive application techniques. **A,** As the wound is adhered, the edges are apposed with forceps or glove fingers.   *Continued*

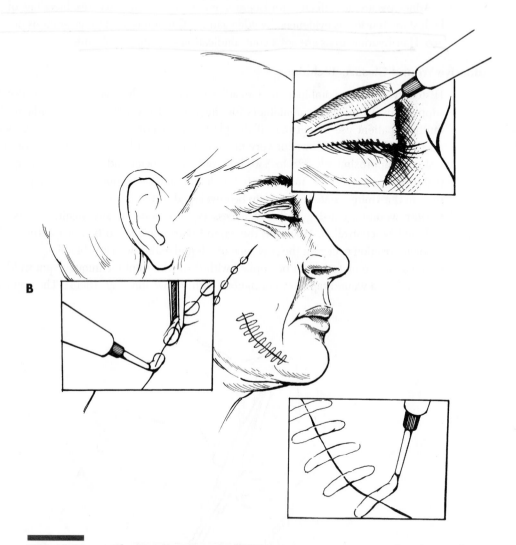

FIG. 13-14, cont'd   **B,** Adhesive can be laid down in a continuous stripe directly over the apposed wound edges, as shown above the eye; or as spot welds, as shown below the eye; or as line welds that are configured like wound tapes.

or needle is held with the bevel facing down or parallel to the wound. Great care is taken to squeeze out just enough adhesive to form the spot weld, line weld, or continuous application.

- During welding, the wound has to be held together with either forceps or fingers. Because polymerization occurs rapidly, in 1 or 2 seconds, fingers or forceps are held in place for 5 seconds after each spot or line, to ensure hardening, before moving to the next one. After the adhesive application is complete, the wound is supported for 30 to 60 seconds to guarantee full polymerization.
- Droplets or lines of adhesive are spaced approximately 0.5 cm apart. Close spacing is necessary to provide for closure security. Because adhesives are not initially as strong as sutures, closure strength is increased by increasing the number of spot or line welds.

Adhesive Closure Aftercare

The patient is instructed to keep the wound clean and dry for 24 hours. After this period, gentle cleansing can be carried out with great care and caution so as not to disrupt the closure. Band-Aids or other dressing can be applied as needed on areas other than the face. Should a wound dehisce, the patient is instructed to return so that delayed primary closure with wound tapes or sutures can be carried out. No follow-up is necessary for glue removal because it will peel off on its own or come off with the natural sloughing of keratinized epidermis.

REFERENCES

1. Bruns TB, McLario DJ, Simon HK, et al: Laceration repair using a tissue adhesive in a children's emergency department, *Acad Emerg Med* 2:427, 1995 (abstract).
2. Conolly BW, et al: Clinical comparison of surgical wounds closed by suture and adhesive tapes, *Am J Surg* 117:318-322, 1969.
3. Dunmire SM, et al: Staples versus sutures for wound closure in the pediatric population, *Ann Emerg Med* 18:448, 1989 (abstract).
4. Efron G, Ger R: Use of surgical adhesive tape (Steri-Strip) to secure skin graft on digits, *Am J Surg* 116:474, 1968.
5. Ellis DAF, Shaikh A: The ideal tissue adhesive in facial plastic and reconstructive surgery, *J Otolaryngology* 19:68-72, 1990.
6. George TK, Simpson DC: Skin wound closure with staples in the accident and emergency department, *J R Coll Surg Edinb* 30:54-56, 1985.
7. Harrison ID, Williams DF, Cuschieri A: The effect of metal clips on the tensile properties of healing skin wounds, *Br J Surg* 62:945-949, 1975.
8. Harvey CF, Hume Logan CJ: A prospective trial of skin staples and sutures in skin closure, *Ir J Med Surg* 155:194-196, 1986.
9. Koehn GG: A comparison of the duration of adhesion of Steri-Strips and Clearon, *Cutis* 26:620-621, 1980.
10. Noordzij JP, Foresman PA, Rodeheaver GT, et al: Tissue adhesive wound repair revisited, *J Emerg Med* 12:645-649, 1994.

11. Quinn JV, Drzewiecki A, Li MM, et al: A randomized, controlled trial comparing a tissue adhesive with suturing in the repair of pediatric facial lacerations, *Ann Emerg Med* 22:1130-1135, 1993.

12. Rodeheaver GT, Spengler MD, Edlich RF: Performance of new wound closure tapes, *J Emerg Med* 5:451-462, 1987.

13. Roth JH, Windle BH: Staple versus suture closure of skin incisions in a pig model, *Can J Surg* 31:19, 1988.

14. Toriumi DM, O'Grady K: Surgical tissue adhesives in otolaryngology-head and neck surgery, *Otolaryngol Clinics North Am* 27:203-209, 1994.

15. Toriumi DM, Raslan WF, Friedman M, Tardy ME: Histotoxicity of cyanoacrylate tissue adhesives, *Arch Otolaryngol Head Neck Surg* 116:546-550, 1990.

16. Trott AT: Alternative methods of wound closure: wound staples. In Roberts JR, Hedges JR, editors: *Clinical procedures in emergency medicine,* Philadelphia, 1985, Saunders.

17. Watson DP: Use of cyanoacrylate tissue adhesive for closing facial lacerations in children, *BMJ* 299:1014, 1989.

18. Windle BH, Roth JH: Comparison of staple-closed and sutured skin incisions in a pig model, *Surg Forum* 35:546-550, 1984.

19. Yaron M, Halperin M, Huffer W, Cairns C: Efficacy of tissue glue for laceration repair in an animal model, *Acad Emerg Med* 2:259-263, 1995.

14 *Bite Wounds*

Animal and human bites are common wounds managed by emergency caregivers. Bites can be from a multitude of sources, but the majority are caused by dogs, cats, and humans.[28, 32] In spite of apparently similar mechanisms of injury, each type of bite has different clinical, microbiologic, and treatment considerations that affect the management of bite-wound patients. With animal bites, there is also the possibility of secondary systemic infectious complications, the most important of which is rabies. It is the responsibility of any person caring for an animal bite victim to thoroughly investigate the biting circumstances and make an appropriate decision about whether or not to administer rabies prophylaxis.

ANIMAL BITE EPIDEMIOLOGY

It is estimated that 500,000 to 2 million animal bites occur in the United States each year, most of which are unreported.[28, 32] Dog bites predominate, accounting for approximately 80% of all animal bites.[48] Of reported bites, 5% to 15% are caused by cats.[48] The occurrence of human bites varies according to the reporting institution with a range of 3.6% to 23%.[19, 28, 39] Urban emergency departments treat a greater proportion of those victims than community ones.[28] Other animals such as rodents, monkeys, large mammals, and marine animals account for a small number of bite wounds.

Bite injuries are more likely to occur in children, with a peak incidence between the ages of 5 and 14 years old.[38] Dog bites are more common in males; cat bites and scratches are seen more often in females.[32, 38] Fortunately, most of the attacking animals are known to the victim and can be easily traced. Wild or possibly untraceable animals are involved in about 3% to 15% of bite incidents.[1, 32] The ability to find, investigate, and quarantine the animal makes the decision to administer rabies prophylaxis to a patient much easier.

MICROBIOLOGY OF BITE WOUNDS

The microbiology of bite wounds can be bewildering. Microorganisms belonging to 30 different genera have been cultured from a dog's mouth.[2] A large variety of microorganisms can be cultured from a normal cat mouth as well.[25] Clinical studies have shown, however, that there is little correlation between these potentially contaminating organisms and the ones that actually cause a wound infection.[8, 9, 24] Attempts to use a Gram stain to correctly predict the presence of infecting pathogens are thwarted by the multiplicity of morphologically similar organisms that can be present merely as contaminants.[1, 24]

Identification of organisms cultured from actual bite wound infections provides more useful information and predictive value with regard to prophylactic antibiotic choices than cultures of noninfected wounds. The number of species of bacteria that is implicated in true infections, although extensive, is much smaller than the total number of species that can be identified in an animal's mouth.[22] The majority of infected bite wounds are polymicrobial with an average of 3 to 4 bacterial species, including anaerobic, recovered from any given dog or cat bite.[22] Up to 5 different bacterial species can be isolated from infected human bite wounds.[19]

For dogs and cats, the clinically relevant infecting bacteria are *Pasteurella* species (*P. multocida ss multocida, P. multocida ss septica, P. canis,* and *P. dagmatis*), *Streptococcus* species (alpha, beta, gamma, hemolytic), *Staphylococcus* species (aureus, intermedius), *Moraxella* sp., and *Enterococcus* sp.[28] A rare but potentially fatal dog bite infection is caused by *Capnocytophaga canimorsus* (CDC group DF-2).[22] It is a gram-negative rod that has been isolated from both dogs and cats although infection from cats is rare. Patients susceptible to this infection often have predisposing factors such as asplenia, immunosuppression, or chronic disabling diseases.

The microbiology of human bites differs from cat and dog bites and is more complex. Aerobic organisms recovered from human bite infections include *Streptococcus* species (alpha, beta, hemolytic), *Staphylococcus* species (aureus, epidermidis) and *Corynebacterium* species. *Eikenella corrodens* has been recovered from up to 29% of human bites including 25% of all clenched fist injuries.[3, 23, 41] *E. corrodens* is a particularly virulent organism that can result in serious, chronic, and indolent infections. Human bite infections in hospitalized or institutionalized patients are often caused by gram-negative organisms such as *Escherichia coli, Proteus* species, and *Pseudomonas* species.

All mammalian bites, but in particular human bites, are at risk for anaerobic infection. Anaerobic organisms are usually isolated in conjunction with other organisms previously described. Species include *Fusobacterium, Bacteroides, Porphyromonas, Prevotella,* and *Peptostreptococcus.* Anaerobic species recovered in dog and cat bite infections commonly produce beta lactamase.

Infectious complications of human bites can also derive from viruses and other organisms.[28] Viruses transmitted through human bite include hepatitis B and C and herpesvirus types 1 and 2. *Mycobacterium tuberculosis* and *Treponema pallidum* have been reported to be transmitted through human bite. To date, while it is biologically possible, no case of human immunodeficiency virus (HIV) infection has been reported from transmittal through a human bite.[28]

BITE RISK FACTORS

An excellent review by Callaham lists the important risk factors that are predictive of bite wound complications.[9] These factors can influence the choice of wound management strategies, such as the decision to close the wound with sutures or to use prophylactic antibiotics.[9, 37] Recommendations for specific biting species are made in subsequent sections; however, all bites should be considered in the context of the Callahan risk factors (see Box 14-1).

Location

Approximately 75% of animal bites occur on the extremities.[8, 32] In children, however, especially those who are under 9 years old, the predominant injury area is the face and head.[8] When examining children, the risk of skull penetration has to be considered. The location of the bite is important because there is a significant difference in the rate of infection per site. The hand appears to be at highest risk, with an incidence of infection in dog bites reported in one study to be as high as 30%.[9] The most resistant anatomic location is the face, which has an infection rate of 1.4% to 5.8%.[8, 30]

All human bites to the hand are considered serious injuries. Approximately 3.6% of all bite injuries are caused by humans with 61.2% of those being inflicted on the hand and upper extremity.[39] The hand is a complex anatomic structure with a high density of movable structures enclosed in limited tunnels and spaces. The hand does not tolerate infection well and can easily be devastated by even trivial injuries that introduce small inocula of bacteria.[33, 42] When the hand comes into contact with the human mouth in a violent manner, it is exposed to a tremendous variety of pathogenic bacteria in high concentrations.[35]

Type of Wound

The mechanism of injury from an animal bite or attack plays an important role in predicting the chance of infection and therefore the choice of management technique. All animal bites are to be considered contaminated with potentially pathogenic bacteria. These injuries are frequently associated with crushing, tearing, and avulsion forces, and devitalized tissue. The combination of bacterial contamination with accompanying devitalized skin and fascia creates a setting ripe for the establishment of infection.

At high risk for becoming infected is the puncture wound caused by fangs.[1, 8, 51] Slender cat fangs are particularly treacherous because they can be driven deep into tissue and deliver an infectious inoculum of bacteria through the small entry site. These wounds are difficult to adequately cleanse, irrigate, and debride and are considered at greater risk for infection. Large open wounds are less likely to develop this complication. Superficial, laceration-like wounds, without devitalized tissue, carry a low rate of infection regardless of the species.

Most bites are occlusional. The hand, however, is subject to another type of bite wound, the clenched-fist injury. A fist struck against the mouth can drive teeth into the lightly padded knuckles. Tendons and their sheaths, as well as underlying joints, are particularly vulnerable. Suppurative complications are common and violation to either tendon, bone, or joint has been reported in up to 75% of cases.[35] These injuries require aggressive intervention with exploration, irrigation, debridement, and early parenteral antibiotic administration. The care is best carried out in consultation with a specialist.

Patient Risk Factors

Any of the patient conditions listed in Box 14-1 require serious consideration for antibiotic prophylaxis in spite of little investigational support for their use.[37]

Biting Species

The overall infection rate of dog and cat bites varies considerably. Between 4% and 10% of dog bites become infected.[8, 32, 38] Sutured dog bites of the face, on the other hand, have been reported to become infected in only 1.4% of cases.[30] Up to 17% to 50% of cat bites become infected.[13, 32, 38] Cat scratches have also been thought to carry an increased rate of infection, but a recent investigation of 14 claw injuries reported no infections.[13]

Because of the preantibiotic era necessity of performing frequent amputations or resultant severe disability, human bites retain a bad reputation among clinicians.[33] In fact, simple occlusional bites, not on the hand, have an infection rate not much higher than common lacerations and dog bites.[22, 34] The overall incidence of infections has been reported to be approximately 17% with a range from 10% to 50%.[1, 9, 34, 45] One investigator reported the incidence of infection following human bites to the face to be 2.5%.[16] Original investigations appeared to have been biased by how much time had elapsed before treatment was administered.[19, 35] This factor would skew the findings toward a higher infection rate. The face and ear, probably because they have a rich vascularity, have a higher innate resistance to infection and tend to become infected less often.[6, 50]

GENERAL BITE WOUND MANAGEMENT

Wound management depends on the type of wound, its severity, and its anatomic location. Simple contusions and superficial bite abrasions, in which no obvious skin puncture, laceration, or avulsion is present, can be treated by thorough cleansing alone. In

BOX 14-1

Animal Bite Risk Factors

HIGH RISK

Location

    Hand, wrist, or foot

    Scalp or face in infants (high risk of cranial
       perforation; skull x-ray examination
       mandatory)

    Over a major joint (possibility of perforation)

    Through-and-through bite of cheek

Type of wound

    Punctures (impossible to irrigate)

    Tissue crushing that cannot be debrided
       (typical of herbivores such as cows and
       horses)

    Carnivore bite over vital structure (artery,
       nerve, joint)

Patient

    Older than 50 years

    Asplenic

    Chronic alcoholic

    Altered immune status (chemotherapy,
       AIDS, immune defect)

    Diabetic

    Peripheral vascular insufficiency

    Chronic corticosteriod therapy

    Prosthetic or diseased cardiac valve
       (consider systemic prophylaxis)

    Prosthetic or seriously diseased joint
       (consider systemic prophylaxis)

Species

    Domestic cat

    Large cat (canine teeth produce deep
       punctures that can penetrate joints,
       cranium)

    Human (hand wounds only, particularly with
       delayed medical care)

    Primates (anecdotal evidence only)

    Pigs (anecdotal evidence only)

LOW RISK

Location

    Face, scalp, ears, and mouth (all facial
       wounds should be sutured)

    Self-bite of buccal mucosa that does not go
       through to skin

Type of wound

    Large clean lacerations that can be
       thoroughly cleansed (the larger the
       laceration, the lower the infection rate)

    Partial-thickness lacerations and abrasions

Species

    Rodents

From Callaham ML, French SP: Bites and injuries inflicted by mammals. In Auerbach P, editor: *Wilderness medicine: management of wilderness and environmental emergencies,* ed 3, St Louis, 1995, Mosby.

spite of the relatively minor appearance of many of these wounds, the patient still is at risk for developing rabies and this possibility has to be addressed.

    For larger wounds that violate the epidermis and dermis, standard wound-care techniques are carried out.

- Povidone-iodine is the wound-cleansing solution that is recommended for periphery cleansing. The standard 10% solution is diluted 10:1 to 20:1 with saline and can serve as both the cleansing agent and irrigant.
- After thorough scrubbing of the wound periphery, copious high-pressure irrigation is the next step, using a 19-gauge needle, catheter, or splash shield attached to a 20- or

35-ml syringe. Delivering diluted povidone-iodine solution directly into the wound enhances its microbicidal action.

- Debridement of all devitalized tissue and wound edges is essential for reducing the possibility of wound infection. Irrigation after debridement is recommended because it provides greater exposure of the wound. Studies, both retrospective and prospective, have demonstrated that wound infection is reduced significantly after debridement.[8, 9, 54]
- For fang wounds, particularly slender cat teeth wounds, there is often minimal devitalization of the skin. Therefore edge debridement might not be necessary. However, the problem of adequate wound cleansing remains. To facilitate effective irrigation, after local infiltration anesthesia, the entry site can be widened with a simple 1 to 1.5 cm incision across the puncture with a #15 knife blade as shown in Fig. 14-1. The new wound is then retracted open with a hemostat or forceps to permit irrigation. These incisions, are left to close without sutures. If the edges are devitalized, they should be trimmed back to viable skin.
- Culture purulence or suspected infection.
- Obtain radiographs when fracture or joint penetration is suspected.
- Ensure proper tetanus immunization.
- Assess and treat for rabies exposure if necessary.

SPECIFIC INJURIES
Dog Bites
Suturing

The issue of whether or not to suture dog bite wounds is controversial. Investigational data and the author's personal experience support the practice of primary suture closure of low-risk dog bite wounds.[8, 9, 14, 30, 49] Suturing, however, is not recommended for wounds greater than 8 to 12 hours old, fang (puncture) wounds, hand lacerations, or those that are high risk as noted in Box 14-1.[22] When closure contraindications exist, delayed primary closure (tertiary union) or open closure (secondary union) can be considered. Because of the cosmetic concerns associated with facial bites, and a low potential for infection, suturing, even after 8 to 12 hours, can be considered.[30] Consultation with a specialist is recommended to assist in the decision. Whenever primary closure of any dog bite is carried out, deep closures are avoided to minimize the potential for infection.[22]

Antibiotics

The use of antibiotics for dog bite wounds is one of the most controversial topics in emergency medicine.[7] This controversy is fueled by the lack of large, definitive, controlled clinical trials without methodological errors. One fact is clear: antibiotics are still no substitute for careful and thorough wound cleansing, irrigation, and debridement. The choice of agents is also complicated by the myriad of potentially infecting organ-

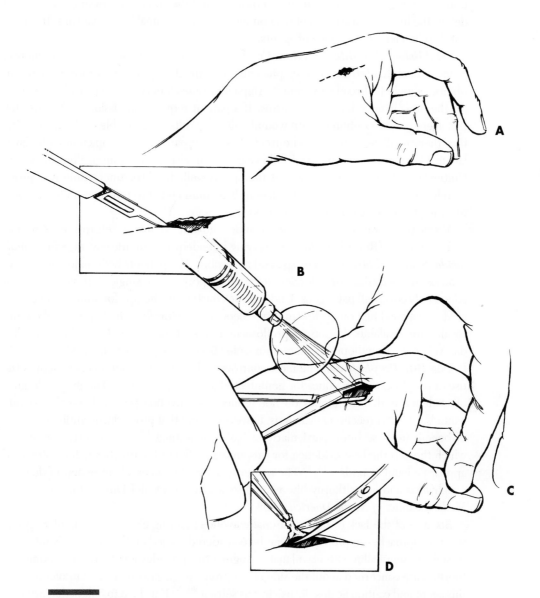

FIG. 14-1   Fang wound management. **A,** A fang wound with a suggested line of incision to open the wound for effective irrigation and debridement. **B,** A small 1 to 1.5 cm incision can be made with a scalpel and #15 blade. **C,** Once incised, the wound can be exposed with forceps and copiously irrigated. **D,** The incision also facilitates wound edge debridement if devitalization or excessive contamination is present.

isms, conflicting results from in vivo clinical studies versus in vitro sensitivity studies, the difference between serum antibiotic levels versus tissue levels, etc. The recommendations following are based on current knowledge and the author's experience. Table 14-1 details the in vitro sensitivities of the common infecting animal bite organisms. It can assist the clinician in the choice of agents.

Established Dog Bite Infection. For wounds with signs of infection (i.e., purulence, redness, heat, tenderness, and lymphangitis) the initial empiric dose of intravenous antibiotics should be broad spectrum.[22] Ampicillin/sulbactam (Unasyn) provides coverage for the most likely infecting organisms. If a patient requires admission to the hospital, this agent can be continued until wound culture results are available to determine further therapy. If the patient can be treated as an outpatient, oral ampicillin with clavulanate (Augmentin) can be used following the initial parenteral ampicillin/sulbactam. Culture results can guide outpatient therapy as well. Total treatment time is approximately 10 to 14 days; however, the patient is recommended to return in 48 to 72 hours for assessment of treatment effectiveness.

Alternative intravenous antibiotics include cefoxitin (Mefoxin), cefuroxime (Zinacef), and ceftriaxone (Rocephin). All have varying but adequate empiric coverage for *P. multocida*, *S. aureus*, *Streptococcus* sp., and anaerobes. For patients with major allergic responses to penicillin or allergies to cephalosporins, no single intravenous agent adequately covers all pathogens. Under these constraints, therapy for adults can be initiated with a combination of clindamycin (Cleocin) and ciprofloxacin (Cipro) until culture results are available. Because ciprofloxacin is not recommended for children, clindamycin plus trimethoprim/sulfamethoxazole (Bactrim, Septra) can be used.

Dog Bite Prophylaxis. The most controversial area of dog bite management is the use of prophylactic antibiotics for noninfected appearing wounds.[7] The preponderance of evidence is that antibiotics do not reduce the infection rate in low-risk dog bite wounds.[8, 15, 46] A recent metaanalysis, however, found that prophylactic antibiotics were of benefit in these bites, particularly in high-risk settings.[12] The high-risk setting for which there is the best evidence for prophylactic effect of antibiotics is for uninfected appearing hand wounds.[8, 14, 18] The reader is referred to an excellent review of dog bite prophylaxis and other thorny bite wound issues by Dr. Daniel Dire in the *Emergency Medical Clinics of North America*, 1992.[14]

Because of the lack of investigational evidence pointing clearly to particular agents, several approaches to prophylaxis can be considered. Based on the potentially infecting organisms, ampicillin with clavulanate (Augmentin) provides good coverage. Some authorities are concerned about the side effect profile (e.g., gastrointestinal intolerance) of this agent and caution against its use in this setting.[26, 27] For the 3 to 5 days that are necessary for prophylaxis, this antibiotic should be well tolerated.

The second approach is based on studies and clinical experience with several inexpensive, low side effect antibiotics that appear to have a prophylactic effect in spite of a limited bite organism sensitivity profile.[14, 46, 54] These include ampicillin, penicillin,

Table 14-1 *Antimicrobial Susceptibilities of Bacteria Frequently Isolated from Animal-Bite Wounds*

Agent	S. aureus	E. corrodens	Percentages of Isolates Susceptible			
			Anaerobes	P. multocida	C. canimorsus	S. intermedius
Penicillin	10	99	50/95*	95	95	70
Dicloxacillin	99	5	50	30	NS	100
Amoxicillin/clavulanic acid	100	100	100	100	95	100
Cephalexin	100	20	40	30	NS	95
Cefuroxime	100	70	40	90	NS	NS
Cefoxitin	100	95	100	95	95	NS
Erythromycin	100	20	40	20	95	95
Tetracycline	95	85	60	90	95	NS
TMP-SMZ	100	95	0	95	V	NS
Quinolones	100	100	40	95	NS	NS
Clindamycin	95	0	100	0	95	95

From Goldstein EJC: Bite wounds and infection, *Clin Infect Dis* 14:637, 1992.
NOTE: Data are compiled from various studies.
TMP-SMZ, Trimethoprim-sulfamethoxazole; *NS*, not studied; *V*, variable.
*Percentage of human-bite isolates/percentage of animal-bite isolates.

dicloxacillin, and cephalexin (Keflex). Ampicillin and penicillin have limited effectiveness against *S. aureus*.[22] Dicloxacillin and cephalexin are not primary agents of choice for *P. multocida*.[22] In spite of these apparent limitations, many practitioners initiate prophylaxis with these agents with apparent success.

Another approach is to use the combination of penicillin and dicloxacillin as an alternative to amoxicillin with clavulanate.[7] Prescribing two antibiotics, however, raises the issue of compliance. For patients with major reactions to penicillins or allergies to cephalosporins, ciprofloxacin alone or in combination with clindamycin can be prescribed. For children, trimethoprim/sulfamethoxazole alone or in combination with clindamycin are reasonable alternatives.

Cat Bites
Suturing

Unless tissue coverage or cosmetics are important considerations, cat-bite and scratch wounds are probably best left open and not sutured. Cat fangs can penetrate deeply into the soft tissues, and because the infection potential of these wounds is great, the most judicious course of action is to cleanse, irrigate, and debride the wound and leave it open.[53] Another option is to open the wound with a simple incision as described previously in the section on bite wound management. Exceptions to this recommendation include large, easily cleansed lacerations that are not on the hand or foot. Most lacerations of the face are protected by the good vascular supply of the face. Whenever suturing is chosen, only percutaneous nonabsorbable sutures are used. Deep closures are avoided because of the increased risk of infection.

Antibiotics

Although cat bites are less common than dog bites, the rate of infection is significantly higher than for dog bites.[1, 17] Because the hand is a frequent site of injury and cats have sharp, slender teeth, the risk for infection is greater. *P. multocida* is more commonly found in a higher proportion of cat bite wounds.[28]

Established Cat Bite Infections. For initial empirical therapy, as with dog bites, an intravenous dose of ampicillin/sulbactam (Unasyn) can be delivered in the emergency department. This agent can be continued during inpatient admission until culture results are known. For outpatient treatment ampicillin with clavulanate (Augmentin) can be prescribed for a full course of 10 to 14 days. Again, this can be modified with culture results and reviewed at the recommended 48 to 72 hour return visit.

Infection with *P. multocida* is often characteristic with onset of symptoms within 24 hours of the bite, prominent pain and swelling, and a serosanguinish and grayish exudate.[52] Because of this organism's exquisite sensitivity to penicillin, it can be initiated parenterally in the emergency department and continued during admission. Alternative intravenous antibiotics include cefuroxime (Zinacef) and ceftriaxone (Rocephin). For adult patients with major allergies to penicillin or allergies to cephalosporins, doxycycline (Vibramicin) can be administered with or without clindamycin (Cleocin). For children, trimethoprim/sulfamethoxazole (Bactrim, Septra) with or without clindamycin can be used.

Cat Bite Prophylaxis. Prophylaxis for uninfected appearing cat bites is less controversial than prophylaxis for dog bites.[1, 14, 17] Most cat bites, unless they are minor scratches or limited to the superficial dermis, are candidates for oral prophylactic antibiotics.[13] For prophylaxis to be effective, the first dose should be delivered in the emergency department and, preferably, in intravenous form. Either ampicillin/sulbactam (Unasyn) or penicillin can be that agent. Amoxicillin with clavulanate (Augmentin) or Penicillin VK are continued orally. Alternatives include cefuroxime (Zinacef) or doxycycline (Vibramicin). Both cefuroxime (Ceftin) and doxycycline (VibraTabs) come in oral preparations. For children allergic to penicillin or cephalosporins, trimethoprim/sulfamethoxazole (Bactrim, Septra) is recommended as the prophylactic agent.

Human Bites
Suturing

As a general rule, closure of human bite wounds has traditionally been avoided.[28] However, a study has cast doubt on the practice of not closing human bite wounds.[5] Sutured versus nonsutured hand lacerations from human bites had the same outcome. Further studies are needed to confirm these results. Large, easily cleansed and irrigated proximal extremity or truncal wounds can be closed with a single layer of nonabsorbable material. Facial human bites can be potentially disfiguring. A fresh facial bite, less than 12 hours old, that does not show signs of infection can be safely closed with sutures.[50] Consultation is recommended when there is doubt about what management steps should be carried out for human bites. All clenched-fist bite injuries, with penetration of the dermis, should be managed in consultation with a specialist.

Antibiotics

Most authorities and clinicians recommend antibiotic prophylaxis for all but the most superficial human bite wounds.[10, 19, 29, 47] Until reliable clinical studies are carried out to clarify the true risk of human bites and the value of prophylaxis, it is best to err on the side of treatment.

Established Hand Infections. For established infections, in addition to extensive wound cleansing, irrigation, and necessary debridement, ampicillin/sulbactam (Unasyn) can be initiated intravenously in the emergency department. It provides excellent coverage against *S. aureus*, *E. corrodens*, and the relevant anaerobic species. Most patients with established hand infections are admitted to the hospital for continued intravenous antibiotics and ampicillin/sulbactam can be continued until culture results are known. An alternative with similar good coverage against the relevant pathogens is cefoxitin (Mefoxin). Patients with major allergic responses to penicillin or allergies to cephalosporins can be treated initially with doxycycline (Vibramicin) alone or in combination with clindamycin (Cleocin). Children can be treated with trimethoprim/

sulfamethoxazole (Bactrim, Septra) in addition to clindamycin. In human bites inflicted by institutionalized patients, coverage for gram-negative organisms should be considered and the addition of an aminoglycoside to one of the above regimens might be indicated.

Hand Bite Prophylaxis. Uninfected nonhand bite wounds can be treated on an outpatient basis. Simple abrasions or superficial occlusional bites can be cleansed and observed. Antibiotics are given at the discretion of the caregiver. Penetrating wounds into the dermis or subcutaneous tissue, are best treated with antibiotics. Any bite of the hand needs careful follow-up in addition to antibiotics. Because of the potential seriousness of these bites, consultative support is recommended. To ensure early and appropriate antibiotic levels, an initial parenteral dose of ampicillin/sulbactam (Unasyn) should initiate prophylaxis. Oral agents are continued for 3 to 5 days. These are discussed in the preceding section on established infections.

Rat Bites

Most reported rat bites occur in a domestic setting. In a recent study of 50 cases, *Staphylococcus epidermidis* was the most common organism cultured from the open, fresh wound.[40] Other organisms included *Bacillus subtilis*, diphtheroids, and alpha hemolytic streptococci. Although 30% of wounds had positive cultures, only one case became infected. No patient was treated with prophylactic antibiotics. Antibiotics are recommended only if wound infection is evident. Dicloxacillin and erythromycin are effective. Rats do not carry rabies, and patients do not need postexposure prophylaxis.

Fish Bites

People who work with or own fish are susceptible to infection by the small gram-positive rod *Erysipelothrix*. This organism causes a slowly spreading cellulitis of the affected area, usually the hand. The organism responds to penicillin.

WOUND AFTERCARE AND FOLLOW-UP

All animal-bite victims or members of their families have to be instructed about the signs of infection: pain, redness, swelling, and purulent drainage. Dressings have to be removed approximately 24 hours after the initial visit so that the wound can be inspected. A wound infection with *P. multocida* usually is apparent by that time.[52] If signs of infection are present, the patient should return to a medical-care facility for treatment. A routine follow-up visit for deep, extensive, face or hand wounds, between 24 (particularly for cat bites) to 72 hours following care, can be a prudent measure to take. Tetanus prophylaxis is administered according to the guidelines outlined in Chapter 18.

RABIES EXPOSURE AND PROPHYLAXIS

Until effective rabies control programs covered the nation by the 1950s, 50 cases of human infection a year were reported, the majority from dog bites.[20, 21] Between 1980 and 1993, only 18 cases were reported to U.S. public health authorities, and only 8 were acquired within the country. Because of the control programs, almost all, 85%, of wildlife rabies occurs in skunks, raccoons and bats.[44] Although canine rabies has been dramatically reduced, it has not been completely eradicated, particularly along the United States/Mexico border. In the rest of the world, including Asia, Africa, and Latin America, dogs remain the most significant threat to humans for rabies transmittal.

Rabies is a neurotropic virus that, on entering the peripheral nervous system, becomes protected from immune response.[43] For this reason, immediate wound care and postexposure prophylaxis should be initiated to prevent that crucial access. The size of the rabies inoculum, the richness of nerve innervation at the bite site, and proximity to nerve terminals are crucial risk factors for active disease susceptibility. Animal wounding studies have shown that thorough wound cleansing using soap and water can significantly reduce a bite victim's risk of contracting rabies.[44]

When confronted with a bite victim, the emergency physician has to consider several factors before initiating postexposure prophylaxis.[36] These include: the animal species involved, the geographic location, type and severity of exposure, status of the animal

Table 14-2 *Rabies Postexposure Prophylaxis Guide, United States, 1991*

Animal Type	Evaluation and Disposition of Animal	Postexposure Prophylaxis Recommendations
Dogs and cats	Healthy and available for 10 day's observation	Should not begin prophylaxis unless animal develops symptoms of rabies*
	Rabid or suspected rabid	Immediate vaccination
	Unknown (escaped)	Consult public health officials
Skunks, raccoons, bats, foxes, and most other carnivores; woodchucks	Regarded as rabid unless geographic area is known to be free of rabies or until animal proven negative by laboratory tests†	Immediate vaccination
Livestock, rodents, and lagomorphs (rabbits and hares)	Consider individually	Consult public health officials. Bites of squirrels, hamsters, guinea pigs, gerbils, chipmunks, rats, mice, other rodents, rabbits, and hares almost never require antirabies treatment

Centers for Disease Control: Rabies prevention—United States, 1991: recommendations of the ACIP, *MMWR* 40(RR-3):1-18, 1991.
*During the 10-day holding period, begin treatment with HRIG and HDCV or RVA at first sign of rabies in a dog or cat that has bitten someone. The symptomatic animal should be killed immediately and tested.
†The animal should be killed and tested as soon as possible. Holding for observation is not recommended. Discontinue vaccine if immunofluorescence test results of the animal are negative.

(captured or not), and the underlying disease status of the patient. Tables 14-2 and 14-3 summarize the current postexposure guidelines and treatment schedule.

Animal Identification

Wild Carnivores and Bats. Approximately 3% to 20% of all bats submitted for rabies testing are positive for the virus.[44] Bats are responsible for the majority of cases of human rabies in the United States and its territories. Skunks, raccoons, foxes, woodchucks, and wild carnivores should be considered rabid unless they are in a geographic area known to be free of wildlife rabies. Postexposure prophylaxis should be initiated

Table 14-3   *Rabies Postexposure Prophylaxis Schedule, United States, 1991*

Vaccination Status	Treatment	Regimen*
Not previously vaccinated	Local wound cleansing	All postexposure treatment should begin with immediate thorough cleansing of all wounds with soap and water.
	HRIG	20 IU/kg body weight. If anatomically feasible, up to one-half the dose should be infiltrated around the wound(s) and the rest should be administered IM in the gluteal area. HRIG should not be administered in the same syringe or into the same anatomical site as vaccine. Because HRIG may partially suppress active production of antibody, no more than the recommended dose should be given.
	Vaccine	HDCV or RVA, 1.0 ml, IM (deltoid area†), one each on days 0, 3, 7, 14 and 28.
Previously vaccinated§	Local wound cleansing	All postexposure treatment should begin with immediate thorough cleansing of all wounds with soap and waer.
	HRIG	HRIG should not be administered.
	Vaccine	HDCV or RVA, 1.0 ml, IM (deltoid area†), one each on days 0 and 3.

Centers for Disease Control: Rabies prevention—United States, 1991: recommendations of the ACIP, *MMWR* 40(RR-3):1-18, 1991.
*These regimens are applicable for all age groups, including children.
†The deltoid area is the only acceptable site of vaccination for adults and older children. For younger children, the outer aspect of the thigh may be used. Vaccine should never be administered in the gluteal area.
§Any person with a history of preexposure vaccination with HDCV or RVA; prior postexposure prophylaxis with HDCV or RVA; or previous vaccination with any other type of rabies vaccine and a documented history of antibody response to the prior vaccination.

when patients are exposed to wild carnivores and bats unless (1) the exposure occurred in an area of the continental United States known to be free of terrestrial rabies and the results of immunofluorescence antibody testing is available within 48 hours, or (2) the animal has already been tested and shown not to be rabid. If the animal cannot be captured or tested, prophylaxis is begun immediately. Because the issue of geographic location and the incidence of wildlife rabies can be complicated, consultation with local public health officials is recommended. It is important to note that if there is any delay in obtaining that consultation or the caregiver has any doubt whatsoever about the nature of the biting species, postexposure prophylaxis should be initiated until clinical clarity is obtained. Treatment can always be discontinued if it is determined that the risk does not warrant prophylaxis.

Dogs and Cats. The likelihood of a dog carrying rabies varies with geographic area. The area of highest risk in the United States is along the Mexican border. Eighty percent of all dogs submitted for testing in that region have been shown to be positive for the rabies virus.[21] Away from the border region, in areas where rabies exists in terrestrial wildlife, only 0.1% to 1% of dogs test positive. That fact underlies the 10 day observation period when a dog is available for observation.

Cats have been reported to have a higher rate of rabies infection than dogs. The region for greatest cat rabies risk is the mid-Atlantic, and transmittal to cats is probably through raccoons.

No case of animal rabies has been reported from dogs that have been fully vaccinated (2 shots).[44] Only 3 cases of rabies have been reported in dogs and cats that have been reportedly vaccinated. In all of these cases, it was discovered that the animals had been incompletely vaccinated and had received only 1 of the 2 recommended immunization shots.

Treatment guidelines are as follows: when the animal is known to be rabid or suspected to be, prophylaxis is initiated without delay. For bites from healthy captured but unvaccinated animals, quarantine for 10 days is recommended. Any illness that develops in that period is followed immediately by initiation of prophylaxis. Treatment is not delayed for animal sacrifice and rabies immunofluorescence testing of the brain. For truly wild, unwanted animals that have been captured, immediate sacrifice and testing can be carried out. If the animal cannot be captured and tested, postexposure prophylaxis is guided by the risk of endemic, wildlife rabies in that area. In these circumstances, consultation with public health officials is recommended. In cases where consultation cannot be obtained within 48 hours of the biting incident, initiation of prophylaxis is recommended if there is any uncertainty regarding the status of the biting animal. When the circumstances are later clarified, termination of the prophylaxis regimen is carried out if the exposure carried negligible risk.

Rodents and Lagomorphs. Rodents include mice, rats, squirrels, hamsters, guinea pigs, gerbils, and chipmunks. Lagomorphs are rabbits or hares. The overall rate of rabies infection in this group is 0.01%. No cases of human rabies have ever been documented following a rodent or lagomorph bite. Woodchucks and groundhogs are an exception because of reported rabies carriage in some regions. In the event of a rodent or groundhog/woodchuck bite, guidance from the local public health officials is recommended.

Exotic Pets. Included in this group are ferrets, exotic wild animals, and domestic animals crossbred with wild ones. The true risk of rabies in these animals is unknown, and it is recommended by authorities that they be sacrificed and tested rather than observed. Rabies prophylaxis can be initiated and terminated should immunofluorescence be negative. On occasion, the animal is of such rarity or value that immunoprophylaxis might be chosen over animal sacrifice. Consultation with public health officials or zoological experts can assist in these rare cases.

Livestock. Livestock, particularly cattle, are susceptible to rabies infection from skunks. Horses, mules, sheep, goats, and swine are also susceptible but at a lower rate than cattle. Because of the logistical problems created by large animal exposure, consultation with a veterinarian or public health official is recommended in these cases.

Type of Exposure

Rabies is almost always transmitted by the saliva of an infected animal through a bite. Bites that cause any interruption of the skin—epidermis or dermis—constitute a significant exposure. Significant nonbite exposures include skin scratches, abrasions, open wounds, or mucous membranes that become exposed to and contaminated by the saliva or tissue from a potentially rabid animal. Saliva or tissue that is dry is considered noninfectious. The risk of contracting rabies through a bite from a known rabid animal ranges between 5% and 80%.[31] On the other hand, the risk of exposure of rabies to a skin scratch is 0.1% to 1%.

Aerosolized rabies, such as what might be found in laboratories or caves with resident bats, has been implicated in rare nonbite cases of human rabies. Animal source responsible for six cases happened through corneal transplantation. Since these cases have come to light, guidelines for corneal harvesting have been modified to significantly reduce that risk. Preexposure rabies prophylaxis is recommended for rabies laboratory workers and spelunkers (Table 14-4).

Concern is often raised about having an incidental contact (lack of skin or mucous membrane exposure) with a potentially rabid animal. These exposures do not constitute a rabies risk. Additionally, contact with body fluids such blood, feces (bat guano), or urine is also considered nonsignificant.

Timing of Postexposure Prophylaxis

In optimal circumstances, and because the stakes can be high, every attempt is made to administer postexposure prophylaxis, if indicated, within 48 hours of contact. This timing is based on the fact that the incubation period of rabies can be as short as 5 days and a margin of safety is desirable.[21] The incubation period can be as long as 2 years with an

Table 14-4 *Rabies Preexposure Prophylaxis Guide, United States, 1991*

Risk Category	Nature of Risk	Typical Populations	Preexposure Recommendations
Continuous	Virus present continuously, often in high concentrations. Aerosol, mucous membrane, bite, or nonbite exposure. Specific exposures may go unrecognized.	Rabies research lab worker;* rabies biologics production workers.	Primary course. Serologic testing every 6 months; booster vaccination when antibody level falls below acceptable level.†
Frequent	Exposure usually episodic, with source recognized, but exposure may also be unrecognized. Aerosol, mucous membrane, bite, or nonbite exposure.	Rabies diagnostic lab workers,* spelunkers, veterinarians and staff, and animal-control and wildlife workers in rabies enzootic areas. Travelers visiting foreign areas of enzootic rabies for more than 30 days.	Primary course. Serologic testing or booster vaccination every 2 years.†
Infrequent (greater than population at large)	Exposure nearly always episodic with source recognized. Mucous membrane, bite, or nonbite exposure.	Veterinarians and animal-control and wildlife workers in areas of low rabies enzooticity. Veterinary students.	Primary course; no serologic testing or booster vaccination.
Rare (population at large)	Exposures always episodic. Mucous membrane, or bite with source unrecognized.	U.S. population at large, including persons in rabies epizootic areas.	No vaccination necessary.

Centers for Disease Control: Rabies prevention—United States, 1991: recommendations of the ACIP, *MMWR* 40(RR-3):1-18, 1991.

*Judgment of relative risk and extra monitoring of vaccination status of laboratory workers is the responsibility of the laboratory supervisor (58).

†Minimum acceptable antibody level is complete virus neutralization at a 1:5 serum dilution by RFFIT. Booster dose should be administered if the titer falls below this level.

average of 30 to 90 days.[44] For this reason, prophylaxis is administered to any patient found to have a rabies risk bite or exposure regardless of the interval from contact to treatment. The average interval between exposure to care is 5 days and that delay has not been found to increase the risk of contracting the disease.[4] Because the risk of canine rabies is low in the United States, other than along the Mexican border, a delay of 10 days is considered acceptable if the animal can be confined for observation. In fact, dogs infected with the rabies virus almost always become clinically rabid well before that 10 day period has elapsed.[21]

Immunosuppression and Pregnancy

Corticosteroid administration, immunosuppressive therapy or disease, and antimalarials can impair the protective immune response of rabies prophylaxis vaccination. Under these circumstances, serum testing for rabies antibody response is recommended. Rabies postexposure prophylaxis provides no risk to a fetus; therefore pregnant mothers are treated the same as other exposed persons.

POSTEXPOSURE PROPHYLAXIS

The currently approved regimen for rabies postexposure prophylaxis includes the administration of human rabies immune globulin (HRIG) and five doses of human diploid cell vaccine (HDCV). An additional vaccine, rabies vaccine, adsorbed (RVA), is available and is equally efficacious to HDVC. Virtually all vaccines undergo an appropriate antibody response and antibody titer testing is not necessary. Alternative vaccine dose schedules (e.g., intradermal or IM 3 doses) are not recommended for use in the United States.

The use of rabies vaccine induces local reactions such as pain, erythema, swelling, or itching at the injection site in 30% to 74% of recipients.[44] Approximately 5% to 40% of vaccinees report systemic reactions, such as headache, nausea, abdominal pain, muscle aches, and dizziness. Extremely rare, with only three cases reported, are neurologic illnesses resembling the Guillain-Barré syndrome. All three cases resolved without sequelae by 3 months. Another reaction, occurring in 6% of recipients, is an immune complexlike illness characterized by urticaria, arthralgia, arthritis, angioedema, nausea, vomiting, and fever. Local pain and low grade fever have been reported with HRIG.

Because of the seriousness of rabies, rabies prophylaxis should not be interrupted or discontinued if at all possible. Attempts are made to manage local or mild systemic reactions with antiinflammatories and antipyretics. Ultimately, in serious reactions, the risk of acquiring rabies must be weighed against the nature of the reaction. In cases such as these, advice and assistance should be sought from public health officials or the Centers for Disease Control in Atlanta.

Postexposure Therapy of Previously Vaccinated Bite Victims

Patients who have previously undergone preexposure or postexposure rabies prophylaxis are treated with 2 doses of the vaccine alone, 1 immediately and the other 3 days later. Human rabies immune globulin is unnecessary because the vaccination booster provides an effective amnestic antibody response.

REFERENCES

1. Aghababian R, Conte J: Mammalian bite wounds, *Ann Emerg Med* 9:79-83, 1980.
2. Bailie W, Stove E, Schmitt A: Aerobic bacterial flora of oral and nasal fluids of canines with reference to bacteria associated with bites, *J Clin Microbiol* 7:223-231, 1978.
3. Basadre JO, Parry SW: Indications for surgical debridement in 125 human bites of the hand, *Arch Surg* 126:65-67, 1991.
4. Beck AM, Felser SR, Glickman LT: An epizootic of rabies in Maryland, 1982-84, *Am J Public Health* 77:42-44, 1987.
5. Bite U: Human bites of the hand, *Can J Surg* 27:616-618, 1984.
6. Brandt F: Human bites of the ear, *Plast Reconstr Surg* 43:130-134, 1969.
7. Callaham ML: Controversies in antibiotic choices for bite wounds, *Ann Emerg Med* 17:1321-1330, 1988.
8. Callaham ML: Prophylactic antibiotics in common dog bite wounds: a controlled study, *Ann Emerg Med* 9:410-414, 1980.
9. Callaham ML: Treatment of common dog bites: infection risk factors, *J Am Coll Emerg Phys* 7:83-87, 1978.
10. Chuinard R, D'Ambrosia R: Human bite infections of the hand, *J Bone Joint Surg* 59 A:416-418, 1977.
11. Deleted in proofs.
12. Cummings P: Antibiotics to prevent infection in patients with dog bite wounds: A mete-analysis of randomized trials, *Ann Emerg Med* 23:535-540, 1994.
13. Dire DJ: Cat bite wounds: risk factors for infection, *Ann Emerg Med* 18:471, 1989 (abstract).
14. Dire DJ: Emergency management of dog and cat bite wounds, *Emerg Med Clin North Am* 10:719-736, 1992.
15. Douglas LG: Bite wounds, *Am Fam Phys* 11:93-99, 1990.
16. Earley MJ, Bardsley AF: Human bites: a review, *Br J Plast Surg* 37:458-462, 1984.
17. Elenbaas RM, McNabney WK, Robinson WA: Evaluation of prophylactic oxacillin in cat bite wounds, *Ann Emerg Med* 13:155-157, 1984.
18. Elenbaas RM, McNabney WK, Robinson WA: Prophylactic oxacillin in dog bite wounds, *Ann Emerg Med* 11:248-251, 1982.
19. Farmer C, Mann R: Human bite infections of the hand, *South Med J* 59:515-518, 1966.
20. Fishbein DB, Arcangeli LS: Rabies prevention in primary care, *Postgrad Med* 82:83-95, 1987.
21. Fishbein DB, Robinson LE: Rabies, *NEJM* 329:1632-1638, 1993.
22. Goldstein EJC: Bite wounds and infection, *Clin Infect Dis* 14:633-640, 1992.
23. Goldstein EJC, Barones MF, Miller TA: *Eikenella corrodens* in hand infections, *J Hand Surg* 8:563-566, 1983.
24. Goldstein EJC, Citron D, Finegold SM: Dog bite wounds and infection: a prospective clinical study, *Ann Emerg Med* 9:508-512, 1980.
25. Goldstein EJC, Citron DM, Wield B: Bacteriology of human and animal bite wounds, *J Clin Microbiol* 8:667-672, 1978.

26. Goldstein EJC, Reinhardt JR, Murray PM, et al: Outpatient therapy of bite wounds *Int J Dermatol* 26:123-127, 1987.

27. Goldstein EJC, Reinhardt JR, Murray PM, et al: A comparative study of Augmentin versus penicillin dicloxacillin: a special report, *Postgrad Med* 56:105-110, 1984.

28. Griego RD, Rosen T, Orengo IF, et al: Dog, cat, and human bites: a review, *J Amer Acad Dermatol* 33:1019-1029, 1995.

29. Guba A, Mulliken J, Hoopes J: The selection of antibiotics for human bites of the hand, *Plast Reconstr Surg* 56:538-541, 1975.

30. Guy RJ, Zook EG: Successful treatment of acute head and neck dog bite wounds without antibiotics, *Ann Plast Surg* 17:45-48, 1986.

31. Hatwick MAW: Human rabies, *Public Health Rev* 3:229-274, 1974.

32. Kizer K: Epidemiologic and clinical aspects of animal bite injuries, *J Am Coll Emerg Phys* 8:134-141, 1979.

33. Koch S: Acute rapidly spreading infections following trivial injuries to the hand, *Surg Gynecol Obstet* 59:277-308, 1934.

34. Lindsey D, Christopher M, Hollenbach I, et al: Natural course of the human bite wound: incidence of infection and complications in 434 bites and 803 lacerations in the same group of patients, *J Trauma* 27:45-48, 1987.

35. Malinowski R, et al: The management of human bite injuries to the hand, *J Trauma* 19:655-658, 1979.

36. Mann J: Systemic decision-making in rabies prophylaxis, *Ped Infect Dis* 2:162-167, 1983.

37. Mann R, Peacock J: Hand infections in patients with diabetes mellitus, *J Trauma* 17:376-380, 1977.

38. Marcy S: Infections due to dog and cat bites, *Ped Infect Dis* 1:351-356, 1982.

39. Marr J, Beck A, Lugo J: An epidemiologic study of the human bite, *Public Health Rep* 94:514-521, 1979.

40. Ordog GJ, Balasubramaniam S, Wasserberger J: Rat bites: fifty cases, *Ann Emerg Med* 14:126-130, 1985.

41. Patzakis MJ, Wilkins J, Bassett RL: Surgical findings in clenched-fist injuries, *Clin Orthop Relat Res* 220:237-240, 1987.

42. Peeples E, Boswick J, Scott F: Wounds of the hand contaminated by human or animal saliva, *J Trauma* 19:655-658, 1979.

43. Plotkin S, Clark H: Prevention of rabies in man, *J Infect Dis* 123:227-240, 1971.

44. Rabies Prevention-United States, 1991, Recommendations of the Immunization Practices Advisory Committee (ACIP), *MMWR Morbid Mortal Wkly Rep* 40(RR-3):1-19, 1991.

45. Rest J, Goldstein ECJ: Management of human and animal bites, *Emerg Clin North Am* 3:117-126, 1985.

46. Rosen RA: The use of antibiotics in the initial management of recent dog-bite wounds, *Am J Emerg Med* 3:19-23, 1985.

47. Shields C, et al: Hand infections secondary to human bites, *J Trauma* 15:235-236, 1975.

48. Strassburg M, et al: Animal bites: patterns of treatment, *Ann Emerg Med* 10:193-197, 1981.

49. Thomas PR, Buntine JA: Man's best friend? a review of the Austin hospital's experience with dog bites, *Med J Aust* 147:536-540, 1987.

50. Thomasetti B, Walker L, Bormby M: Human bites of the face, *J Oral Surg* 37:565-568, 1979.

51. Thomson H, Svitek V: Small animal bites: the role of primary closure, *J Trauma* 13:20-23, 1973.

52. Tindall J, Harrison C: *Pasteurella multocida* infections following animal injuries, especially cat bites, *Arch Dermatol* 105:412-416, 1972.

53. Vietch J, Omer G: Case report: treatment of cat bite injuries of the hand, *J Trauma* 19:201-202, 1979.

54. Zook EG, Miller M, Van Beek AL, et al: Successful treatment protocol for canine fang injuries, *J Trauma* 20:243-246, 1980.

15 *Common Wound Care Problems*

Common nonlaceration problems lend themselves to emergency wound care techniques. These include retained foreign bodies and fishhooks, plantar puncture wounds, and abrasions. Although they can appear trivial, each of these problems presents special challenges and, occasionally, requires sophisticated diagnostic and management procedures. In addition, certain anatomic areas of the body, particularly the structures of the face, hand, and foot, can be fraught with unique difficulties that are best managed by a thorough understanding of the issues and application of proper technique.

FOREIGN BODIES

Any object becomes a foreign body when it penetrates the skin and lodges in the soft tissue. In a clinical study of foreign bodies retained in the hand, the most common objects, in order of frequency, were wood splinters, glass fragments, various metallic objects, and needles.[1] Included in the list were pencil leads, thorns, nails, and plastic objects. Generally, foreign bodies are classified by material—inert, nonreactive; and organic, reactive.

Inert (Nonreactive) Objects

Inert objects include bullets, needles, and other metallic items. Although they do not provoke inflammation, they can cause chronic pain and discomfort, especially in weight-bearing areas or near joints. Metals that oxidize, that is, rust, can cause a mild to moderate tissue reaction. The clinical decision to remove an inert object has to be weighed against the potential damage that could be created during a search for the object. Inert objects can be left in place if they are inaccessible and will not cause tissue damage or a functional deficit. If left alone, noncritical inert foreign bodies encapsulate within soft tissue and cause no further problem.

Although glass is considered inert, glass foreign bodies are often symptomatic. Removal is recommended if accessible except for small, insignificant fragments. Pencil "lead," graphite, is inert but can cause tattooing. It can also be accompanied by wood fragments during injury. For these reasons, even though it is inert, graphite should be removed from the injury site.

Organic (Reactive) Objects

Objects that are not inert, wood, bone, soil, stones, rubber, and other organic materials such as thorns, must be removed in their entirety. These materials can cause a variety of bacterial and fungal infections.[4, 26] Synovitis from joint penetration, periosteal reactions, foreign body granulomas, draining fistulas, and pseudotumors of the soft tissue have all been reported with noninert foreign objects.[1, 6, 19] Retained wood objects have been reported to cause chronic inflammation, drainage, and pain for up to 7 years following penetration.[6] Therefore a missed diagnosis or failure to remove all fragments of a noninert object can lead to prolonged disability and patient discomfort.

Clinical Evaluation

When a foreign object penetrates the skin, patients cannot reliably report its presence. In glass wounds, reliance on the patient's history alone would lead to 50% missed fragments.[28] In cases where no foreign body is reported, certain clinical settings carry a higher risk for one being present. Any injury with glass should raise the suspicion of a retained fragment. In glass injuries, the head and foot are more likely to have retained fragments.[23] In lip or perioral injuries, where there is traumatic loss of dentition, a tooth fragment might be embedded in the soft tissue. Injuries to the feet or hands with needles, nails, or splinters should be suspected of retention if the patient cannot account for the entirety of the injuring object. If the suspicion is strong, then the caregiver is obligated to carry out a diagnostic evaluation and local exploration to rule in or rule out the possibility of a retained foreign object.

Before anesthetic is administered, gently running a gloved finger over the suspected foreign body site can elicit in a patient the characteristic sensation. In the anesthetized wound, gently probing and drawing a closed hemostat in and through the wound can alert the operator to the presence of a wood, glass, or metallic foreign body. The hemostat will transmit a distinct "grating" sensation. Probing can reveal the presence of an inert object or a wood splinter before it has been softened by the absorption of tissue fluids.

Plain Radiography

For the most part, radiographs are ordered when there is patient belief or clinical suspicion of a foreign object. Most objects, 80%, can be visualized, either directly or indirectly, with the use of radiographs.[1] Radiodense objects, even the size of a pinpoint, are easily seen. Metallic objects, with the exception of aluminum, can be visualized in almost all cases. A common misconception is that glass is not visible by radiograph.[10] Virtually all types of glass, up to 95% as small as 2 mm in size, can be seen by x-ray.[29] Fragments as small as 0.5 mm can be visualized as well, but only in 50% to 60% of cases. Other radiodense objects include pencil graphite, some plastics, and gravel.

Nonradiodense objects include wood, thorns, chicken bones, and some plastics. Radiodensity of wood and organic objects, to some degree, depends on the time in tissue and absorption of body fluids. Wood has been reported to be visible by radiography in 15% of cases; however, after 48 hours, fluid absorption renders it not visible.[1] Nonradiodense objects, such as splinters or plastic fragments, can be revealed as a filling defects or outlined by air drawn into the wound during the injury.

Ultrasonography, Computed Tomography, and Magnetic Resonance Imaging

If an object cannot be visualized by plain radiography or retrieved easily through direct visualization, other imaging techniques are available. Ultrasonography can detect nonradiodense foreign bodies as small as 1×2 mm or larger.[20] Whenever a foreign object consists of vegetative matter and removal is necessary, ultrasound can be used not only to localize the object but also as a guidance technique for the operator just before exploration. Tendons, deep scar tissue, fresh hematoma, and tissue calcifications can produce false positive ultrasound readings. Ultrasonography for foreign bodies requires experience and skill to maximize its usefulness.

Computed tomography (CT) scans offer an alternative to ultrasound.[25] Not only can a CT scan identify vegetative objects such as splinters and thorns, it can localize objects in relationship to the surrounding anatomic structures. Magnetic resonance imaging (MRI) has similar capabilities to CT scans but should never be used to locate objects that contain metal.[2] Both CT scans and MRIs are expensive alternatives and require a high degree of patient cooperation, often not possible for the pediatric patient.

Techniques for Removal

Once the diagnosis is made, localizing and retrieving the foreign body are carried out. These steps are often frustrating and attended by unanticipated difficulties. It seems a simple matter to make a small incision and retrieve an object that appears to be close to the surface of the skin. However, simple retrieval is not always possible. As a rule, if attempts at retrieval exceed 30 minutes, serious consideration should be given to terminating the procedure and obtaining consultation.

Radiodense objects: For objects that are located below the surface and out of direct sight, careful localization is necessary before proceeding with exploration. Radio-dense objects can be localized by a variety of techniques using markers and radiographs. A simple technique recommended by this author is to bend a paper clip to form a flat plane with an extended arm. The extended arm is placed directly over the skin entry wound created by the foreign object, and the paper clip is secured with a small piece of tape (Fig. 15-1). Two radiographs are taken *exactly* at an angle of 90 degrees to each other (anteroposterior and lateral views) using the plane of the clip as a geometric point of reference (Figs. 15-2 and 15-3). In this manner, both the location and depth of the object relative to the extended arm of the paper clip can be determined. Magnification by this technique occurs and the distance between the object and the clip on the radiograph is greater than the actual distance. After appropriate cleansing and the administering of an anesthetic, a small incision is made and exploration is carried out until the object can be removed. The radiographs are needed in the care area for reference during the removal.

Nonradiodense objects: Because radiographs are not usually helpful, nonradiodense objects are best approached through a more generous incision and thorough exploration

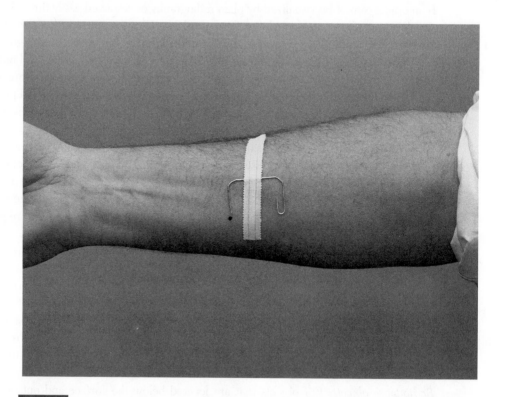

FIG. 15-1   Technique for placing a reconfigured paper clip with the extended arm directly over the entry point of a foreign-body penetration.

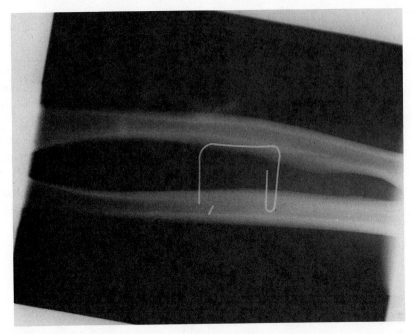

FIG. 15-2 Direct anteroposterior view of the paper clip and foreign body.

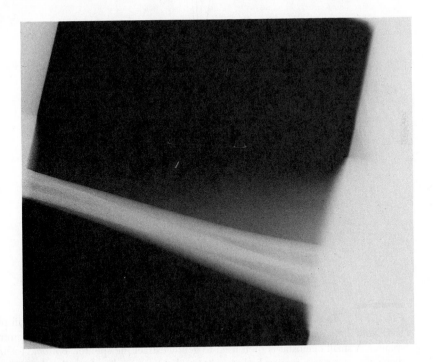

FIG. 15-3 Direct lateral view of the paper clip and foreign body. Note that these two radiographs can be used to accurately locate the position of the foreign body relative to the extended arm by the anteroposterior view and its depth by the lateral view.

by direct visualization. Incisions permit debridement and removal of tissue that is embedded with foreign material. When the foreign body is located in the hand or foot, the exsanguination tourniquet technique as described in Chapter 8 is recommended. Even a small amount of bleeding can make visualization impossible.

Protruding objects: For objects that are partially protruding from the skin, the temptation to "grab and yank" has to be resisted. If a wood splinter is pulled out injudiciously through a small, tight, entry wound, small fragments can be stripped off the splinter and left behind to cause future difficulty.[20] The technique illustrated in the finger shown in Fig. 15-4 demonstrates how a small incision is made parallel to the course

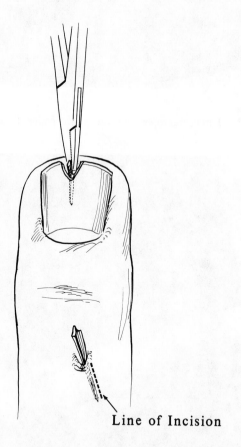

Line of Incision

FIG. 15-4 *Top,* Technique for removing small splinter from between the nail plate and nail bed. Note that a small wedge of nail has been removed to gain exposure of the protruding of the splinter. A small hemostat is then used to gently extract the splinter. *Bottom,* Technique for removing a penetrating foreign body, a splinter, that is protruding from the skin. Note that a small incision is made directly away from the entry point, parallel to the shaft of the foreign body. The splinter can be removed in its entirety without leaving smaller splinters.

and angle of the object. By creating an incision, the splinter can be removed without leaving behind smaller splinters. In addition, the wound can be copiously irrigated to decrease the level of bacterial contamination. It is important to note that these small incisions must not be closed with sutures. They should be left open to drain the site, if necessary, and prevent the accumulation of purulence that might lead to the formation of an abscess.

Objects under nail plates: A common problem is a splinter or other object that is lodged under a nail plate. If the object can be grasped by a hemostat, then it can be carefully pulled out from under the nail. Again, care has to be taken not to strip fragments off a wooden object. For a splinter that cannot be grasped, removal of a small part of the nail plate in a wedge-shaped fashion can be carried out to expose the splinter, as shown in the top half of Fig. 15-4.

A simple technique for removing small splinters lodged under the nail plate is to bend the tip of a 25- or 27-gauge needle so that a small barb equal in size to the diameter of the needle is created.[7] The shaft of the needle is then introduced adjacent and parallel to the splinter and carried back to the most proximal portion of the object. Then the barb is raked along the splinter, and both the needle and the foreign object are pulled out from under the nail. Removing objects from under nails is best carried out when the patient is anesthetized. The anesthetic is usually delivered via a digital block as described in Chapter 5.

Thorns/cactus spines: Particularly troublesome are small thorns and cactus spines that can accidentally become embedded in the skin in large numbers, usually in children. In a controlled rabbit experiment, Elmer's Glue-All was applied under a single layer of gauze and allowed to dry. Gentle peeling successfully removed 95% of all spines.[21] The next most effective method was manual removal with tweezers, with a 76% rate of spine removal. The combination of tweezer removal of large spines followed by glue application is very effective.

When to consult: Occasionally, a foreign body cannot be successfully retrieved by attempts at localization and exploration in an emergency wound care setting. The most common situation in which this eventuality arises is deep foreign objects of the foot. These foreign bodies are best removed in radiology department suites where ultrasound, image intensifiers, and stereotaxic localization can be applied while a consultant explores the affected area.[22, 30]

PLANTAR PUNCTURE WOUNDS

Plantar puncture wounds are a common presenting complaint. The vast majority, 90% or more, is caused by stepping on nails.[12] In many cases, the patient seeks only a tetanus shot and not care for the wound itself. Because many patients do not seek care at all for punctures, the true complication rate is unknown. The complication rate for patients who do seek care ranges from 2% to 8%.[12, 15] The time from injury to presentation is significant because patients who present after 48 hours are more likely to have complications.[5] In actuality, they are brought to care because of persistent or worsening symptoms.

In addition to delay of presentation, there are other circumstances that increase the risk for infection and other complications. Punctures suffered outdoors are more likely to be contaminated or caused by rust covered nails. Remnants of socks or shoes can be carried into wounds with tennis shoes creating an increased risk for osteomyelitis secondary to *Pseudomonas aeruginosa*.[11, 16] The forefoot, including the metatarsals heads and toes, are far more vulnerable than the midfoot or heel to complications, particularly pyarthrosis and osteomyelitis. In one study, 34 of 35 serious plantar puncture injuries occurred in the forefoot.[24] Deep punctures can penetrate bone, tendon, or joints. Finally, patients with diabetes, peripheral vascular disease, or immunosuppression carry a greater risk for complications.

Treatment of Puncture Wounds

The management of puncture wounds is controversial and ranges from doing minimal skin cleansing to complete coring of the puncture wound site. The following are guidelines based on different clinical presentations:

Simple punctures: Most patients present with benign appearing puncture wounds caused by clean objects such as tacks; needles; or small unrusted, exposed, nails. These patients often present in less than 24 hours from the injury.[27] Realistically, to clean and irrigate the length and depth of the actual wound might cause more complications than it would prevent. If there are no indications of retained foreign material, the wound edges are clean and not devitalized, and the puncture site is not indurated or excessively tender to palpitation, skin cleansing and a small application of antibiotic ointment, followed by a Band-Aid, should suffice.

Puncture with suspected retained material: In these wounds, the puncture is often larger than the very small sites noted previously. The wound edges are contaminated, stellate, or shredded appearing. Old nails, exposed bolts, and miscellaneous sharp objects are causes of these punctures. By history, the puncturing object is not clean, has broken during the puncture, or has possibly forced sock or shoe fragments into the wound. These patients are more likely to complain of significant pain or a foreign body sensation on palpation of the puncture site. They often present more than 48 hours after the injury after having tried to treat themselves or having ignored the symptoms, without success.[27]

After providing anesthesia, either through a foot block or by local infiltration, a transverse incision (parallel to the wrinkle line of a curled foot) is made through the puncture site, long enough to provide good exposure of the puncture site and proximal wound track (Fig. 15-5). Any foreign material or devitalized tissue can be debrided. With the wound edges retracted, thorough irrigation is carried out. No attempt is made to suture this wound. The wound edges will close without difficulty following

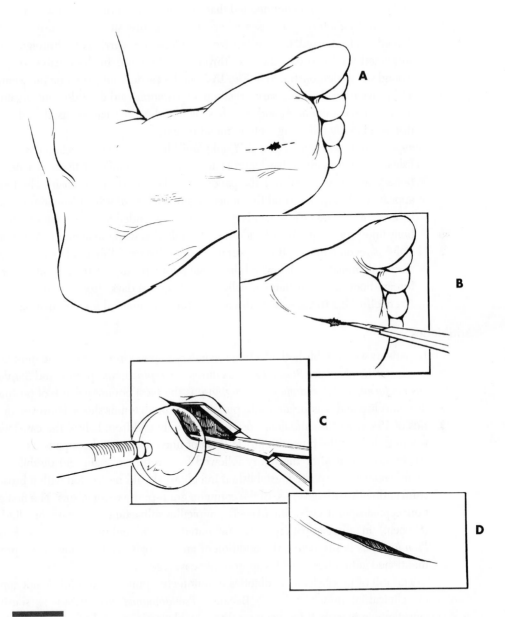

FIG. 15-5   Plantar puncture wound management. **A,** A suggested incision line, parallel to the wrinkle lines, through the puncture wound. **B,** The incision can be made with a scalpel and #15 blade through the thick dermis. **C,** A hemostat is used to expose the wound for exploration and irrigation. **D,** The wound edges can be debrided if necessary and left unsutured to heal by secondary intention.

application of a small amount of an antibiotic ointment and a Band-Aid. For comfort and protection, it is recommended that the patient use crutches for 2 to 3 days.

Complicated punctures: In cases where the puncture site is obviously infected, inflamed, or devitalized, more extensive debridement is carried out. Foreign material is suspected until proven otherwise through exploration. In these cases, opening the wound site as demonstrated in Fig. 15-5 can be carried out to expose the wound track and provide for the necessary irrigation, exploration, and debridement. Again, suturing is not recommended and crutches, as noted earlier, can be used. Antibiotics, as discussed in the following section, might be indicated.

Complicated puncture with deep foot symptoms: In cases where infection has been established, foreign material has had a chance to create significant tissue reaction, or the bone/joint has been violated, the patient complains of deep foot pain. The foot might appear swollen well beyond the puncture site itself and/or lymphangitic streaks could be evident. In these cases, a radiograph is recommended to screen for foreign objects, bony injury, or gas pockets. In addition, consultation with the appropriate surgical specialist is recommended. It is important to note that established infection or significant tissue inflammation well beyond the actual puncture site is often a result of a retained foreign body. These patients usually present several days after the original puncture. Every effort has to be made to discover or rule out retained foreign material.

Antibiotics

In patients with established infection secondary to puncture wounds, the most common organisms involved are *Staphylococcus aureus*, *Streptococcus* species, and *Staphylococcus epidermitis*.[18] *Pseudomonas aeruginosa* is the most common cause of postpuncture osteomyelitis and is associated with punctures through tennis shoes. However, in one series of 15 cases of *Pseudomonas* osteochondritis in children, half of the cases were not wearing shoes at the time of injury.[17] It is not uncommon for these patients to have initial improvement after the injury followed by a return of pain and disability. Unless *Pseudomonas* is suspected, established infections should be treated with a broad spectrum antibiotic with coverage of the common gram-positive organisms. The first generation cephalosporin cefazolin (Ancef), ampicillin/sulbactam (Unasyn), or clindamycin (Cleocin) in allergic patients, can be initiated until culture results are known. If *Pseudomonas* is suspected, the addition of an aminoglycoside to any of the previously mentioned antibiotics provides appropriate coverage.

The use of prophylactic antibiotics in uninfected puncture wounds is not supported by clinical studies.[5, 9, 17, 18] Because *Pseudomonas aeruginosa* is sensitive to ciprofloxacin in vitro, it has been used as a prophylactic agent. In fact, this agent is not a first line agent for the treatment of *Pseudomonas*; and it is contraindicated in children, the group most at risk for this type of infection.[17] Reliance on prophylactic antibiotics is undercut by a study in which cellulitis was shown to occur in 9 patients in spite of receiving appropriate antibiotic coverage.[12] The most important finding of this study was that 5 of those cases had a retained foreign object. In uninfected puncture wounds of the foot, careful instructions to the patient regarding the signs of infection and the arrangement of appropriate follow-up is the recommended course of action. Should an infection occur, a well-informed patient returns for appropriate treatment. It cannot be overemphasized that, if an infection develops, retained foreign material is the cause until proven otherwise.

FISHHOOKS

A number of techniques have been described to remove fishhooks. As a rule, hooks with small barbs can be removed with retrograde techniques, and hooks with large barbs are often best managed by the push-through and cut method. In a 1991 study of 97 patients with fishhook injuries, the most common and therefore successful removal technique was the push-through and cut.[9] Several methods for fishhook removal are described in the following section and their success rates, based on this study, accompany the descriptions.

Retrograde Removal

Hooks with small barbs or hooks that are only very superficially embedded can often be backed out through the original site of penetration. Gentle pressure is applied to the eye and shank to push the barb away from tissue. Simultaneously, a hemostat is applied to the curved portion of the shaft. Traction with the hemostat "backs" the hook out. This technique was successful in 17 of 97 cases in the previously mentioned study.

Experienced fishermen sometimes make a small incision in the dermis at the entry site and pull the hook out retrograde with needle-nose pliers. Dermis is the most likely layer to resist removal of the hook and barb because of its naturally tough consistency. This extraction procedure can easily be duplicated in an emergency wound-care facility. After basic cleansing with an appropriate solution like povidone-iodine, a small amount of anesthetic is injected adjacent to the penetrating shaft. With a #11 or #15 blade, a small incision is made in line with the barb, inside the concave portion of the hook (Fig. 15-6). The portion of the shaft at skin level is grasped with a hemostat; and the hook is removed with a sharp, rapid pulling motion. The pulling motion is in direct line with length of the shaft closest to the barb of the hook.

String Traction

Another method for removing a hook with small barbs requires the use of some string with good tensile strength like umbilical tape or 0-silk suture (Fig. 15-7). The string is looped around the curved portion of the shaft of the hook and is gently drawn parallel to and in the opposite direction of the straight portion of the shaft. The straight shaft and eyelet portions are depressed against the skin to slightly rotate the barb from its point of attachment in the skin. The string is given a sharp pull to release the hook. Caution is suggested as bystanders might find themselves in the pathway of the hook. This method

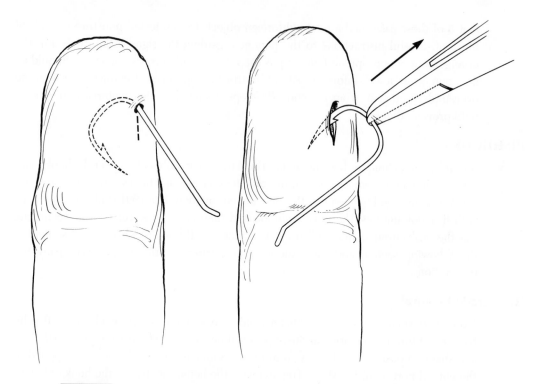

FIG. 15-6 Technique for removing a fishhook with a small barb. Note that a small incision is made in line with the concavity of the curve of the hook. The needle is then gently backed out through this incision.

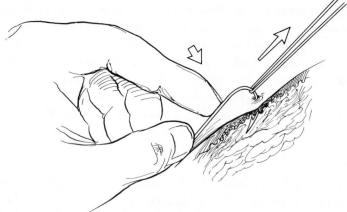

FIG. 15-7 Technique for removing a fishhook with a small barb by using traction with 0 silk or umbilical tape. Note that pressure is applied to the shaft of the hook towards the skin as a swift "yank" of the cord is applied in the direction opposite the barb. Care is taken to warn bystanders that the fishhook could fly across the room. Placing a small piece of adhesive tape around the hook and string might help avoid this hazard.

of hook removal does not require the administration of an anesthetic. This method was successful in 17 of 97 cases.

Barb Cover Technique

Another removal method is carried out with the use of an 18- or 16-gauge needle. As illustrated in Fig. 15-8 the needle is introduced into the skin through the original wound entry site. It is passed adjacent to the shaft until the hollow portion of the needle point can be placed over, or "cover" the barb. While both are held firmly together, the needle and hook are brought back out through the wound site. The needle effectively sheaths the barb and prevents it from snagging on tissue during removal. In 7 of 97 cases hooks were removed with this technique.

Hook Push-Through

For deeply embedded hooks or those with large barbs, the push-through method is recommended. With 56 of 97 hook removals, this method was the most commonly used technique. Trying to back out a deeply penetrated or large barbed hook can cause excessive tissue damage. Basic skin preparation is carried out, and a small amount of local anesthetic is injected at the site through which the hook point is to be extruded. Using a hemostat as a grasping instrument, the hook shaft is manipulated in such a manner so as

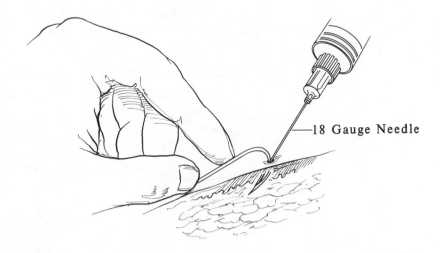

18 Gauge Needle

FIG. 15-8   Technique for removing a fishhook by placing an 18-gauge needle on the barb of the hook and backing it out through the puncture wound.

to push the hook point out through the dermis (Fig. 15-9). The hook is then clipped off with wire cutters, and the shaft is backed out of the wound.

Certain anatomic sites deserve separate mention. Hooks embedded in cartilage, most commonly the ear or nose, cannot be successfully backed out. The push-through method is recommended for these sites. Hooks that penetrate into joint capsules are also best removed by the push-through method because barbs can break off in the joint space when backed out. Violation of a joint space can lead to serious complications;

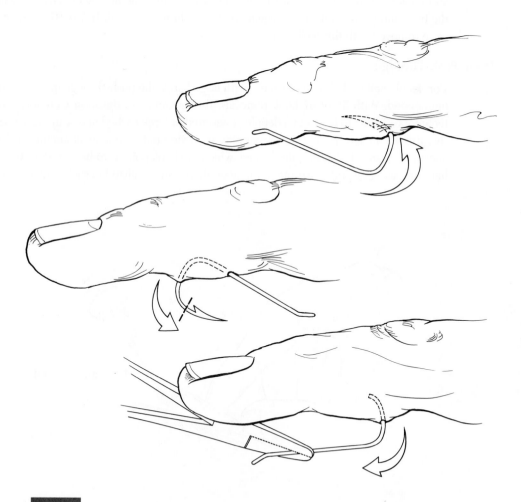

FIG. 15-9   The push-through technique for removing hooks with large barbs or hooks that are lodged in cartilage or joint spaces. The anesthetic is infiltrated in the area of the hook and the projected exit site. Once the exit has been accomplished, the barb is removed, and the shaft is backed out through the original puncture site.

therefore consultation is encouraged. Occasionally, fishhooks penetrate the cornea or other part of the globe. This complication constitutes an emergency. No attempt is made to remove the hook in an emergency wound-care area. Ophthalmologic consultation is mandatory. If the patient has to be transferred to another facility for hook removal, he or she should be placed in a semirecumbent position to decrease eye pressure. A metal eyeshield is taped gently over the eye, avoiding any direct contact or pressure on the eye. Pressure-patching with gauze sponges is absolutely contraindicated to avoid extrusion of intraocular contents through the eye wound.

ABRASIONS AND TATTOOING

Abrasions are skin wounds caused by tangential trauma to the epidermis and dermis, the "skinned knee." The skin is forced against a resistant surface in a rubbing or scraping fashion. The resultant injury is analogous to a burn. Varying thicknesses of epidermis and dermis can be lost, including tissue as deep as the superficial fascia and even bone. Abrasions can be very small or can cover large body surface areas. Frequently these injuries are impregnated with dirt, debris, and road tar. The principles for management include prevention of infection, promotion of rapid healing, and prevention of "tattooing" from the retained foreign material. This latter problem is of special cosmetic importance because, once the healing process traps unsightly debris in the epidermis and dermis, it cannot easily be removed by later surgical intervention.

Most abrasions are small and relatively clean. Like burns, however, they are extremely sensitive and painful to the touch. Cleansing has to be gentle, yet thorough. An appropriate wound-cleansing solution will suffice to remove surface contaminants and to prepare the wound for dressing. Povidone-iodine solution, without detergent, or chlorhexidine, as described in Chapter 6, are effective in cleaning abrasions.

Cleansing of contaminated and debris-laden abrasions can be tedious and difficult. If the abrasion is small, a local anesthetic can be injected around the area in a "field" or circumferential pattern. Once the pain is eliminated, scrubbing with a sponge or soft surgical brush can take place, using an appropriate cleansing solution. If necessary, meticulous removal of all particulate debris can be aided by using a needle, a #11 surgical blade, or a small-jaw tissue forceps. If all ground-in particulate matter cannot be removed in the emergency department with these steps, consultation is recommended to manage this potential cosmetic problem.

Large abrasions that are heavily contaminated are difficult to manage in an emergency wound-care area because the volume of local anesthetic necessary to achieve anesthesia would exceed toxic limits. In these cases, parenteral sedation is recommended, and in extreme cases, the patient might be better served in an operating suite.

One of the most common foreign contaminants of abrasions is road tar or asphalt. If permanently impregnated in skin, tar is a cosmetic disaster because of its dark color. All tar or asphalt particles must be removed during initial wound cleansing and debridement. A cleansing adjunct that is very useful for tar removal is polyoxyethylene sorbitan, a nonionic surface-active agent with both hydrophilic and lyophilic properties.[3] It is an emulsifying agent that is virtually nontoxic to tissue. This substance is most commonly available as a component of Neosporin G antibacterial cream. Neosporin or Polysporin ointments, with a petrolatum base, are also helpful in dissolving tar and can be substituted for the cream when it is not available.[8] However, the ointment is not as effective and is not water soluble like the cream. The water-solubility of the cream makes it easy to wash off after it has been applied to the tar-laden abrasion. Another effective commercial tar removal agent is Medi-Sol, a high-purity hydrocarbon that contains limonene, lanolin, and aloe vera. It is also an adhesive remover.

Once an abrasion is initially cleansed and debrided, follow-up management is usually the patient's responsibility. The abrasion must be kept clean to prevent secondary infection. Nature's dry "dressing," the scab, ultimately does the job and most abrasions heal without event, neither infectious or cosmetic. Wound desiccation, however, has been demonstrated experimentally in humans to slow wound healing and impede epithelial cell covering of the injured surface.[14] Dressings provide a moist environment that promotes rapid and effective healing.

For wounds that can be easily covered with a dressing, any nonadherent dressing can be applied over a thin coating of an ointment, such as Neosporin or Polysporin. A bewildering variety of dressing materials are available. Adaptic, Telfa, and Vaseline gauze are the least expensive. Other options include products such as membrane (Tegaderm), foam (Epilock), and hydrocolloid (Duoderm) dressings. The dressing can be removed every 2 or 3 days for gentle cleansing and redressing.

Experimentally, topical antibiotic ointments alone have been demonstrated to increase the rate of wound reepithelialization.[13] Therefore it is recommended that wounds that cannot be easily dressed should be kept moist with a thin coating of an antibiotic ointment like Neosporin or Polysporin.[12] The ointment is usually applied 2 or 3 times a day to maintain the moist wound environment.

REFERENCES

1. Anderson M, Newmeyer W, Kilgore E: Diagnosis and treatment of retained foreign bodies in the hand, *Am J Surg* 144:563-565, 1982.
2. Bodne D, Quinn SF, Cochran CF: Imaging foreign glass and wooden bodies of the extremities with CT and MRI, *J Comput Assist Tomogr* 12:608-611, 1988.
3. Bose B, Tredget T: Treatment of hot tar burns, *Can Med Assoc J* 127:21-22, 1982.
4. Byron T: Foreign bodies found in the foot, *J Am Pod Assoc* 71:30-35, 1981.
5. Chisholm CD: Plantar puncture wounds: controversies and treatment recommendations, *Ann Emerg Med* 18:1352-1357, 1989.
6. Cracchiolo A: Wooden foreign bodies in the foot, *Am J Surg* 140:585-587, 1980.
7. Davis L: Removal of subungual foreign bodies (letter), *J Fam Pract* 11:714, 1980.

8. Demling R, Buerstatte W, Perea A: Management of hot tar burns, *J Trauma* 20:242, 1980.

9. Doser C, Cooper WL, Ediger WM, et al: Fishhook injuries: a prospective evaluation, *Am J Emerg* Med 9:413-415, 1991.

10. Feldman AH, Fisher MS: The radiographic detection of glass in soft tissue, *Radiology* 92:1529-1531, 1969.

11. Fischer MC, Goldsmith JF, Gilligan PH: Sneakers as a source of *Pseudomonas aeruginosa* in children with osteomyelitis following puncture wounds, *J Pediatr* 106:607-614, 1985.

12. Fitzgerald R, Cowan J: Puncture wounds of the foot, *Orthop Clin North Am* 6:965-972, 1975.

13. Geronemus R, Mertz P, Eaglestein W: Wound healing: the effects of topical antimicrobial agents, *Arch Derm* 115:1311-1314, 1979.

14. Hinman C, Maibach H: Effect of air exposure and occlusion on experimental human skin wounds, *Nature* 200:377-378, 1963.

15. Houston A, et al: Tetanus prophylaxis in the treatment of puncture wounds of patients in the deep South, *J Trauma* 2:439-450, 1962.

16. Jacobs RF, Adelman L, Sack CM: Management of *Pseudomonas* osteochondritis complicating puncture wounds of the foot, *Pediatrics* 69:432-435, 1982.

17. Jarvis JG, Skipper J: Pseudomonas osteochondritis complicating puncture wounds in children, *J Pediatr Orthop* 14:755-759, 1994.

18. Joseph WF, LeFrock JL: Infections complicating puncture wounds of the foot, *J Foot Surg* 26:S30-S33, 1987.

19. Kahn B: Foreign body (palm thorn) in knee joint, *Clin Orthop* 135:104-106, 1978.

20. Lammers RL: Soft tissue foreign bodies, *Ann Emerg Med* 17:1336-1347, 1988.

21. Martinez TT, Jerome M, Barry RC, et al: Removal of cactus spines from the skin: a comparative evaluation of several methods, *Am J Dis Child* 141:1291-1292, 1987.

22. McFadden J: Stereotaxic pinpointing of foreign bodies in the limbs, *Ann Surg* 175:81-85, 1972.

23. Montano JB, Steele MT, Watson WR: Foreign body retention in glass-caused wounds, *Ann Emerg Med* 21:1365-1368, 1992.

24. Patzakis MJ, Wilkins J, Brien WW, et al: Wound site as predictor of complications following deep nail punctures of the foot, *West J Med* 150:545-547, 1989.

25. Rhoades C, Saye I, Levine E, et al: Detection of a wooden foreign body in the hand using computed tomography: case report, *J Hand Surg* 7:306-307, 1982.

26. Rudner E, Mehregan A: Implantation dermatosis, *J Cutan Pathol* 7:330-331, 1980.

27. Schwab RA, Powers RD: Conservative therapy of plantar puncture wounds, *J Emerg Med* 13:291-295, 1995.

28. Steele MT, Tran LV, Watson WA, et al: Patient perception of retained foreign body in wounds caused by glass, *Acad Emerg Med* 1:A47, 1994 (abstract).

29. Tanberg D: Glass in the hand and foot, *JAMA* 248:1872-1874, 1982.

30. Wayne R, Carnazzo A: Needle in the foot, *Am J Surg* 129:599, 1975.

16 *Minor Burns*

The treatment of burns is a common activity for facilities and personnel who care for emergency wounds and injuries. A thorough understanding of the treatment requirements of burns is necessary to properly select those patients who can be managed appropriately on an outpatient basis and those who need referral for specialized care. The depth, type, and extent of the burn; anatomic location; and underlying patient condition are all important factors in making that decision. Although individual treatment aspects of minor burns remain somewhat controversial, basic management principles do not vary greatly. The three main principles for treating the patient with burns are: relief of pain, prevention of infection and additional trauma, and minimization of scarring and contracture.[2]

INITIAL MANAGEMENT AND PATIENT ASSESSMENT

No matter how small or trivial a burn appears, the patient must be assessed for more severe associated problems and injuries. If the patient sustained the burn at the scene of a fire or explosion, immediate evaluation for inhalation injury, carbon monoxide exposure, and other trauma is mandatory. Inhalation injury is the most common cause of mortality in fire victims.[20] Clinical signs of inhalation injury include burned nasal hairs, soot on the face, hoarseness, coughing, shortness of breath, and wheezing. Even if these signs are not present at the outset, an inhalation injury must be suspected in patients who were trapped in an enclosed, smoke-filled space. Respiratory tract injury is often delayed, and observation of the patient for 24 hours may be indicated.[1] Carbon monoxide exposure is suspected in any patient who is alert and has a headache or in a patient with confusion or other alteration of mental status.

Once the patient is initially stabilized, vital signs have been taken, and unnecessary articles of clothing removed from the burned area, attention can be turned to the burn itself. The most salient clinical symptom of minor burns is pain. Epidermal (first-degree) and superficial partial-thickness (superficial second-degree) burns can be extremely painful and require immediate pain relief. The simplest and most rapid manner in which to abolish burn pain is by placing moist, cool towels over the burned area.[8] There is clinical and experimental evidence demonstrating that the cooling of burned surfaces can decrease the eventual damage to burned tissues.[4, 6, 13, 16] The water should not be very cold because excessive cold itself can compound the burn injury. A water temperature of 8° C (45° F) to 23° C (75° F) appears to be optimal to obtain both pain relief and some measure of protection for burned tissue.[6] Cooling can be effective for up to 60 minutes postburn. Care must be taken to ensure that large burn areas are not covered with cool, moist towels for excessive periods of time because hypothermia can set in. In addition to cool towels and sponges, parenteral pain medicine such as morphine sulfate or meperidine can be used; especially for patients who have a significant component of anxiety associated with their burns.

While the patient is being stabilized and pain relief is being administered, a thorough history is taken. Items of importance in the history include the age of the patient, any associated conditions and illnesses, psychosocial considerations, and drug allergies. Patients under 2 years old have thin dermis and immature immune systems.[7, 9] These children are rarely treated on an outpatient basis. Likewise, patients over 65 years old tolerate burns poorly and often need inpatient care. Patients with underlying diseases such as diabetes, pulmonary disease, severe cardiac problems, and disorders requiring chronic immunosuppressive therapy are at higher risk with burns and require special consideration for hospital management.

Frequently, burn victims have significant psychosocial problems. Like automobile trauma victims, burn victims often have alcohol- or drug-related disorders. Although these impairments may have nothing to do with the treatment of the burn itself, a severe alcohol or drug dependency may preclude outpatient management, even for minor burns. The worst psychosocial problem associated with burns is child abuse. Experienced burn-care personnel see this catastrophe all too frequently and tend to think of all children with burns as potential victims of child abuse, until proven otherwise. Finally, during the history, a thorough detailing of allergies is necessary because a large number of drugs can be administered or applied to a burn victim during the course of his or her management.

BURN ASSESSMENT
Cause of the Burn

Knowing the cause of a burn can make a difference in predicting its depth and extent. Brief scalding burns, which occur with the spilling or splashing of hot water, usually result in epidermal or superficial partial-thickness burns. Burns caused by immersion into a hot liquid and/or flame contact more frequently cause deep partial-thickness or full-thickness burns. These burns can be complicated and serious, especially when important anatomic parts such as the hands or face are involved. Electrical burns almost always cause full-thickness injuries at the burn site. In addition, electrical injuries can be associated with muscle necrosis, fractures, and cardiac arrhythmias.[15]

Body Location

The anatomic location of a burn is an important factor in determining management. Because of the complexity and crucial function of the hands, extensive partial-thickness or full-thickness burns on the hands are best managed, at least at the outset, in a controlled setting. Not only do hand burns require careful cleansing, debridement, and dressing, but there is also a danger of joint stiffening secondary to the immobility caused by pain and edema. Patients must observe strict elevation of the burned extremity in addition to early motion exercises to prevent "freezing" of the hand. This complication occurs more frequently in patients over the age of 50. Partial-thickness burns of the face not only raise the possibility of airway obstruction and inhalation injury, but they also can be very difficult to manage surgically.

Burns of the perineum are technically difficult to manage and are extremely uncomfortable for the patient. It is beyond the capabilities of most patients or families to care for these problems at home. Among the most frustrating burns to manage on an outpatient basis are those of the foot. The dependent nature of this anatomic part and its weight-bearing function cause frequent failure of outpatient management. It is very difficult for patients to voluntarily maintain the necessary strict elevation of their legs, a failure that can lead to edema, pain, and tissue breakdown at the burn site.

Depth of the Burn

Burns are traditionally divided into three depths of tissue injury: epidermal (first-degree burns); partial-thickness (second-degree burns); and full-thickness (third-degree burns). Partial-thickness or second-degree burns are further subdivided into superficial and deep partial-thickness burns.

Epidermal or first-degree burns are the most common type of burns. Heat induces dermal vasodilation, giving the epidermis its characteristic red color. Blistering does not occur and these burns heal without treatment. The superficial epidermis sloughs or peels about 5 to 7 days after the burn is sustained and the vasodilation gradually disappears. Sunburn is the most common example of an epidermal burn. Occasionally, if the heat exposure was especially intense or prolonged, what appears to be an epidermal burn blisters and becomes a superficial partial-thickness burn after 12 to 24 hours.

Partial-thickness or second-degree burns are so designated because the epidermis and part of the dermis are destroyed. However, dermal appendages such as pilosebaceous units and eccrine sweat glands survive, giving the skin a chance to regenerate epidermis from these preserved dermal foci. These remaining appendages are crucial to eventual healing and recovery.

Clinically, it is important to distinguish between superficial and deep partial-thickness burns. There are important differences in the time they require to heal and in eventual cosmetic appearance. Superficial partial-thickness burns classically blister and are extremely painful. When the necrotic epidermis is removed, the injured dermis is homogeneously pink and moist in appearance. It is extremely sensitive to touch, but will heal without scarring in a 2- to 3-week period. Deep partial-thickness burns are not as painful to touch and they appear drier and whiter when debrided. Sometimes the surface of these burns is interspersed with reddish spots, indicating underlying dermal plexus. However, there still is some awareness of pinprick and some of the dermal appendages are preserved. These burns take longer than 3 weeks to heal.

With full-thickness or third-degree burns the dermis, as well as the dermal appendages, are totally destroyed. A dry, taut, leatherlike surface that is insensitive to examination or pinprick characterizes the appearance of these burn injuries. The color of these burned areas can vary from white to brown to outright black. There is frequent difficulty in distinguishing between deep partial-thickness and full-thickness burns on initial presentation of a patient to a wound-care facility. Often these two types of burns are treated in the same manner and require grafting for final coverage of the damaged area.

Extent of the Burn

Proper estimation of the extent of body surface area affected is crucial to burn management. Only partial-thickness (second-degree) and full-thickness (third-degree) injuries are considered in the calculation. Epidermal (first-degree) burns are not included. The "rule of nines" is adequate for initially estimating burn size in adults (Fig. 16-1). Surface anatomy can be divided into areas that represent 9% or multiples of 9% of the body surface. The head and each arm constitute a 9% surface area apiece, whereas one leg is 18%. The entire surface area of the thorax and abdomen combined, anterior and posterior, is 36%.

Greater precision in estimating burn size can be obtained by using standard, more detailed charts that subdivide the anatomic parts. These diagrams also take into account the variations in surface area that occur with age (Fig. 16-2). In young children the surface area of the head constitutes a much greater area relative to the rest of the body than in adults. As an individual grows, the lower extremities get proportionately larger, while the trunk and arms stay relatively the same throughout life. Final surface area proportions are not reached until after the age of 15.

GUIDELINES FOR HOSPITALIZATION

Box 16-1 lists suggested criteria for hospital management of burns. Patients not meeting these criteria can be considered to be minor, partial-thickness burn victims and can be

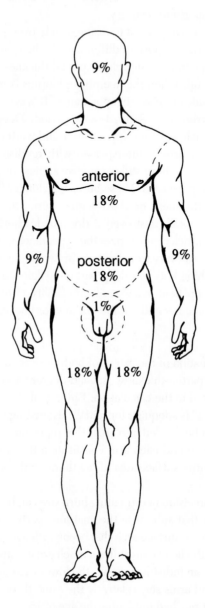

FIG. 16-1   Rapid estimation of burn extent can be determined by the "rule of nines." This rule is illustrated above. Only partial-thickness (second-degree) and full-thickness (third-degree) burns are considered for percentage area determination.

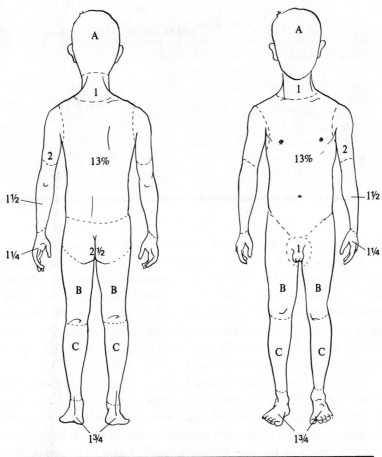

AREA	Age 0	1 yr.	5 yrs.	10 yrs.	15 yrs.
A = ½ of head	9 ½%	8 ½ %	6 ½ %	5 ½ %	4 ½ %
B = ½ of one thigh	2 ¾	3 ¼	4	4 ¼	4 ½
C = ½ of one leg	2 ½	2 ½	2 ¾	3	3 ¼

FIG. 16-2   Estimation of burn size in children. Note that the relative area sizes change significantly with age.

BOX 16-1

Guidelines for Hospital Admission of Burn Victims

Partial-thickness burns >15% surface area (>10% surface area of child)
Full-thickness burns >3% surface area
Suspected inhalation injury
Age <2 or >65
Partial- or full-thickness burns of hands, face, perineum, or feet
Electrical burns
Severe underlying systemic disease
Acute alcohol or drug abuse
Suspected child abuse

---

treated as outpatients. Different authorities vary on what constitutes an appropriate burn size that can be treated without having to admit the patient to a hospital. The total extent of burn limit for outpatient management varies between 10% to 15% of the area that has sustained a superficial-thickness burn.[4,9] The author, who advocates 10% burn-surface area as the cut-off point, believes that pain relief, initial cleansing, debridement, and patient education are best accomplished in a controlled patient setting. Highly motivated, responsible adults with good family support systems probably will do well on an outpatient basis with burns approaching the 15% range.

Children are best managed on an inpatient basis with any partial-thickness burn that is greater than 10%. Again, pain relief, wound cleansing, debridement, and dressings are easier to manage in the hands of experienced personnel. After the parents recover from the trauma, they can be properly educated in the care of the burn before the child is discharged. Except for the most trivial burn, children under 2 years old should be managed in-house. On the other end of the age scale, it is recommended that patients over the age of 65 be considered for similar treatment.

As previously discussed, burns in crucial anatomic locations such as the hands, feet, face, and perineum are best managed in an inpatient setting. Full-thickness burns of greater than 3% of the body surface area require surgical management and grafting. Even smaller full-thickness burns, if initially treated out of the hospital, need to be referred to a specialist for continued management and possible later skin grafting.

If there is any suspicion of inhalation or airway injury, no matter how small or superficial the burn, the patient must be admitted for observation. Inhalation injury can be insidious, and overt signs and symptoms often do not appear for several hours postexposure.[1] Finally, the decision to treat patients in the hospital is often determined by the extent of underlying disease, alcohol or drug abuse, and suspicion of potential child abuse.

TREATMENT OF MINOR BURNS

The large majority of burns that are treated on an outpatient basis are epidermal or superficial partial-thickness burns. Because these burns tend to have an overwhelmingly favorable outcome irrespective of treatment, some of the controversies over management are not crucial. However, for the sake of completeness, these controversies are mentioned in context with each management step.

Epidermal Burns

Epidermal or first-degree burns usually are called to the attention of medical care personnel only if the burns are extensive or very painful. A gentle cleansing with a nonirritating soap, such as Ivory Flakes or Dreft soap, mixed in a solution of cool saline is recommended. Diluted (with 2 to 4 parts cool saline) chlorhexidine (Hibiclens) can also be used.[2] For home symptom relief, the patient can apply any number of commercial preparations containing at least 60% aloe vera. Not only does this compound have some antimicrobial activity, but it provides local pain relief as well.[7, 9] Analgesia can be supplemented with aspirin, ibuprofen, acetaminophen, or codeine for up to 48 to 72 hours, after which the acute pain eventually subsides.

These burns usually heal within 5 to 7 days after going through epidermal desquamation. Occasionally, epidermal burns convert to superficial-thickness injuries with blistering 12 to 24 hours after heat exposure. Should this occur, returning to a medical-care facility or contacting the primary-care physician is recommended.

Partial-Thickness Burns
Cleansing

Partial-thickness burns are also best managed by an initial cleansing with a nonirritating soap, Dreft, or with chlorhexidine (Hibiclens) diluted in 2 to 4 parts of cool saline. Ice chips can be mixed into the solution to provide a cooling effect. Hair can be clipped but should not be shaved with a razor in the burn site to prevent any further damage to the remaining dermal appendages from which new epidermis arises.[17] To effectively clean and debride a partial-thickness burn, which is extremely sensitive to touch or manipulation, a parenteral narcotic is often recommended for the patient.

Blisters and Debridement

Once cleansing has taken place, the next step is debridement. Obviously necrotic and partially sloughed epidermis and dermis are removed by using forceps and tissue scissors. This skin is dead and insensitive. Therefore local anesthetics are not required. A controversy in burn management is whether to remove intact blisters. Proponents for blister removal point to the ideal culture media that blister fluid represents with a concomitant risk of burn infection.[9] There is clinical and experimental evidence, however, that leaving blisters intact has several beneficial effects on burn wounds.[11, 12, 22] Intact blisters tend to prevent capillary stasis and retard necrosis within burn injury sites, as well as decrease desiccation of the burn wound. It is also believed that retention of blisters aids in the control of pain, a benefit that is especially important over joint surfaces where pain can limit active movement, thereby leading to potential joint stiffness.[18] As a general rule, large confluent blisters are likely to break easily and should be removed. Small intact blisters on the hands, feet, and over joints should be left intact. It can be argued that blisters on noncompliant patients should be removed to prevent infection from neglect or improper home care.

Burn Dressing

Preferences for burn dressing vary widely among practitioners who care for burns. Topical treatments range from no agent at all to a variety of topical antibiotics and several newer synthetic wound coverings. Because the eventual outcome of limited superficial partial-thickness burns is uniformly good, there is no clear preference for one agent or dressing over another. In fact, small partial-thickness burns, if kept clean and protected, heal without ointments or specialized dressings.

Uncomplicated, partial-thickness burns of the head and neck, for practical reasons, are best left open during treatment. Gentle cleansing 1 to 2 times a day followed by application of antibacterial ointment leads to complete healing in a 2 to 3 week period.

The open method is an alternative for small burns of the hand. The advantages are maintenance of mobility and flexibility of the hand, freedom from dressing changes, and continued partial use. Because of continued wound exudate and the need to maintain antibacterial ointment on the burn, the open method can be somewhat problematic.

Most other partial- and full-thickness burns are treated with burn dressings (Fig. 16-3). After cleansing and debridement, the burned area is covered with an antibacterial ointment or cream with a gloved finger or sterile applicator. Petroleum-based ointments such as Bacitracin or Polysporin are preferred for ease of application, enhanced wound healing, and good suppression of bacterial colonization.[7] Silver sulfadiazine (Silvadene) is an effective antibacterial but is impractical for open treatment and can form a pseudomembrane over partial-thickness burns that is difficult and painful to remove. The ointment is followed by a single layer of fine-mesh gauze or a nonadherent material such as Adaptic. Gauze "fluffs," created by unfolding gauze 4 × 4 sponges, are packed over the fine gauze layer. The fluffs absorb copious drainage created by the fresh wound. The dressing is anchored with gauze bandage roll and tape strips.

The interval between dressing changes varies among practitioners. Many burn authorities recommend twice daily changes to maintain the effectiveness of the antibacterial ointment or cream. In practicality, once daily changes are probably sufficient for the limited partial-thickness burn. Patients are sent home with specific instructions and burn supplies as listed. The follow-up interval can vary based on the compliance and motivation of the patient and the extent and location of the burn. Burns of the hand need close follow-up with a visit to a caregiver within 48 to 72 hours of the injury. Further visits are individualized.

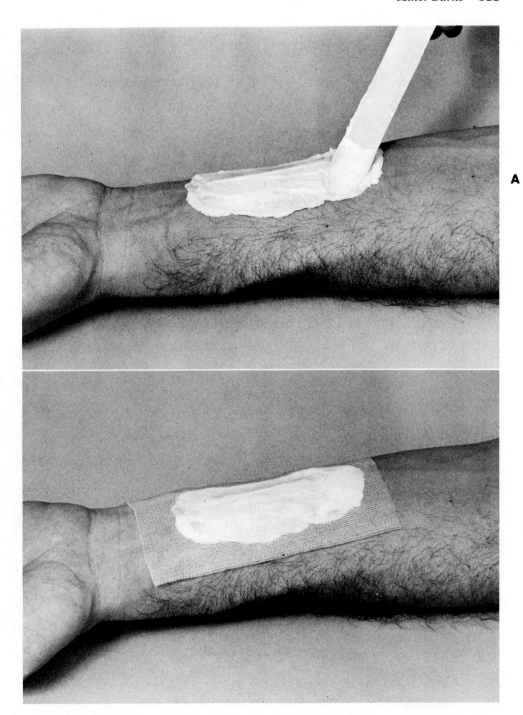

FIG. 16-3   Burn dressing application. **A,** Burn ointment of choice is applied with a sterile blade. **B,** A nonadherent dressing material is placed directly over the cream.   *Continued*

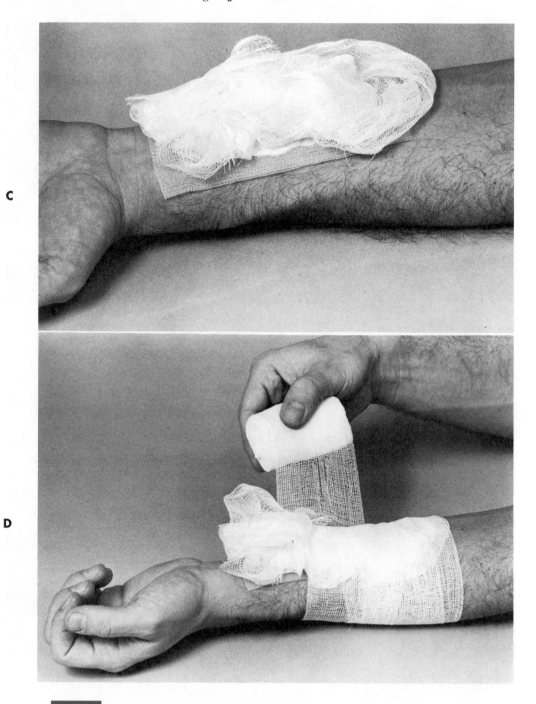

C

D

FIG. 16-3, *cont'd* **C,** Gauze sponges or gauze "fluffs" are placed over the nonadherent base. **D,** Gauze wrapping completes the dressing.

Synthetic dressings offer another alternative for the limited partial-thickness burn patient. There are many products on the market including Duoderm, Opsite, Vigilon, and Biobrane. These dressings can be applied to fresh burns that have been cleaned and debrided of dead skin or any debris.[5] The dressing is cut in a customized manner to correspond to the burn site with approximately a 1 to 2 cm marginal overlap. An outer gauze wrap is applied to maintain dressing adherence and absorb excessive exudate. These dressings afford good pain relief and can be left on for the duration of the healing. They are, however, time consuming and somewhat difficult to apply. They can dry, crack, and peel at the edges.[21] These dressings are not suitable for covering joints or large areas. Use of these dressings should be in consultation and agreement with the caregiver responsible for follow-up and ongoing care once the patient leaves the emergency department.

Home Management and Follow-Up

Burn supplies, including gauze sponges, gauze wrap, antibacterial soap, and a sterile tongue depressor are dispensed or prescribed along with written and verbal instructions on how to use them. A small jar or tube of topical antimicrobial agent is also dispensed or prescribed. The patient is instructed to remove the first dressing the morning after his or her first wound-care visit. The burned area is gently washed with the soap and two or three of the sterile sponges provided. A topical agent is spread over the wound and gauze wrapping is applied. Some authorities believe that the first dressing can remain in place for 2 or 3 days. At the University of Cincinnati it is believed that once- or twice-a-day changes prevent the exudate buildup and crusting that can disrupt epithelization when infrequent dressing changes are made. Again, there is no clear evidence to support any specific dressing change interval for minor burns.

All minor burn victims are seen in follow-up 48 hours after initial treatment. From that time on, individualized treatment regimens are prescribed. Strict elevation of the burned part is essential to proper healing. The use of slings for upper-extremity and hand burns can accomplish this goal while the patient is in an upright position. Gentle but frequent motion of joints within the burn-injured anatomic parts is also mandatory. Pain often deters a patient from this activity, so appropriate oral medication like aspirin, ibuprofen, acetaminophen, or codeine may be required early during convalescence. Usually, however, if the patient thoroughly understands the need for joint motion, cooperation with burn-care personnel quickly follows in spite of some wound discomfort.

Full-Thickness Burns

Full-thickness burns that cover less than 3% of the body surface area and that are in a noncritical site (hand or face) can be treated in the manner described previously for partial-thickness burns. However, before proceeding it is best to discuss the case with a consultant. These patients require close follow-up care, and initial treatment decisions are best made in concert with a consultant.

TETANUS AND ANTIBIOTIC PROPHYLAXIS

Finally, there are the considerations of tetanus prophylaxis and the possibility of wound infection. Tetanus toxoid and tetanus immune globulin should be given to all burn wounds in accordance with the recommendations in Chapter 20. Currently, there are no studies that support the use of prophylactic oral or parenteral antibiotics in the minor superficial burn setting.[3, 12, 19] Control and antibiotic-treated groups consistently yield the same infection rate of approximately 3% to 4%. Should a burn-wound infection develop, it is best managed with local wound care and appropriate antibiotics at that time.[14]

REFERENCES

1. Achauer B, et al: Pulmonary complications of burns, *Ann Surg* 177:311-319, 1973.
2. Baxter CR, Waeckerle JF: Emergency treatment of burn injury, *Ann Emerg Med* 17:1305-1315, 1988.
3. Boss WK, et al: Effectiveness of prophylactic antibiotics in the outpatient treatment of burns, *J Trauma* 25:224-227, 1985.
4. Cone JB: Minor burns: standards for outpatient treatment, *Consultant* 27:37-42, 1987.
5. Curreri W, et al: Safety and efficacy of a new synthetic burn dressing, *Arch Surg* 115:925-927, 1980.
6. Davies J: Prompt cooling of burned areas: a review of benefits and the effector mechanisms, *Burns* 9:1-6, 1983.
7. Griglak MJ: Thermal injury, *Emerg Clin North Am* 10:369-383, 1992.
8. Gruber RP, Laub DR, Vistness LM: The effect of hydrotherapy on the clinical course and pH of experimental cutaneous chemical burns, *Plast Reconstr Surg* 55:200-203, 1975.
9. Heimbach D, Engrav L, Marvin J: Minor burns, *Postgrad Med* 69:22-32, 1981.
10. Leyden JJ, et al: Comparison of antibiotic ointments, a wound protectant, and antiseptics for the treatment of human blister wounds contaminated with *Staphylococcus aureus*, *J Fam Pract* 24:601-604, 1987.
11. Moserova J, Runtova M, Broz L: The possible role of blisters in dermal burns, *Acta Chir Plast* 25:51-53, 1983.
12. Moylan J: Outpatient treatment of burns, *Postgrad Med* 73:235-242, 1983.
13. Pushkar N, Sandorminsky B: Cold treatment of burns, *Burns* 9:101-110, 1983.
14. Richards R, Mahlangu G: Therapy for burn wound infection, *J Clin Hosp Pharm* 6:223-243, 1981.
15. Sances A, et al: Electrical injuries, *Surg Gynecol Obstet* 149:97-108, 1979.
16. Saranto J, Rubayi S, Zawacki B: Blisters, cooling, antithromboxanes, and healing in experimental zone-of-stasis burns, *J Trauma* 23:927-933, 1983.
17. Shuck J: Outpatient management of the burned patient, *Surg Clin North Am* 58:108-117, 1978.
18. Swain AH, et al: Management of blisters in burns, *Br Med J* 295:181, 1987.
19. Timmons M: Are systemic prophylactic antibiotics necessary for burns? *Ann R Coll Surg Engl* 65:80-81, 1983.
20. Trunkey D: Inhalation injury, *Surg Clin North Am* 58:1133-1140, 1978.
21. Warren R, Snelling C: Clinical evaluation of the Hydron gel burn dressing, *Plast Reconstr Surg* 66:361-368, 1980.
22. Zawacki B: Reversal of capillary stasis and prevention of necrosis in burns, *Ann Surg* 180:98-102, 1974.

17 Cutaneous and Superficial Abscesses

Clinical Presentations
Microbiology of Abscesses
Management of Abscesses
   Technique for Incision and Drainage
   Special Treatment Settings

Follow-Up Care
Antibiotic Use in Abscess Care

Cutaneous and other superficial abscesses are commonly diagnosed and treated in emergency departments. The procedural nature of abscess care makes it a problem with similar technical requirements as wounds and lacerations. Although drainage is the key therapeutic intervention for all abscesses, significant differences exist between types and locations that necessitate individualized treatment. Most cases can be managed in the emergency department with routine outpatient follow-up care. A few, however, require specialist consultation for possible operative intervention or inpatient management.

CLINICAL PRESENTATIONS

A cutaneous abscess can be defined as a "localized collection of pus causing a fluctuant soft tissue swelling surrounded by firm granulation tissue and erythema." Abscesses can begin as furuncles, which are firm, red, tender nodules that go on to become fluctuant, and if left untreated, drain spontaneously. Cutaneous abscesses can occur on any body surface but tend to be more common in certain areas.[6] The most common sites are head, neck, axillae, and the buttock and perineal areas. Carbuncles are deep abscesses, with multiple loculations, that occur at the nape of the neck, back, and thighs. Any interruption of the protective layers of the skin, even trivial, with subsequent invasion of exogenous or endogenous microflora, can lead to abscess formation. Abscesses are commonly a result of an obstruction of the apocrine and sebaceous glands. Sebaceous glands are widely distributed over the body, and apocrine glands are found most commonly in axillae and anogenital regions. These glands frequently form cysts that are prone to abscess formation.

Of special note are abscesses that arise on the upper lip and nose. Infections in these sites drain through the facial and angular emissary veins to the cavernous sinus. As discussed in the following section, antibiotics are indicated in the treatment of these lesions.

A common and difficult condition to manage that predisposes to abscess formation is hidradenitis suppurativa.[8] This is a chronic, relapsing, inflammatory involvement of apocrine glands of the axillae and pubic regions. Abscess formation is followed by extensive, and excessive, scarring. Recurrent abscess formation also predisposes to fistula tracks, skin, and subcutaneous induration and inflammation in various stages of progression. Emergency management is limited to incision and drainage of the discrete abscesses. These patients require long-term care and a program of management best coordinated and carried out by specialists such as dermatologists or surgeons.

Although breast abscesses are commonly associated with the postpartum period, more than 90% occur outside of that period.[10] Postpartum mastitis, which can occur in nursing mothers within 2 to 6 weeks from delivery, predisposes to abscess formation. It is caused by an invasion of *Staphylococcus aureus* through sore, abraded nipples. These patients are often quite sick from extensive local involvement, pain, and chills and fever. Nonpuerperal abscesses can occur in superficial, as well as deep tissues, of the breast. Superficial abscesses can be cutaneous or periareolar. Periareolar abscesses arise from occluded ducts and are associated with multiple organisms including anaerobes. They involve mammary, as well as ductal tissue. Superficial abscesses, most often resulting from *S. aureus,* are less complicated.

Deep breast abscesses are either intramammary or retromammary. As is the case for periareolar abscesses, fluctuance can be difficult to detect. Fluctuance is also difficult to diagnose when overlying cellulitis is deep and extensive. In these cases, needle aspiration may be required to ensure the proper treatment, that is, incision and drainage.

Bartholin's glands, located in the vestibule of the vagina, can form cysts from ductal occlusion. These cysts can go on to abscess formation secondary to infection from *Neisseria gonorrhea*, enteric organisms, and anaerobic bacteria. In addition to the abscess, the labia is usually inflamed and very tender. These abscesses can be confused with periovular cutaneous abscesses arising from an infected pubic hair. In addition to drainage and catheter placement as described in the following, it is recommended that sexually active patients be considered for treatment with antigonorrheal and antichlamydial antibiotics.

Pilonidal abscesses arise from cysts that form within embryologic remnant sinuses in the sacrococcygeal area. Patients often present with painful induration of the buttock crease. Fluctuance may not be appreciated; therefore needle aspiration is sometimes necessary to diagnose purulence. Cultures reveal gram-negative enteric organisms and anaerobes. These abscesses often recur unless the sinuses are excised after initial drainage.

Buttock abscesses are common but must be clinically distinguished from perianal and perirectal infections. Buttock abscesses occur cutaneously and do not involve the anus. Perianal abscesses arise from anal crypts and impinge on the anal sphincter. Unlike patients with buttock abscesses, rectal examination is very painful for patients with peri-anal abscesses. Perianal abscesses are often associated with fistula in ano. The presence of a perianal abscess might also point to other serious, related, abscesses and infections of the ischiorectal, intersphincteric, and pelvirectal areas. Patients with these abscesses complain of deep rectal or pelvic pain. They often have fever and appear toxic as mani-fested by diaphoresis and tachycardia. A rectal exam reveals marked tenderness of the anal sphincter and rectum. Masses can be palpated with the examining finger. This con-dition requires urgent intervention by a consultant in an operative setting.

A common problem seen by emergency physicians is abscess formation in parenteral drug users. Not only are the patients at risk for bacterial tissue invasion but also chemi-cal irritants that can provoke intense and extensive involvement. These abscesses are often extensive and often involve the thighs, buttocks, or forearms. Parenteral drug users have a high incidence of other infectious complications like hepatitis, endocarditis, and HIV-related disorders. Caregivers are urged to observe strict blood and body fluid precautions when draining the patient's abscesses.

MICROBIOLOGY OF ABSCESSES

A large variety of bacteria can be cultured from abscesses. Most lesions are polymicro-bial with an average of one aerobic and two anaerobic species per abscess.[7] Staphylococ-cus aureus is the most common aerobe.[3, 6, 7] It can be found in most sites with the axilla and upper extremity predominating. Anaerobes, including *Bacteroides* species, are more likely to be recovered from the vulvovaginal, buttock, and perirectal areas. For reasons that are not clear, Proteus mirabilis is commonly associated with abscesses in the head and neck regions, trunk, and axilla.[6]

Because incision and drainage alone are effective for treating abscesses, Gram stains and cultures are not routinely necessary.[6] They are recommended for patients with sys-temic symptoms (indicating extensive involvement), diabetics, parenteral drug users, and patients with conditions causing immunosuppression. In parenteral drug users with fever, blood cultures are recommended before the drainage procedure. The treatment manipulation of incision and drainage of an abscess can cause transient bacteremia in 30% of cases.[2] This bacteremia uncommonly lasts more than 20 minutes and is of no clinical consequence in otherwise healthy patients.

MANAGEMENT OF ABSCESSES

When confronted with a suspected abscess, palpation does not always reveal fluctuance. Abscesses on the back of the neck, sacrococcygeal area, buttocks and thighs can be deep or accompanied by significant overlying tissue induration. Whenever an abscess is sus-pected but clinically not evident, needle aspiration can be carried out with an 18-gauge needle attached to a 5- or 10-ml syringe. The presence of aspirated pus provides the ev-idence needed to carry out a full incision and drainage.

In patients with cardiac valvular disease, prophylactic antibiotics as recommended by the American Heart Association should be administered before incision and drainage.[9] Antibiotic prophylaxis should also be considered in patients with implanted orthopedic or other medical devices.

Technique for Incision and Drainage

Once the presence of pus has been established, either by the palpation of fluctuance or aspiration, the abscess site is briefly cleaned with a wound cleansing solution. Wound cleansing of these obviously contaminated sites is carried out to render the field clear of gross contaminants and to prevent extraneous microflora from contaminating any wound cultures should they be indicated.

Incision and drainage manipulations are exceedingly painful. For small abscesses, less than 5 cm in diameter, a field block followed by injection of the abscess roof often suffices for pain control. Parenteral narcotics and intravenous sedation techniques, as described in Chapter 5, can bring considerable relief to the patient. Even with parenteral pain relief or sedation, the incision site is always anesthetized with a local anesthetic.

The instruments and items needed to drain an abscess include a knife handle and #11 blade, a hemostat, gauze packing, and an irrigation syringe mated to a #16 or #14 gauge plastic intravenous catheter (Fig. 17-1). Once the field of local anesthesia is created, an

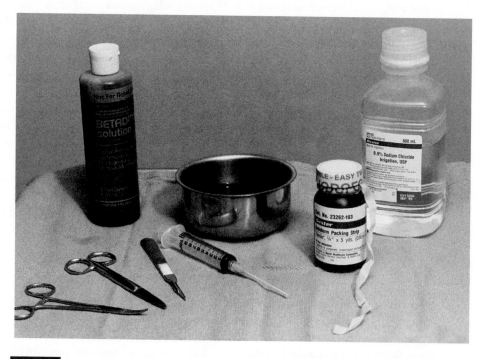

FIG. 17-1   Instruments and materials commonly used to lance, drain, and pack a cutaneous abscess.

incision is made that is the full length of the fluctuance or, at minimum, two thirds the diameter of the abscess cavity itself (Fig. 17-2). It is a common mistake to make a small, stablike incision. Wide incisions are necessary to provide for adequate cavity probing and loculation disruption, irrigation, and packing placement.

After the incision, the operator gently probes the abscess cavity with either a hemostat or finger. Once all of the abscess cavity surfaces have been explored and loculations broken up, irrigation with saline is carried out through the catheter until all purulence is evacuated. Drainage is considered adequate when the saline effluent is free from pus and appears blood tinged.

The final step in the procedure is to gently and loosely pack the abscess cavity with plain or medicated gauze. For small abscesses drained in the emergency department, ¼- or ½-inch wide gauze strips are adequate. The purpose of the gauze packing is to promote continued drainage from the abscess cavity. Excessive packing of the cavity can create the direct opposite of the intended outcome. Packing at the incision opening can become encrusted with dried purulence causing an iatrogenic obstruction to further drainage.

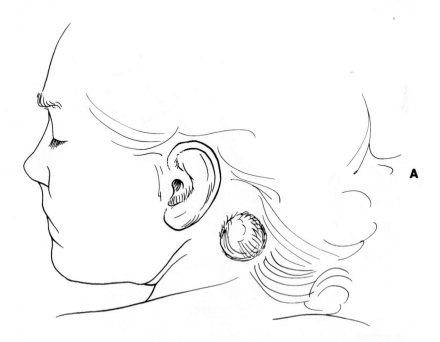

FIG. 17-2 Procedure for abscess drainage. **A,** Typical cutaneous abscess.
Continued

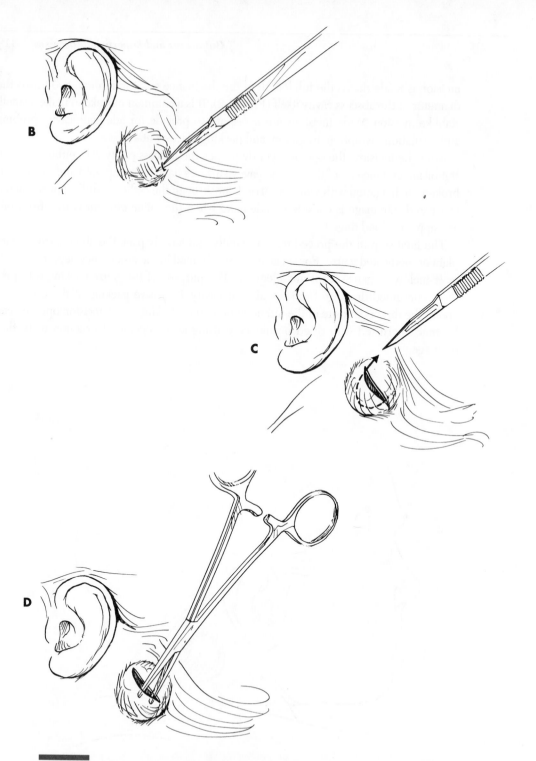

FIG. 17-2, cont'd   **B,** A scalpel with #11 blade is used to "lance" fluctuant mass. **C,** The incision should be generous and, at least, two third the diameter of the cavity. **D,** A hemostat is used to probe the cavity and gently break up loculations.

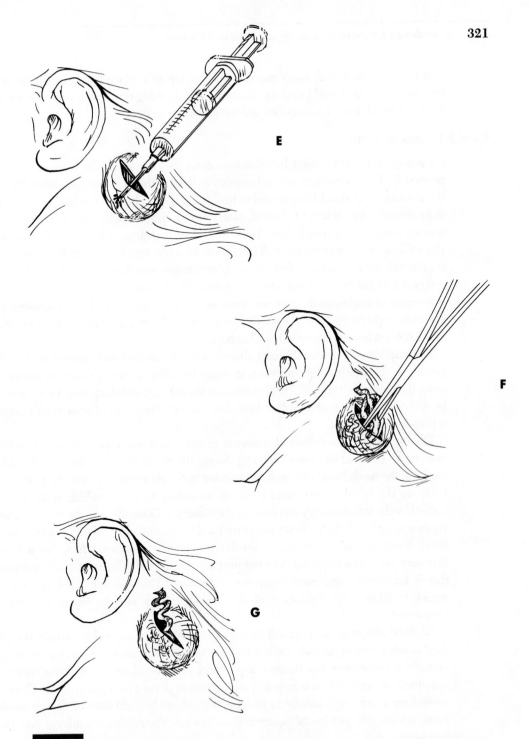

FIG. 17-2, cont'd **E,** The cavity is irrigated until the effluent is clear of purulence. **F,** Gauze tape is used to pack the cavity. Caution is taken not to overpack and obstruct subsequent flow and drainage of remaining purulence. **G,** A 2- to 3-inch tail is left to prevent incision site closure and to aid in packing removal at a later time, 2 to 3 days postprocedure.

A bulky dressing, with many gauze sponges or layers, is placed over the site to absorb the inevitable continued purulent drainage. This dressing remains in place for 48 to 72 hours, at which time it is removed and the abscess is inspected.

Special Treatment Settings

Cutaneous abscesses caused by sebaceous cysts are drained in the manner described previously. These abscesses recur, however, as long as the cyst remains. After drainage, the abscess cavity should be allowed to heal completely. The cyst can easily be removed in its entirety when it is not inflamed. Attempts to remove it at the time of abscess intervention are only met with failure. The cyst wall, at that time, is friable and easily tears. Even if a small fragment of the wall is left behind, a new cyst forms with the resultant return in risk for new abscess formation. After incision and drainage, patients should be referred for later cyst removal after all inflammation has subsided.

Because of the cosmetic concerns involved in the treatment of facial abscesses, consultation might be required. When draining a facial abscess, any incision has to conform to the tension lines as discussed in Chapter 2.

Uncomplicated superficial breast abscesses can be incised and drained as described previously. It is important, however, to make the skin incision in a radial orientation using the nipple as the "hub." Periareolar, intramammary, and deep breast abscesses can be difficult to drain and are often best done under general anesthesia in an operative setting by a consultant.

The drainage of Bartholin's abscesses is carried out using a specially designed Word catheter.[11] To avoid excessive bleeding during the procedure, the drainage incision is made on the medial wall of the abscess closest to the introitus. Incisions carried out laterally on the labial surface tend to bleed secondary to the vasodilation in that area caused by the inflammatory response to the infection. Once the incision is made and irrigation completed, the catheter is inserted and inflated. Unlike other abscesses, the incision for Bartholin's abscesses is smaller so that the catheter, which has a narrow diameter, remains secure and does not prematurely fall out. Sitz baths can begin immediately for comfort and encouragement of drainage. The catheter is left in for 4 to 6 weeks to allow epithelialization of the drainage track and to lessen the risk for recurrence.

Pilonidal abscesses are drained through generous incisions and packed in the standard manner. These patients are referred for definitive treatment by a consultant, particularly if recurrence has become a problem. Buttock abscesses are also treated as described earlier. Caution is urged in attempting to drain a perianal abscess. These abscesses are exceedingly painful to manipulate and can be indicative of deeper involvement within the pelvirectal spaces. Consultation should be considered for these abscesses.

FOLLOW-UP CARE

Most small cutaneous abscesses treated in the emergency department require a single packing that stays in place 2 to 3 days. On the first return follow-up visit, the dressing and packing are removed. With successful drainage, the patient reports significant pain relief and there is minimal continued drainage. For these patients, a regimen of daily wound soakings for 20 to 30 minutes for approximately 1 week suffices to maintain any further drainage until the abscess heals. Abscess cavities heal within a 1- to 2-week period. If the abscess is large and there is continued drainage, repacking can be carried out at 2- to 3-day intervals as necessary. If the patient complains of unremitting pain and discomfort at the drainage site on the first return visit, an undrained cavity or loculation should be considered.

ANTIBIOTIC USE IN ABSCESS CARE

For common, uncomplicated cutaneous abscesses, incision and drainage is curative. Antibiotics offer no advantage.[1, 4, 5] Under certain conditions, however, they are recommended. When the abscess is surrounded by cellulitis that extends well beyond the margins that might be accounted for by the abscess alone, antibiotics are prescribed as an adjunct. Other indications include: systemic toxicity as indicated by fever and chills, underlying comorbid condition (diabetes, disease- or drug-induced immunosuppression), face location, and cardiac valve disorder. First generation cephalosporins (Keflex, Velosef), clindamycin (Cleocin), or erythromycin provide coverage for the common organisms. Cardiac prophylaxis is administered as noted under management of abscesses.

REFERENCES

1. Blick PWH, Flowers MW, Marsden AK, et al: Antibiotics in surgical treatment of acute abscesses, *Br Med J* 281:111, 1980.
2. Fine BC, Sheckman PR, Bartlett JC: Incision and drainage of soft-tissue abscesses and bacteremia (letter), *Ann Int Med* 103:645, 1985.
3. Ghoneim ATM, McGoldrick J, Blick PWH, et al: Aerobic and anaerobic bacteriology of subcutaneous abscesses, *Br J Surg* 68:498-500, 1981.
4. Llera JL, Levy RC: Treatment of cutaneous abscess: a double-blind clinical study, *Ann Emerg Med* 14:15, 1985.
5. Macfie J, Harvey J: The treatment of acute superficial abscesses: a prospective clinical trial, *Br J Surg* 64:264, 1977.
6. Meislin HW, Lerner SA, Graves MH, et al: Cutaneous abscesses: anaerobic and aerobic bacteriology and outpatient management, *Ann Int Med* 87:145-149, 1977.
7. Meislin HW, McGehee MD, Rosen P: Management and microbiology of cutaneous abscesses, *JACEP* 7:186-191, 1978.
8. Paletta C, Jurkiewicz MJ: Hidradenitis suppurative, *Clin Plast Surg* 14:383, 1987.
9. Sanford JP, Gilbert DN, Sande MA: *Guide to antimicrobial therapy*, Dallas, 1995, Antimicrobrial Therapy.
10. Scholefield JH, Duncan JL, Rogers K: Review of a hospital experience of breast abscesses, *Br J Surg* 74:469, 1987.
11. Word B: Office treatment of cysts and abscess of Bartholin's gland duct, *South Med J* 61:514, 1968.

18 *Wound Dressing and Bandaging Techniques*

The choice of a dressing for an emergency wound is subject to the preference of the caregiver who is applying it. There are no hard and fast rules that can be followed when selecting a dressing. What follows is a discussion of the general principles of wound dressing and some recommendations for dressing and bandaging depending on the type of wound, body location, and other factors. A discussion of specialized dressings for burns is found in Chapter 16.

WOUND DRESSING PRINCIPLES

The first decision to be made after repairing a wound is whether to apply a dressing at all. Uncomplicated lacerations of the face and scalp are often left open. The head and face are very vascular, and wounds in these areas are very resistant to infection. If the patient is careful and keeps the wound clean, a sutured laceration heals without event. These wounds need the regular application of a petrolatum-based antibacterial ointment to maintain a moist environment and to help prevent crusting that can interfere with suture removal.[13] Petrolatum-based antibacterial ointments, such as Neosporin and Silvadene, have been shown experimentally to effectively encourage epithelialization when compared with other ointments such as Furacin and Pharmadine, which contains povidone-iodine.[4] Neosporin is easier to apply to the face than Silvadene, which needs to be laid down in a relatively thick layer. Other agents that can be used for this purpose are Polysporin and Bacitracin.

The generally accepted practice for wounds and lacerations that are not on the head and face is to apply a wound covering, although there is little evidence that a dressing improves the eventual outcome of sutured lacerations. One study of uncovered surgical incisions that were sutured postoperatively could not document an increase in the rate of infection when compared to dressed incisions.[6] When the decision is made to apply a dressing, the following principles should be observed.

Tidiness

A dressing must be neat and uncomplicated. Sloppy or poorly applied dressings and bandages do not convince a patient that good wound care has been delivered. A great number of small wounds are best served by a simple Band-Aid or two. This dressing remains one of the most versatile and appropriate wound coverings yet devised.

Nonadherent, Porous Base

The base of a dressing, the portion in direct contact with the wound surface, should not be adherent.[8] Plain, fine-mesh gauze is an example of a dressing that sticks to wounds by becoming incorporated in the coagulum. When it is removed, it can disrupt healing by disturbing the delicate epithelial covering. A good wound covering also has to allow for the passage of exudate so that excessive accumulation does not occur.

Moist Environment

At the same time, the wound has to remain moist. Experimental studies convincingly show that desiccation by exposure can significantly delay epithelial layer formation.[5, 8] Fig. 18-1 illustrates the pathways for epidermal healing in moist and dry environments. In

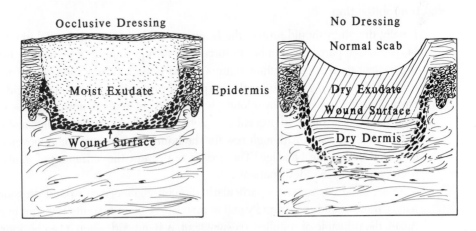

FIG. 18-1   Note the different pathways necessary for epithelial cells to migrate to provide an epithelial cell covering of an open wound. The moist environment experimentally appears to provide for more rapid healing than a dry environment as seen in open, uncovered wounds.

a nonoccluded wound, epithelial cells are forced to find a pathway beneath dry coagulum/exudate and dermal remnants.

In practice, synthetic dressings like Adaptic, Xeroform, and Telfa are traditional nonadherent, porous coverings that allow for the drainage of exudate, but do not permit excessive desiccation.

A point of controversy that has yet to be resolved is whether the application of antibacterial creams or ointments under dressings has any value.[7] Claims against the use of these agents include excessive maceration of tissue and the emergence of resistant bacteria.[1, 11] Suppression of infection and improved wound-edge healing, particularly for flaps, are reasons given in support of the use of topicals.[3, 4, 9] Currently, these agents are recommended for facial wounds (e.g., lacerations, abrasions, burns) or any other wound that is treated without dressing and bandaging. For dressed wounds, any antibacterial effect is lost unless dressings are changed at frequent intervals, at least 2 to 3 times a day.[3] This makes application of these ointments impractical for wound protection against infection.

Protection

Protection from contamination is best accomplished by ensuring that in addition to the nonadherent base, the wound is also well covered with gauze sponge material and an appropriate gauze wrap. Gauze sponges help meet this requirement of wound dressing. Most minor wounds and lacerations produce very little exudate; therefore a simple 2×2 or 4×4 gauze sponge or even a Band-Aid suffices for this purpose. Complicated or contaminated wounds with a potential for infection are likely to exude freely and copiously. In addition to several layers of gauze sponges, frequent dressing changes are often necessary.

Partial Immobilization

Finally, dressings should protect the healing wound and provide partial immobilization of the injured part. Any number of forces can disrupt a suture line, ranging from clothing contact to accidental minor trauma to the wound. Gauze sponges in combination with gauze wrapping suffice for the purpose of protection. Occasionally, rigid splinting, particularly for lacerations over joints, is necessary. In general, however, excessive wrapping should be avoided to prevent complete immobilization of a moving anatomic part, particularly the hand. Although rest for the injury is necessary, some movement is encouraged within the bandage. The goal is to prevent the stiffening of joints that can occur, especially in elderly patients.

Young children present a particularly difficult challenge in wound dressing. Fortunately, their wounds heal rapidly and in practice, seem to be quite resistant to infection. Again, the principle of simplicity is important. A Band-Aid, when it can be appropriately used, is the dressing of choice for small wounds. If the Band-Aid is removed by the child, it can easily be replaced by a parent. Children are more likely to leave Band-Aids in place because this dressing is recognized as a "badge" for other children to appreciate. When more complicated dressings have to be used, as on the hand, a "mittenlike" bandage that encompasses the entire hand is often recommended. If the laceration or wound is serious, most older children seem to have an instinctive understanding that prevents them from removing dressings.

BASIC WOUND DRESSING

The basic wound covering consists of four materials: a nonadherent base, absorbent gauze sponges, gauze wrapping if needed, and tape to secure the dressing. Standard nonadherent bases include Adaptic (a porous synthetic mesh), Telfa, and Xeroform (a treated fine-mesh gauze).

In recent years there has been a proliferation of several semipermeable, occlusive, nonadherent wound dressings that can been applied to lacerations, burns, and abrasions.[10] In a study of a modified polyurethane foam on those three types of wounds, it was found that wounds tended to heal faster, were less painful, and were easier to care for when compared to standard dressing controls.[14] Although this study was encouraging, the investigators terminated their comparison after only 20 days of observation. Final healing outcome, after scar maturation, may have been no different. Other parameters that remain to be fully explored before these new dressings can be routinely recommended for general use include bacterial growth potential at the wound site and effect on wound tensile strength.[2,8] There are conflicting data concerning possible adverse effects in these two areas. Some of these dressing materials are also considerably more expensive than older, standard materials.[14]

Dressing Application

After repair, an antibacterial ointment can be thinly and gently spread over the wound. Based on the preceding discussion, application of a topical agent for sutured lacerations can be considered optional. If one is chosen, Neosporin is commonly used. For patients sensitive to the neomycin in Neosporin, Bacitracin or Polysporin can be substituted. Although sensitivity to neomycin is a concern, an actual allergic response to patch testing is very low. Of a total of 3,333 patients reported in a review of topical agents, only 14, or 0.3%, were found to be sensitive to neomycin.[9]

In a sterile fashion, the nonadherent base is cut to conform with the general wound area as shown in Fig. 18-2. Depending on the potential for wound drainage and exudation, one or more gauze sponges are placed over the base. On an extremity, a gauze wrap is applied, followed by tape. On flat surfaces where gauze wrapping is not appropriate, the tape is placed directly over the gauze sponges.

A common tape adhesive adjunct is tincture of benzoin. This substance is very effective in keeping tape adherent to the skin for the duration of the dressing. Precautions have to be taken, however, not to spill benzoin directly into the wound. Under experimental conditions, this compound has been shown to increase the potential for wound infection when it comes into direct contact with the raw wound surface.[12]

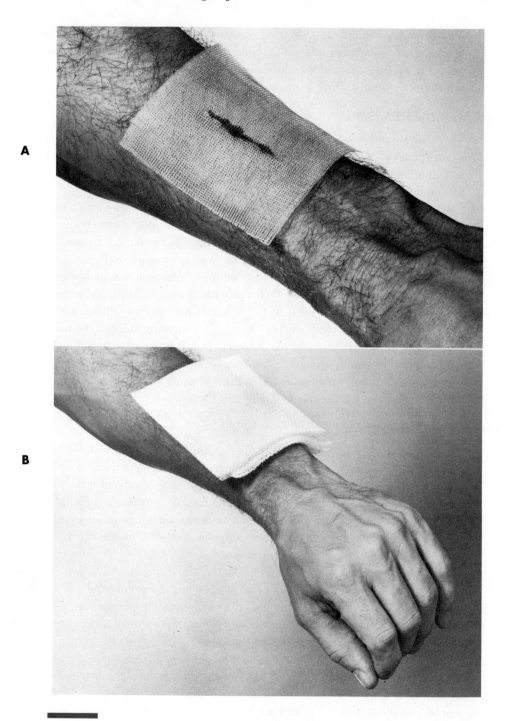

FIG. 18-2   Basic components of a wound dressing. **A,** A nonadherent base. **B,** Gauze sponge covering.

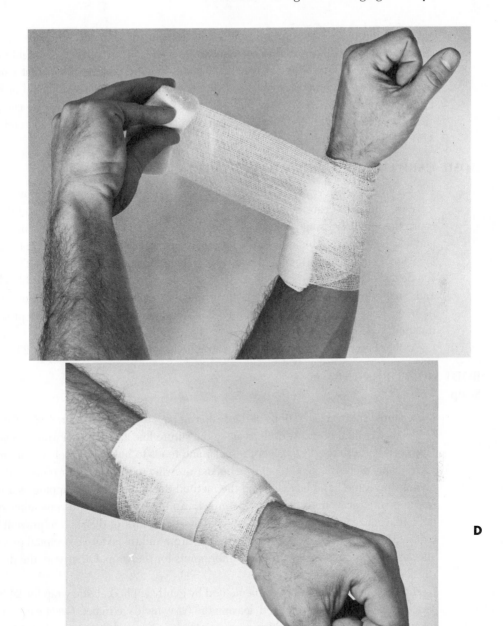

FIG. 18-2, *cont'd*   **C,** Gauze wrap. **D,** Tape application to secure dressing.

One of the most important precautions in dressing and bandaging is never to wrap tape circumferentially around an extremity or digit (Fig. 18-3). Tape, if brought around the finger or wrist to adhere to itself, becomes a nonexpanding band that causes a tourniquet effect on the vascular blood supply to the distal regions of a hand or finger. Pressure builds up as congestion and edema develop. In fact, this pressure can cause complete cessation of blood flow with attendant ischemic necrosis of the anatomic part. This is one of the worst potential complications of wound care.

HOME CARE AND DRESSING CHANGE INTERVALS

Dressing change intervals vary considerably and depend on the patient, wound characteristics, and home care plan. In general, dressings should be kept clean and dry. Because the initial dressing is placed while the wound might be oozing blood or exudate and may be somewhat bulky, it is often useful to instruct the patient to change the dressing 24 to 48 hours following the repair. This change serves several purposes. The wound can be inspected for early signs of infection; the new dressing is exudate and blood free; and, finally, it will be less bulky than the original one. Dressing changes thereafter can be individualized based on the patient's ability to maintain its integrity and protective function.

Further home care information and instructions are contained in Chapter 20.

BODY AREA DRESSINGS
Scalp

Most simple sutured lacerations of the scalp can be left open to the air. A small amount of blood coagulum quickly develops along the suture line and acts as a wound covering. However, because the scalp is very vascular and tends to bleed profusely when injured, occasionally there is a need to apply a bulkier dressing to the area after repair. Fig. 18-4 demonstrates the basic bandage and the method to continue that wrapping as a recurrent dressing for wounds closer to the crown. An important point to remember is that the initial gauze wrap should include the greatest diameter of the skull to prevent inadvertent slippage. The forehead just above the brow and the external occipital protuberance are the landmarks that are the center points for the wrap. Otherwise, the dressing slips over the crown and falls off.

This dressing can often be supplemented by gently applied elastic wrap for 24 hours. The elastic wrap is then removed, leaving the basic bandage intact. Great care must be taken when applying a scalp dressing, particularly with an elastic support, not to cause excessive pressure on the ears. Whenever possible, the ears should be brought out from underneath the bandage to prevent the complication of an ischemic necrosis of the skin of the ear or of the cartilage skeleton.

Face

As mentioned previously, facial lacerations can be left uncovered following repair. Small, uncomplicated lacerations of the ear, eyelid, nose, and lip are included in this recom-

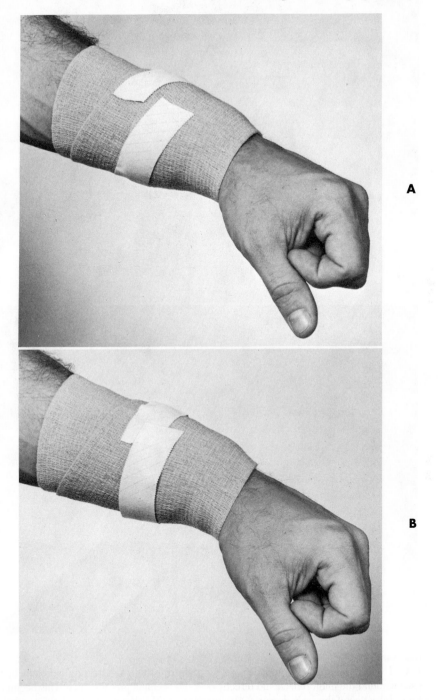

FIG. 18-3   Technique for correct taping of a bandage. **A,** Correct: tape does not overlap if it surrounds an extremity. **B,** Incorrect: overlapping tape can cause unwanted constriction and distal edema.

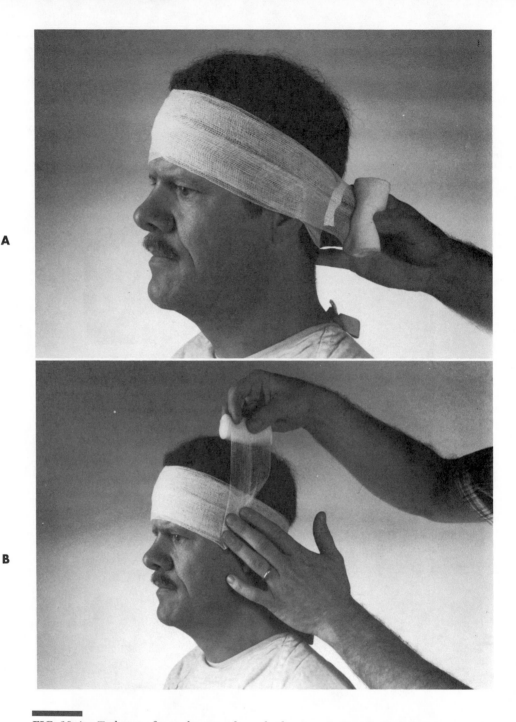

FIG. 18-4   Technique for application of a scalp dressing. **A,** Dressing is begun by wrapping gauze around the midforehead and directly over the occipital protuberance. This beginning allows for stabilization of the scalp dressing. Attempts to wrap the dressing higher on the scalp lead to inevitable loosening of the dressing. **B,** If a recurrent portion of the dressing is necessary to cover lacerations or wounds on the top of the head, or vertex, the recurrent portion is begun as illustrated.

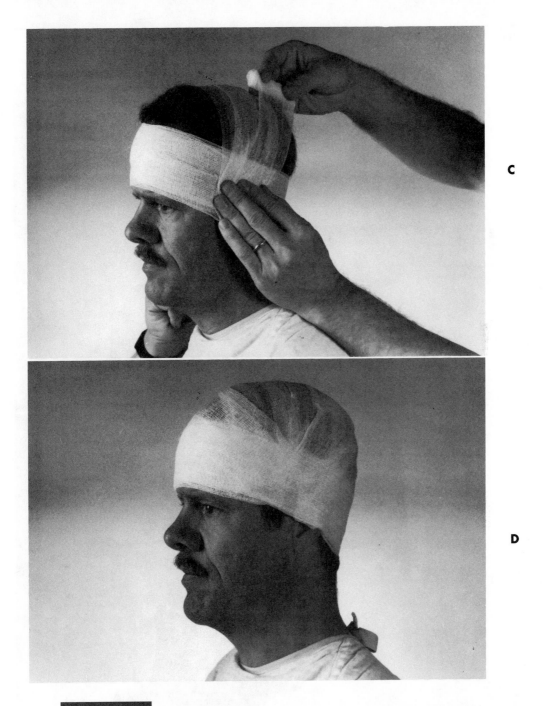

C

D

FIG. 18-4, cont'd **C,** The recurrent portion is brought back and forth over the area of concern. **D,** The recurrent portion is then anchored by continued circumferential wrapping of the gauze around the forehead and external occipital protuberance. *Continued*

FIG. 18-4, cont'd **E,** Tape is applied to secure the scalp dressing. It is important to remove the ears from underneath the circumferential portion of the dressing to avoid ischemia of the ear skeleton. **F,** View of a completed recurrent scalp dressing.

mendation. A very thin film of an antibacterial ointment such as Neosporin can be applied daily by the patient. The antibiotic nature of this ointment is of questionable value at best, but the ointment base is useful in preventing the crusting of coagulum around the wound. By preventing crusting, sutures are much more easily removed with minimal wound disruption. When a facial wound needs covering to protect it from the environment, Band-Aids are recommended. Bulky bandages of the face are poorly tolerated by patients and tend to come off quickly.

Ear and Mastoid

Complicated ear injuries that are at risk for forming perichondral hematomas require a more involved dressing that applies pressure evenly over all of the contours of the ear. One or two 4 × 4 gauze sponges are cut in the contoured fashion shown in steps *A* through *G* of Fig. 18-5. They are placed around and behind the ear to provide support and a "bed" for the cartilaginous skeleton. The area within the helix is filled with petrolatum gauze and "molded" over the antihelix, antitragus, and external canal. Two more intact sponges are placed over the entire ear and 3- or 4-inch gauze bandage is brought

Text continued on p. 338

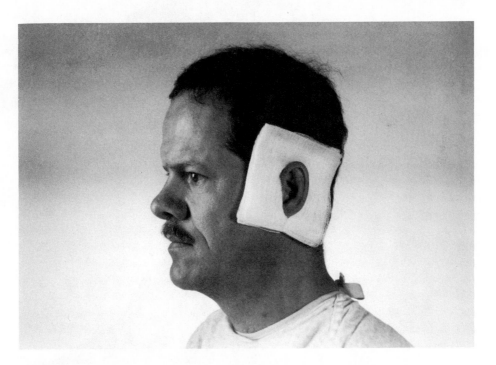

A

FIG. 18-5   Technique for application of a mastoid dressing. **A,** With bandage scissors, cut a center portion out of two or three 4 × 4 gauze sponges so that they fit behind the cartilaginous skeleton of the ear. It is important that the cartilaginous skeleton is well supported and not "crushed" against the scalp.   *Continued*

FIG. 18-5, cont'd   **B,** Petrolatum gauze packing is placed and molded within the cartilaginous skeleton. **C,** Fresh sponges are placed over the molded petrolatum gauze.

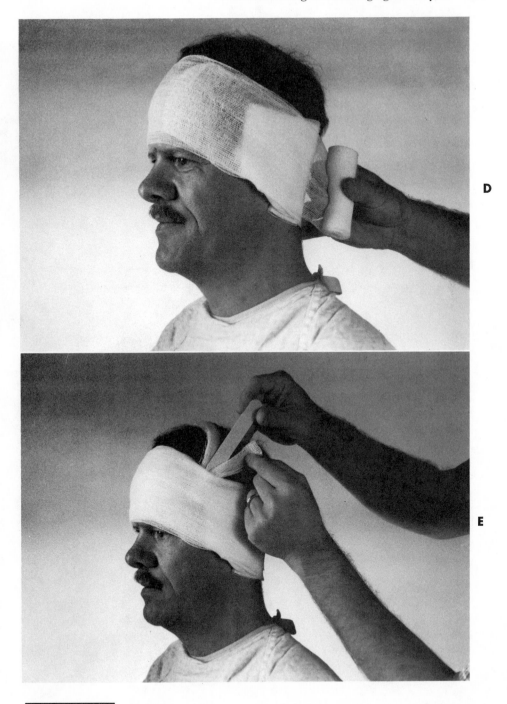

FIG. 18-5, cont'd   **D,** Circumferential gauze wrapping is placed from the midforehead directly over the external occipital protuberance. This portion is then secured with tape. **E,** A gauze tie is inserted anterior to the affected ear using a tongue blade.   *Continued*

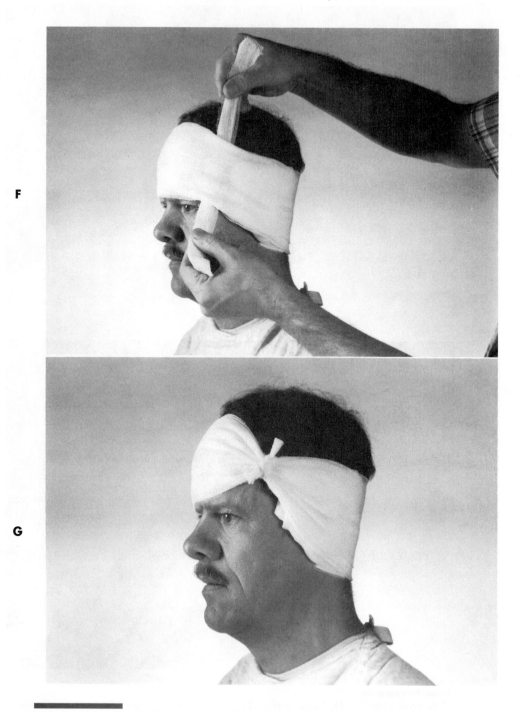

FIG. 18-5, cont'd   **F,** This gauze is firmly tied in a square knot to provide even pressure over the ear. **G,** The final appearance of a mastoid dressing.

around the head and over the ear several times. After the bandage is taped, it is tightened by placing a gauze tie just anterior to the ear. The net effect is to provide even pressure over the ear without compromising its blood supply.

Neck

The neck is an uncommon site for lacerations and other wounds. Dressings need to be effectively secured without compromising the airway or venous return through the jugular system. Simple wrapping with a gauze bandage over the dressing base suffices in most cases. For wounds of the posterior neck in the region of the occiput, the gauze bandage can be wrapped around both the head and the neck to provide for adequate coverage and security (Fig. 18-6).

Shoulder

The shoulder can be a difficult area to dress, especially if the wound is large, in the axilla, or directly over the articular surfaces. The dressing illustrated in Fig. 18-7 takes advantage of the trunk to anchor the shoulder portion. The wrap is brought alternately around the trunk and shoulder/upper arm until it is complete. This dressing configuration is also useful for the upper arm, an area in which bandages tend to slip down with arm motion and gravity. For clarity, a schematic of the shoulder dressing is illustrated in Fig. 18-8.

Truncal

Most wounds on the trunk can be covered with the standard base described previously and taped over benzoin. Larger wounds, such as burns, need larger bandages. The dressing described earlier to cover the shoulder can be extended downward over the trunk and will not slip toward the abdomen. Another method to dress the trunk is illustrated in Fig. 18-9.

Groin, Hip, and Thigh

The groin, hip, and thigh are also difficult regions to properly cover. The technique illustrated in Fig. 18-10 is all-purpose and protects most large wounds in those areas. Like the shoulder, the gauze wrap is brought alternately around the trunk and thigh until it is complete.

Hand and Finger

Fingers can be bandaged in one of two ways: gauze wrapping or tube gauze application. After applying ointment and a nonadherent base, 2 × 2 sponges are placed over the actual wound. One or two layers of 2-inch gauze bandage are then placed over the finger in the manner illustrated in Fig. 18-11. The bandage is then turned to circumferentially wrap the entire finger from finger base to tip and back to the base again. To complete the bandaging, the gauze is carried in a figure-eight pattern down around the palm and is finally anchored at the wrist. Gauze bandaging of the finger alone tends to be inade-

Text continued on p. 344

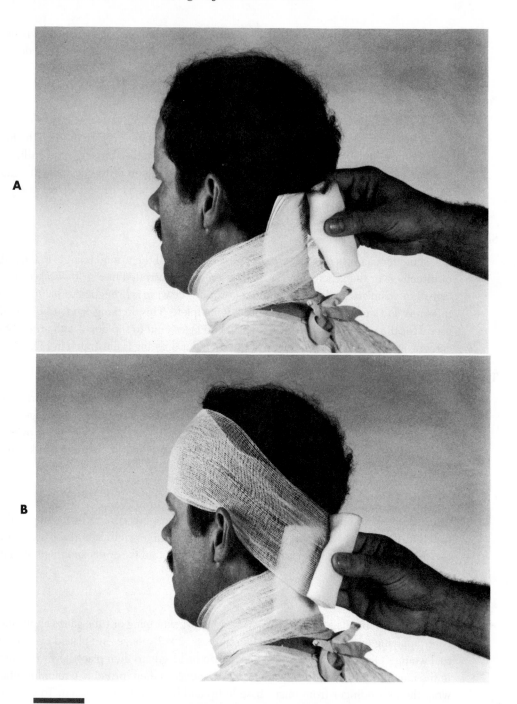

FIG. 18-6 Technique for application of dressing of posterior neck area. **A,** After placement of 4 × 4 sponges, gauze wrapping is gently brought around the neck to secure the gauze. **B,** In a recurrent manner, the dressing is then continued around the frontal area and neck in a figure-eight fashion to secure the dressing completely. Note that the ear is clear of the dressing.

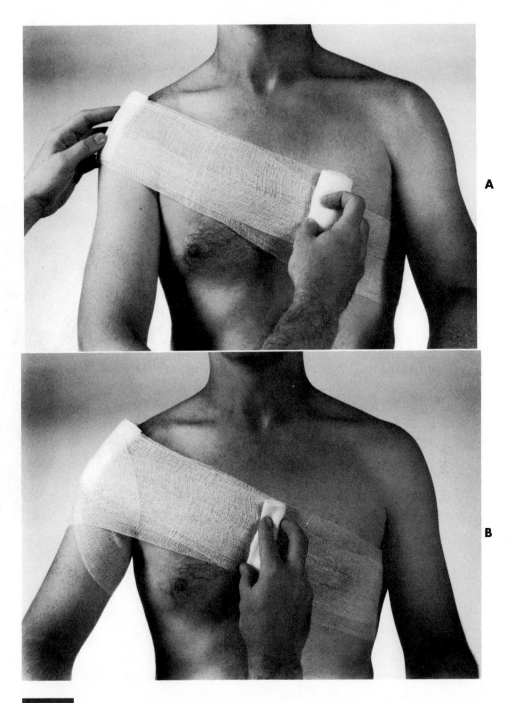

FIG. 18-7 Technique for application of shoulder and upper arm dressing. **A,** Note that the gauze base is placed in the area of injury and the gauze wrapping is begun by circumferentially placing it around the trunk and shoulder area. **B,** The gauze is then continued around the upper arm and the chest in an alternating manner.

Continued

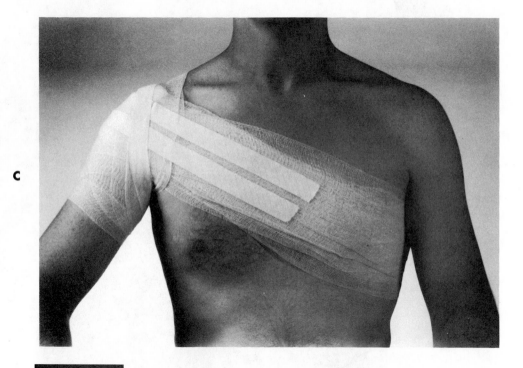

FIG. 18-7, cont'd   **C,** The final appearance of a shoulder dressing.

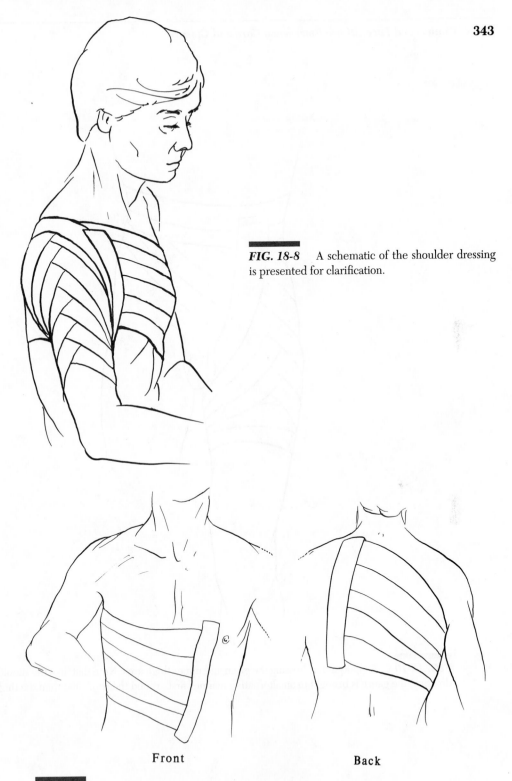

FIG. 18-8   A schematic of the shoulder dressing is presented for clarification.

Front

Back

FIG. 18-9   Technique for application of truncal dressing. Note that gauze wrapping is brought around the hemithorax and secured with benzoin and tape.

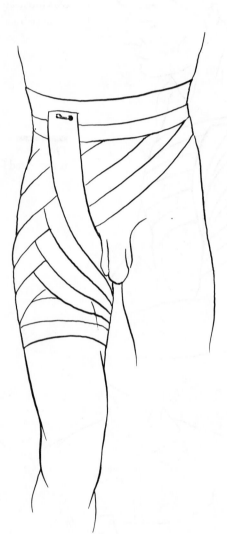

FIG. 18-10   Technique for dressing the groin and upper thigh area. Note that, like the shoulder dressing, the gauze is brought in an alternating manner first around the trunk and then the thigh.

quate, and the dressing can come off prematurely. The basic technique of tube gauze bandages is illustrated in Fig. 18-12.

Injuries of the hand itself are bandaged as illustrated in Fig. 18-13. Depending on the size of the hand, 2- or 3-inch gauze wrapping is placed over the nonadherent base and sponge covering. The gauze wrap includes the wrist to ensure proper anchoring. When two or more fingers are incorporated in a hand dressing, they have to be separated by gauze or sponge strips to prevent skin-to-skin contact and subsequent maceration (Fig. 18-14).

Elbow and Knee

The elbow and knee can be wrapped circumferentially with 4-inch gauze. Although the dressing is adequate, it limits motion of the joint. When placed with the joint in some flexion, the figure-eight technique allows for more freedom of movement (Fig. 18-15). Incorporated into the bandaging are 4 × 8 gauze sponges that are placed over the extensor surfaces. These large sponges allow for "travel" as the joint is flexed and extended.

Text continued on p. 357

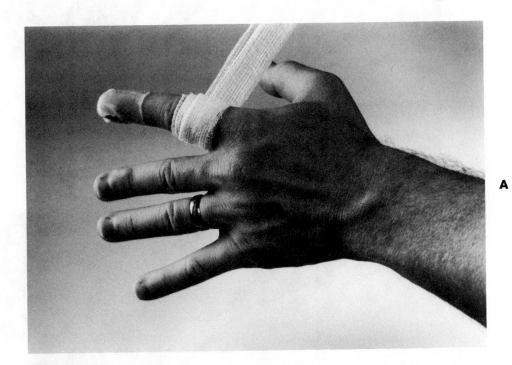

A

FIG. 18-11   Technique for dressing a finger and fingertip. **A,** Note that the nonadherent base is placed over the fingertip. This base can be supplemented by 2 × 2 sponges. The gauze is begun around the base of the finger to initially secure the bandage.   *Continued*

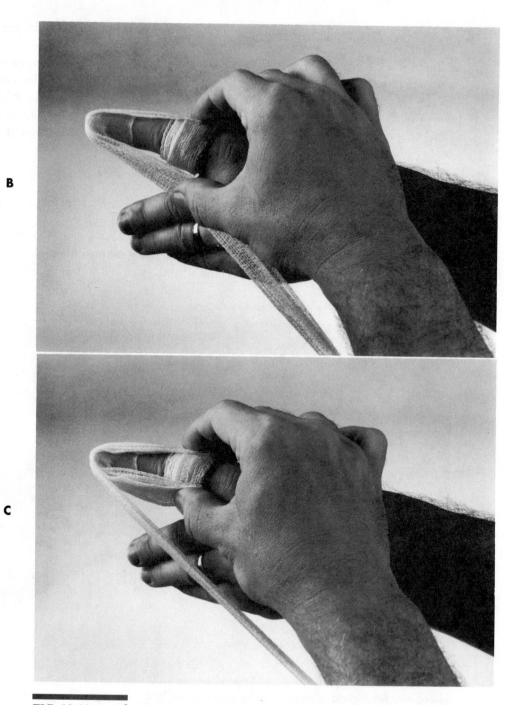

B

C

FIG. 18-11, cont'd   **B,** In a recurrent manner, several layers of gauze are brought back and forth over the tip of the finger to ensure coverage of the distal portion of the digit. **C,** These layers are continued until deemed sufficient.

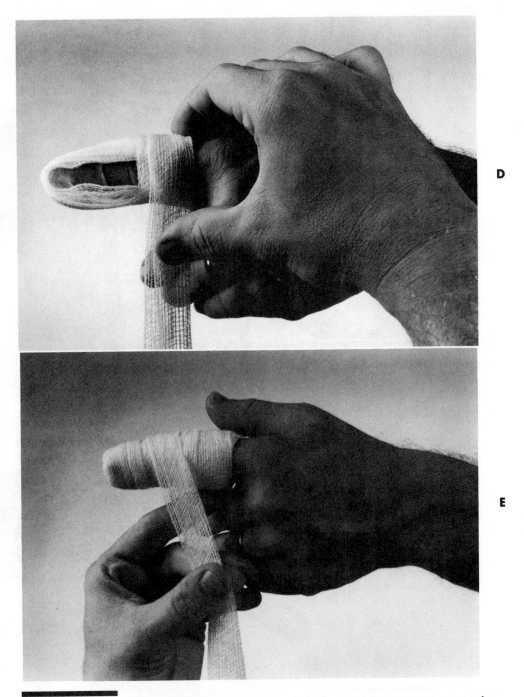

FIG. 18-11, cont'd   **D,** The gauze wrap is then brought back around the finger at its proximal point. **E,** The wrapping is continued to cover the entire digit.   *Continued*

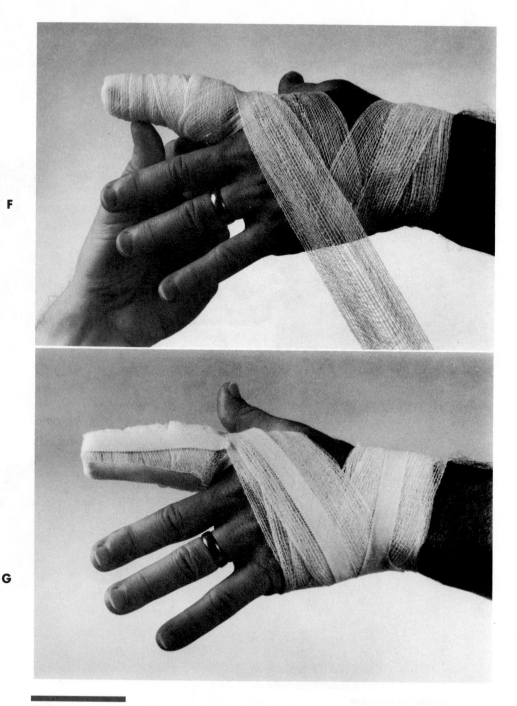

FIG. 18-11, cont'd   **F,** To secure the digit bandage properly, the gauze is continued around the palm and the wrist to secure the bandage firmly. **G,** Final appearance of a proper finger bandage. Note that tape has been applied to secure all elements of the gauze. Also note that none of the tape is wrapped in a circumferential manner.

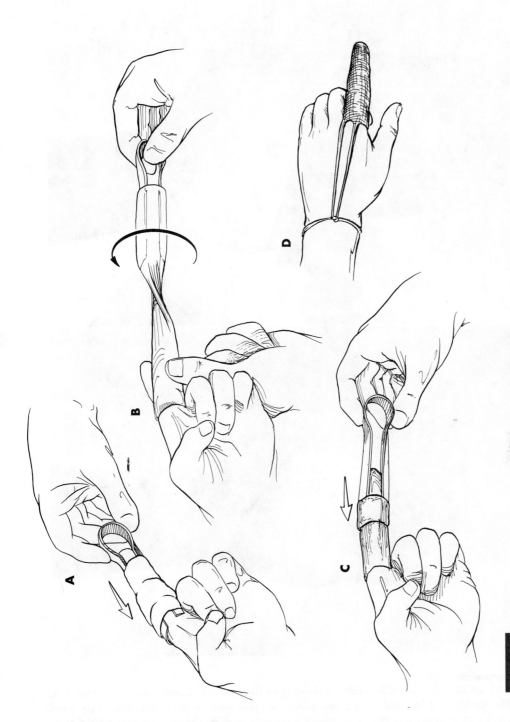

FIG. 18-12 Technique for placement of a tube gauze finger bandage. **A,** Note that sufficient tube gauze is slid onto the applicator and then brought over the finger. **B,** The first layer of tube gauze is secured as the applicator is brought distally from the finger and rotated 180°. **C,** The next layer of tube gauze is placed by the applicator over the digit. **D,** This process is repeated until an adequate number of layers of tube gauze have been applied.

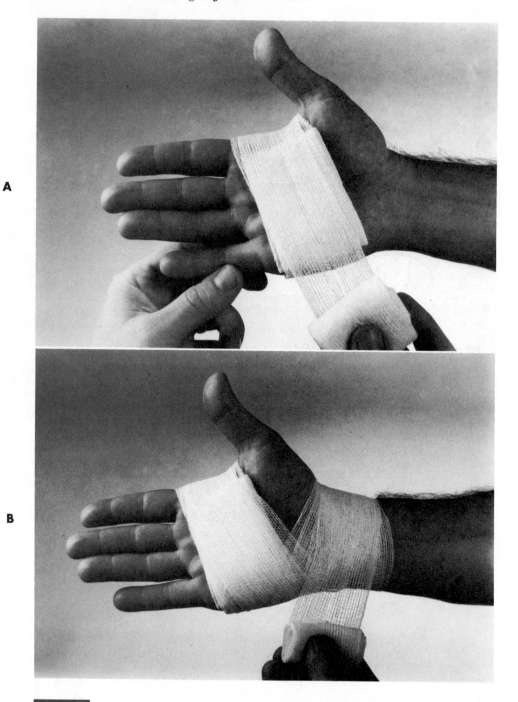

FIG. 18-13 Technique for placing a dressing on the palmar or dorsal surface of the hand. **A,** The nonadherent base and 4 × 4 gauze sponges are placed on the palm or dorsum of the hand. The gauze wrapping is begun by securing this dressing base. **B,** The dressing is completed by alternate wrapping of both the palm and the wrist with the gauze wrap. Tape is applied in a noncircumferential manner to complete the dressing.

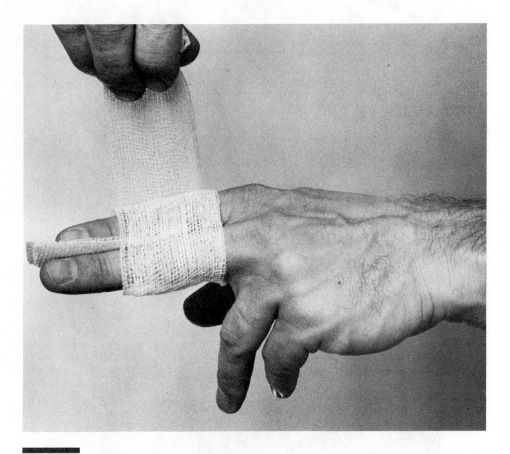

FIG. 18-14 Always place gauze between skin-to-skin contact areas to prevent maceration.

FIG. 18-15 Technique for elbow or knee dressing. **A,** Note that the gauze sponge is placed over the extensor surface of the knee or elbow and secured with the beginnings of a gauze wrap. **B,** The gauze wrap is then brought over to the opposite side of the gauze dressing base.

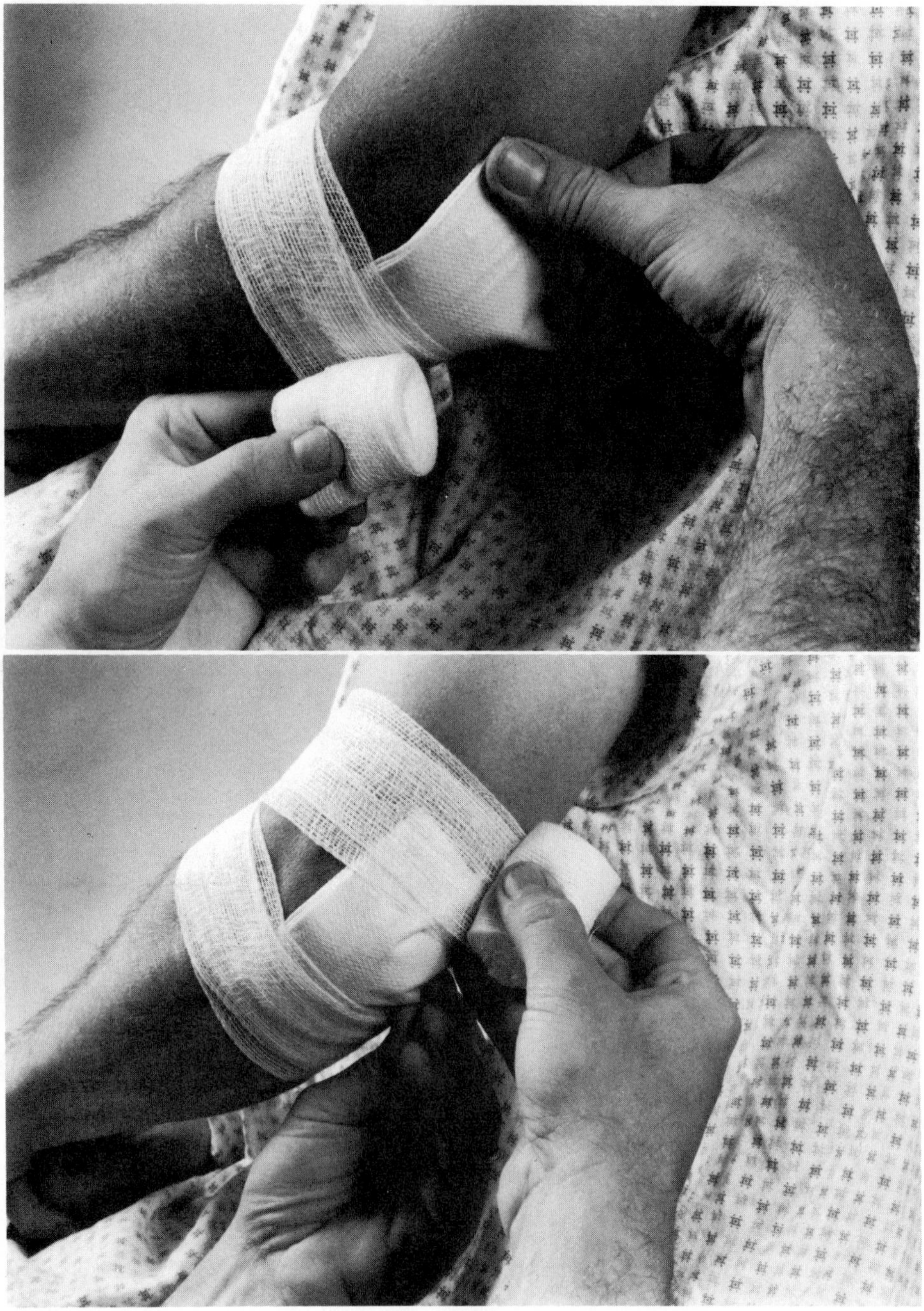

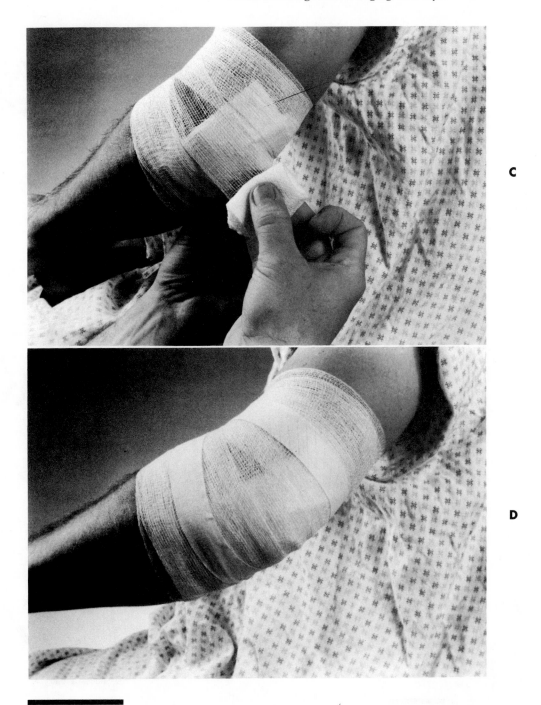

C

D

FIG. 18-15, cont'd   **C,** The gauze wrapping is then continued over the center portion of the dressing base. **D,** An example of a completed dressing. Most elbow and knee dressings are fashioned with the knee or elbow in a slightly flexed position to provide for better patient mobility.

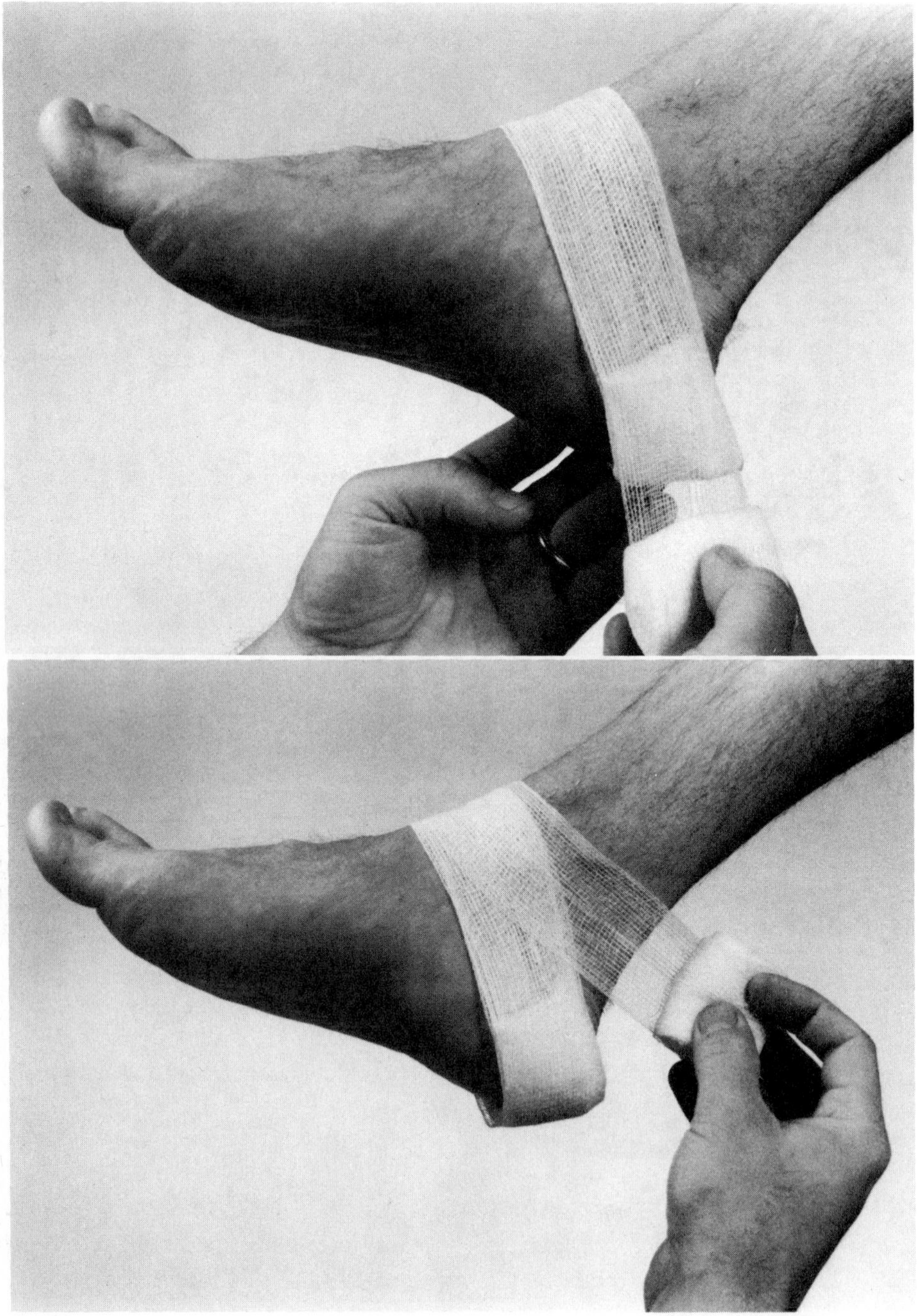

FIG. 18-16   Technique for heel dressing. **A,** The dressing base is placed over the area of concern of the heel, and the initial gauze wrap secures that base. **B,** The gauze wrap is continued around the ankle.

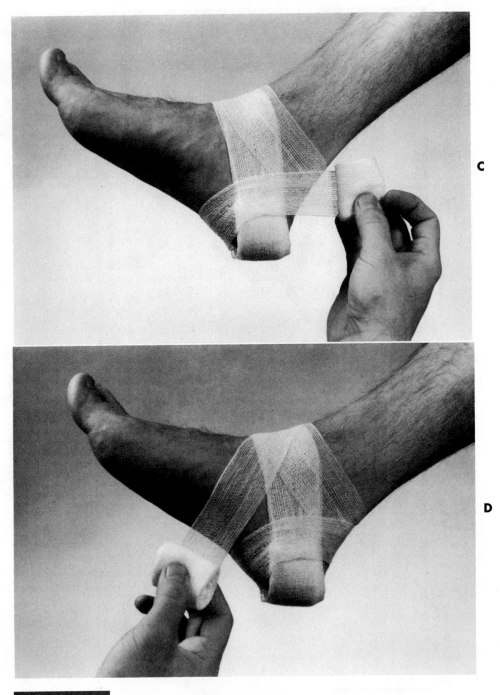

FIG. 18-16, cont'd   **C,** The gauze wrap is then brought directly across and around the heel.
D, Once it has crossed the heel, it is brought over the ankle and then around the foot.

Continued

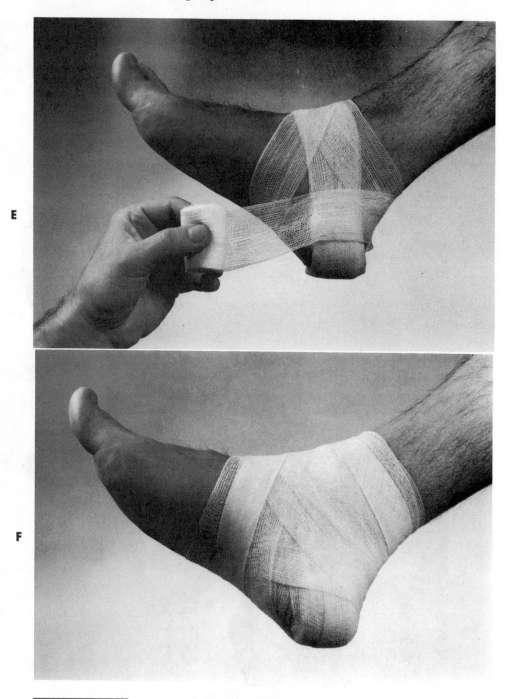

FIG. 18-16, cont'd   **E,** After being brought around the ankle and then around the foot, it is brought back in the reverse manner over the heel. **F,** Completed example of heel dressing.

Ankle, Heel, and Foot

Ankle and foot dressings are straightforward. The gauze bandage wrapping is in the same figure-eight style used for the knee and elbow. When bandaging the foot, always include the ankle as the anchoring point. The difficult area to cover is the heel. The wrapping starts around the heel and anterior portion of the ankle (Fig. 18-16). After three or four wraps, the bandage is brought around the heel alone, then around the foot. This process is continued until the foot, heel, and ankle are all part of the dressing.

REFERENCES

1. Ayliffe GA, Green W, Livingston R, et al: Antibiotic-resistant *Staphylococcus aureus* in dermatology and burn wounds, *J Clin Path* 30:40-44, 1977.
2. Bothwell JW, Rovee DT: The effects of dressings on the repair of cutaneous wounds in humans. In Harkiss KJ, ed: *Surgical dressings and wound healing*, London, 1971, Bradford University Press.
3. Dire DJ, Coppola M, Dwyer DA, et al: Prospective evaluation of topical antibiotics for preventing infections of soft-tissue wounds repaired in the ED, *Acad Emerg Med* 2:4-10, 1995.
4. Eaglestein WH, Mertz PM: Effect of topical medicaments on the rate of repair of superficial wounds. In Dineen P, editor: *The surgical wound*, Philadelphia, 1981, Lea & Febiger.
5. Hinman C, Maibach H: Effect of air exposure and occlusion on experimental human skin wounds, *Nature* 200:377-378, 1963.
6. Howells C, Young H: A study of completely undressed surgical wounds, *Br J Surg* 53:436-439, 1966.
7. Lammers RL: Principles of wound management. In Roberts JR, Hedges JR, editors: *Clinical procedures in emergency medicine*, Philadelphia, 1991, WB Saunders.
8. Lawrence J: What materials for dressings? *Injury* 13:500-512, 1981-1982.
9. Leyden JJ, Sulzberger MB: Topical antibiotics and minor skin trauma, *Am Fam Physic* 23:121-125, 1981.
10. Millikan LE: Wound healing and dermatologic dressings, *Clin Dermatol* 5:31-36, 1987.
11. Norton LW: Trauma. In Hill GJ, editor: *Outpatient surgery*, Philadelphia, 1980, WB Saunders.
12. Panek P, Prusak MP, Bolt D, et al: Potentiation of wound infection by adhesive adjuncts, *Am Surg* 38:343-345, 1972.
13. Stuzin J, Engrav LH, Buehler PK: Emergency treatment of facial lacerations, *Post Grad Med* 71:81-83, 1982.
14. Wayne MA: Clinical evaluation of Epi-Lock: a semiocclusive dressing, *Ann Emerg Med* 14:20-24, 1985.

19 *Tetanus Immunity and Antibiotic Wound Prophylaxis*

. . . .

Tetanus Prophylaxis
    Immunization Schedules
    Complications of Tetanus Toxoid

Prophylactic Antibiotics for Emergency
    Wounds

Two issues of prophylaxis arise for virtually all patients with wounds and lacerations. A careful history is taken to establish the tetanus immune status of every patient. Although nurses in most emergency department settings are required to document that status in their notes, the ultimate responsibility lies with the physician to ensure the patient's tetanus prophylaxis is up to date. Far more controversial and problematic is the issue of antibiotic prophylaxis. Despite that 90% to 95% of all patients with uncomplicated lacerations do not acquire an infection, there remains an excessive use of prophylactic antibiotics.[10, 17, 20, 26, 29] As discussed in the following material, multiple large studies have failed to support the use of prophylactic antibiotics, and, in fact, they may actually increase the risk for infection.

TETANUS PROPHYLAXIS

For all patients with an emergency wound or laceration, a decision has to be made about whether or not to administer tetanus prophylaxis. Although contaminated wounds with extensive devitalized tissue are considered more tetanus-prone than clean minor wounds, up to one third of documented cases of tetanus have originated from seemingly trivial injuries.[4, 15] A common portal of entry for tetanus is a puncture wound to the foot.[15] Tetanus occurs almost exclusively in patients who have never been immunized or who never completed a proper immunization program.[25] Probably for this reason, most cases are reported in patients who are over the age of 50.[25] A high proportion of older adults, when tested for serum tetanus antibody, have been shown to have inadequate levels of protection.[1,9] Young adults and children are more likely to have appropriate levels of protection because of widespread immunization programs that have been put into place in recent years. Irrespective of the circumstances, a careful immunization history is taken for every patient with a minor wound. This history should establish whether initial immunization has been properly completed and the date of the last tetanus toxoid dose.

Immunization Schedules

The guidelines for the administration of tetanus prophylaxis in Table 19-1 are those recommended by the Immunization Practice Advisory Committee (ACIP) of the Centers for Disease Control.[12] The currently recommended preparation of tetanus toxoid includes the diphtheria toxoid and is designated Td. The risk of contracting diphtheria in adulthood is of sufficient magnitude that, as a public measure, prophylaxis against this disease is recommended.[15] The trivalent diphtheria, tetanus, and pertussis (DTP) is administered to children under 7 years old who have not been fully immunized (Table 19-2).[24] It is important to be aware that there is a DT preparation with a higher concentration of diphtheria toxoid. This preparation is not recommended for patients over 7 years and is only occasionally administered to patients under 7 years who cannot tolerate the pertussis (P) component of DTP.

For patients 7 years or older who have never been immunized and who received their first dose of Td at the time of their wound repair, follow-up care should include subsequent visits to a medical care facility to complete immunization.[12] Table 19-3 summarizes the time guidelines for administration of the second, third, and booster doses of Td.

Complications of Tetanus Toxoid

Occasionally, a patient reports an allergic reaction to a prior tetanus shot. In a study of 740 patients who claimed to be allergic to tetanus shots, the true incidence of allergy, on

Table 19-1 *Summary Guide to Tetanus Prophylaxis in Routine Wound Management, 1991*

History of Adsorbed Tetanus Toxoid (Doses)	Clean, Minor Wounds		All Other Wounds*	
	Td[†]	TIG (250 U)	Td[†]	TIG (250 U)
Unknown or <3	Yes	No	Yes	Yes
≥3[§]	No[¶]	No	No[‖]	No

(From ACIP: Diphtheria, tetanus, and pertussis: recommendations for vaccine use and other preventative measures, *MMWR* 40(RR-10):1-50, 1991.)

*Such as, but not limited to, wounds contaminated with dirt, feces, soil, and saliva; puncture wounds; avulsions; and wounds resulting from missiles, crushing, burns and frostbite.

[†]For children <7 years old; DTP (DT, if pertussis vaccine is contraindicated) is preferred to tetanus toxoid alone. For persons ≥7 years of age, Td is preferred to tetanus toxoid alone.

[§]If only 3 doses of *fluid* toxoid have been received, then a fourth dose of toxoid, preferably an adsorbed toxoid, should be given.

[¶]Yes, if >10 years since last dose.

[‖]Yes, if >5 years since last dose. (More frequent boosters are not needed and can accentuate side effects.)

Table 19-2   *Routine Diphtheria, Tetanus, and Pertussis Vaccination Schedule Summary for Children <7 Years of Age—United States, 1991*

Dose	Customary Age	Age/Interval	Product
Primary 1	2 Months	6 Weeks old or older	DTP[†]
Primary 2	4 Months	4-8 Weeks after first dose*	DTP[†]
Primary 3	6 Months	4-8 Weeks after second dose*	DTP[†]
Primary 4	15 Months	6-12 Months after third dose*	DTP[†]
Booster	4-6 Years old, before entering kindergarten or elementary school (not necessary if fourth primary vaccinating dose administered after fourth birthday)		DTP[†]
Additional boosters		Every 10 years after last dose	Td

(From ACIP: Diphtheria, tetanus, and pertussis: recommendations for vaccine use and other preventative measures, *MMWR* 40(RR-10):1-50, 1991.)
*Prolonging the interval does not require restarting series.
[†]Use DT if pertussis vaccine is contraindicated. If the child is ≥ 1 year of age at the time that primary dose 3 is due, a third dose 6-12 months after the second completes primary vaccination with DT.

Table 19-3   *Routine Diphtheria, Tetanus, and Pertussis Vaccination Schedule Summary for Persons ≥ 7 Years of Age—United States, 1991*

Dose	Age/Interval	Product
Primary 1	First dose	Td
Primary 2	4-8 Weeks after first dose*	Td
Primary 3	6-12 Months after second dose*	Td
Booster	Every 10 years after last dose	Td

(From ACIP: Diphtheria, tetanus, and pertussis: recommendations for vaccine use and other preventative measures, *MMWR* 40(RR-10):1-50, 1991.)
*Prolonging the interval does not require restarting series.

skin challenge testing, was very low.[21] Of the 740 patients, 7 developed local reactions that were self-limited. One patient became syncopal, and one developed a fever that lasted for 4 days. Only 1 of 740 patients had a true urticarial response but still tolerated a full immunizing dose. In spite of these reassuring figures, the possibility of a serious reaction still must be considered.[21] For patients considered at high risk for a reaction, tetanus immune globulin (TIG; 250 to 500 units) is given in the emergency department. TIG confers immunity for that injury but not for future exposures. This preparation consists only of antitetanus antibody and does not cross-react with the toxoid. Referral to an allergist for skin testing, and subsequent immunization with toxoid, is recommended as prudent follow-up.

Local and systemic reactions to Td are not common but do occur in up to 7% to 9% of pediatric patients.[8] Pain, swelling, and erythema can occur at the injection site but are usually self-limited. Preparations containing the pertussis vaccine (DTP), on the other hand, are associated with a much higher rate of adverse reactions. Fever can occur in up to 50% of infants receiving DTP.[12] It can last for 24 to 48 hours and can be accompanied by somnolence, nausea, vomiting, and irritability. Other rare reactions that have been reported include Arthus-type hypersensitivity, urticaria, anaphylaxis, and neurologic complications.

PROPHYLACTIC ANTIBIOTICS FOR EMERGENCY WOUNDS

For small, uncomplicated, minor, nonbite wounds and lacerations, there is no convincing clinical evidence that systemic antibiotics provide protection against the development of wound infection.[18, 19, 20, 29] In a study in which intramuscular penicillin was administered to alternate patients with lacerations treated in an emergency department, there was no difference in the rate of infection between the study and control groups.[20] A randomized, controlled study using oral cephalexin for prophylaxis also demonstrated no efficacy of the antibiotic for minor lacerations.[29] In two randomized, controlled studies using oral or parenteral cephalosporins for minor hand lacerations, there was no increase in the infection rate of nonantibiotic treated patients when compared with those treated with antibiotics.[10, 18, 19] In a study of 2834 pediatric patients, not only was there no protective effect, but there was significant increase in the infection rate in the antibiotic treated patients.[2] Other studies support this contradiction as well.[19, 20, 29, 30] It is thought that selection for resistant organisms, rebound bacterial proliferation after the initial effect, or impairment of host defenses by the drugs might account for this paradox.

Although not all authorities agree, nor is there strong scientific evidence underlying any specific set of recommendations for wound antibiotic prophylaxis, clinical and empirical experience suggests that there are wound characteristics and circumstances that warrant antibiotic intervention.[5, 6, 13] If antibiotics are indicated, there is some evidence that the initial dose has to be administered as soon as possible to obtain an effect.[5, 13, 22] Delays in treatment beyond 3 to 5 hours from injury have been shown in some studies to lead to an increase in the infection rate.[5] On the other hand, other investigators have found little correlation between the interval from injury to antibiotic delivery and the ultimate risk of wound infection.

The following are guidelines for which antibiotics should be considered. The initial dose, preferably parenteral, is administered as soon as the decision is reached.[2, 3, 10, 23]

- Wound age: Relative indications include hand and foot wounds greater than 8 hours, facial wounds greater than 24 hours, and other site wounds greater than 12 hours.
- Wound condition: Crushing mechanism wounds for which extensive debridement and tissue revision is needed.
- Contamination: Wounds initially contaminated with soil, vegetative matter, and other particulates that require extensive cleaning and irrigation.
- Mammalian bites: Chapter 14 lists the indications for wound prophylaxis in dog, cat, and human bites.
- Vulnerable anatomic sites: Wounds of cartilage (ear, nose), tendon, bone, and joint.
- Circulatory impairment: Wounds in impaired areas of drainage such as lymphedema secondary to venous disease or surgical procedure (radical mastectomy).
- Impaired host defenses: Diabetes, immunosuppressive agents (corticosteroids, anticancer agents), diseases with altered immune status.
- Cardiac valvular disease: Guidelines published by the American Heart Association should be followed relative to wounds in patients with cardiac valvular disease. Prophylaxis is not indicated in patients who have clean, uncomplicated lacerations.
- Orthopedic implants: Prophylaxis should be considered in patients with orthopedic implants who have contaminated wounds. Prophylaxis is not indicated for clean, uncomplicated wounds.

The choice of antibiotics for nonbite wound prophylaxis is based on the likely infecting organisms. Multiple studies have shown that for common, uncomplicated wounds and lacerations, *Staphylococcus aureus* and *Streptococcal* species are the infecting agents in over 90% of cases.[11, 19, 27, 30] More extensive wounds, involving contamination with soil, increase the spectrum to include gram-negative organisms and *Clostridium* species.[14] Wounds involving fresh water, including lakes, streams, and swimming pools, may be contaminated with *Aeromonas hydrophila*.[16, 28] Injuries occurring in salt water can be infected with *Vibrio vulnificus*.[7]

For prophylaxis to be effective, the initial dose should be delivered as soon after the injury as possible, preferably in parenteral form, to ensure an adequate level of antibiotic activity. For the common, uncomplicated, nonbite wound requiring prophylaxis, the first-generation cephalosporin, cefazolin (Ancef), can be administered parenterally followed by a 3- to 5-day course of cephalexin (Keflex), cephradine (Velosef), cefadroxil (Duricef), or dicloxacillin. Cefadroxil has the advantage of once or twice a day dosing, which may encourage greater compliance. For patients allergic to penicillin and cephalosporins, an intravenous dose of clindamycin (Cleocin) followed with oral clindamycin provides coverage of the known, common, infecting organisms. Because of the short course, the risk of diarrheal complications from clindamycin is negligible. A commonly prescribed prophylactic alternative is erythromycin. Should *Aeromonas hydrophila* be suspected, ciprofloxacin (Cipro), trimethoprim/sulfamethoxazole (Bactrim, Septra), or an aminoglycoside provides adequate coverage. *Vibrio vulnificus* is more difficult to treat but is sensitive to doxycycline (Vibramycin) and chloramphenicol, as well as ceftazidime (Fortaz).

REFERENCES

1. Alagappan K, Rennie WP, McPherson P, et al: Seroprevalence of antibody levels to tetanus in adults over 65 years of age, *Acad Emerg Med* 2:373, 1995 (Abstract).
2. Baker MD, Lanuti M: The management and outcome of lacerations in urban children, *Ann Emerg Med* 19:1001-1005, 1990.
3. Berk WA, Osborne DD, Taylor DD: Evaluation of the "golden period" for wound repair: 204 cases from a third world emergency department, *Ann Emerg Med* 17:496-500, 1988.
4. Brand DA, Acampora D, Gottlieb LD, et al: Adequacy of anti-tetanus prophylaxis in six hospital emergency departments, *N Eng J Med* 309:636-640, 1983.
5. Burke JF: The effective period of preventive antibiotic action in experimental incisions and dermal lesions, *Surgery* 50:161-168, 1961.
6. Cardany CR, Rodeheaver G, Thacker J, et al: The crush injury: The high risk wound, *J Amer Coll Emerg Phys* 5:965-970, 1976.
7. Chuang YC, Young C, Chen CW: *Vibrio vulnificus* infections, *Scand J Infect Dis* 21:721, 1989.
8. Cody CL, Baraff LJ, Cherry JD, et al: Nature of adverse reactions associated with DTP and DT immunizations in infants and children, *Pediatr* 68:650-660, 1981.
9. Crossley K, Irvine P, Warren JB, et al: Tetanus and diptheria immunity in urban Minnesota adults, *JAMA* 242:298-230, 1983.
10. Cummings P, Del Beccaro MA: Antibiotics to prevent infection of simple wounds: a meta-analysis of randomized studies, *Am J Emerg Med* 13:396-400, 1995.
11. Day TK: Controlled trial of antibiotics in minor wounds requiring suture, *Lancet* 2:1174-1176, 1975.
12. Recommendations of the Immunization Practices Advisory Committee (ACIP): Diptheria, tetanus, and pertussis: recommendations for vaccine use and other preventative measures, *Morbid Mortal Week Rep* 40(RR-10):1-50, 1991.
13. Edlich RF, Kenny JG, Morgan RF, et al: Antimicrobial treatment of minor soft tissue lacerations: a critical review, *Emerg Clin North Am* 4:561-580, 1986.
14. Fitzgerald RH, Cooney WP, Washington JA, et al: Bacterial colonization of mutilating hand injuries and its treatment, *J Hand Surg* 2:85-89, 1977.
15. Furste W: Fifth international conference on tetanus, Ronneby, Sweden, 1978, *J Trauma* 20:101-105, 1980.
16. Gold WL, Salit IE: *Aeromonas hydrophila* infections of the skin and soft tissue: report of 11 cases, *Clin Infect Dis* 16:69-74, 1993.
17. Gosnold JK: Infection rate of sutured wounds, *Practitioner* 218:584-585, 1977.
18. Grossman JA, Adams JP, Kunec J: Prophylactic antibiotics in simple hand lacerations, *JAMA* 245:1055-1056, 1981.
19. Haughey RE, Lammers RL, Wagner DK: Use of antibiotics in the initial management of soft tissue wounds, *Ann Emerg Med* 10:187-190, 1981.
20. Hutton PA, Jones BM, Law DJ: Depot penicillin as prophylaxis in accidental wounds, *Br J Surg* 65:549-550, 1978.

21. Jacobs RL, Lowe RS, Lanier BQ: Adverse reactions to tetanus toxoid, *JAMA* 247:40-42, 1982.

22. Morgan WJ, Hutchinson D, Johnson HM: The delayed treatment of wounds of the hand and forearm under antibiotic cover, *Br J Surg* 67:140-141, 1976.

23. Nylen S, Carlsson B: Time factor, infection frequency and quantitative microbiology in hand injuries: a prospective study, *Scand J Plast Reconstr Surg* 14:185-189, 1980.

24. Recommended Childhood Immunization Schedule: United States 1995, *Morbid Mortal Week Rep* 44(RR-5):1-8,1995.

25. Richardson JP, Knight AL: The management and prevention of tetanus, *J Emerg Med* 11:737-742, 1993.

26. Rutherford WH, Spence R: Infection in wounds sutured in the accident and emergency department, *Ann Emerg Med* 9:350-352, 1980.

27. Samson RH, Altman SF: Antibiotic prophylaxis for minor lacerations, *NY State J Med* 77:1728-1730, 1977.

28. Skiendzielewski WH, O'Keefe KP: Wound infection due to freash water contamination of *Aeromonas hydrophila, J Emerg Med* 8:701-703, 1990.

29. Thirlby RC, Blair AJ, Thal ER: The value of prophylactic antibiotics for simple lacerations, *Surg Gynecol Obstet* 156:212-216, 1983.

30. Worlock P, Boland P, Darrell J, et al: The role of prophylactic antibiotics following hand surgery, *Br J Clin Pract* 34:290-292, 1980.

20 Suture Removal and Wound Aftercare

. . . .

Suture Removal
    Timing of Removal
    Technique for Removal
Analgesia
Instructions to the Patient
    Wound Protection

Dressing Change and Follow-Up Intervals
Wound Cleansing and Bathing
Signs of Wound Infection
Written Instructions
Understanding Wound Healing

Wound aftercare includes return scheduling for suture removal, aftercare instructions to the patient, and information on what to expect as the wound heals. When carefully and fully informed, most patients take good care of their wounds and dressings. Written instructions are best followed when reinforced with unhurried verbal explanations. Because each wound and patient differ, information about dressing care, limitations of activity, bathing, and suture removal has to be individualized. Patients often expect that healing is complete when the sutures are removed. If educated about the changes that a wound undergoes over a period of months, patients are more likely to understand and accept its appearance.

SUTURE REMOVAL
Timing of Removal

The recommended intervals between wound repair and suture removal are detailed in Table 20-1. In the face, where cosmetic appearance is paramount, sutures are removed as early as possible. This is done, however, with the knowledge that a facial wound has barely begun to gain tensile strength. Minimal accidental force can cause disruption and dehisce the laceration. Therefore the application of wound tapes for continued support over healing lacerations is recommended. A return visit for tape removal and wound adhesive closure is not necessary. If wound tapes are the primary method of wound closure, they can be left in place for up to 10 days without causing complications. Adhesives will flake off with time. At minimum, these alternative closures should support the wound for the time period recommended for sutures.

Table 20-1 *Recommended Intervals for Removal of Percutaneous (Skin) Sutures*

Location	Days to Removal
Scalp	6-8
Face	4-5
Ear	4-5
Chest/abdomen	8-10
Back	12-14
Arm/leg*	8-10
Hand*	8-10
Fingertip	10-12
Foot	12-14

*Add 2 to 3 days for joint extensor surfaces.

It is important to understand that suture punctures are small wounds. Epithelial cells invade these small wounds leaving keratinized epithelial "plugs" caught in the healing suture wound. This phenomenon produces unsightly "railroad tracks" that can be avoided if sutures are removed in less than 7 days.[1] The use of skin tapes and wound adhesives as the wound closure methods are alternative techniques to avoid suture tracking. The subcuticular and pull-out dermal closures described in Chapter 10 are other closure options.

In other areas of the body, where cosmetics are not as important and wound healing is not quite as rapid as in the highly vascular face, sutures are left in for longer periods. Extensor surfaces of joints require somewhat longer times before removal because of the mechanical forces brought to bear on the healing wound. Because of the dependency of the lower extremities and their relatively slower rate of healing, sutures are also left in place for longer in those sites as well.

Technique for Removal

The technique for suture removal is illustrated in Fig. 20-1. The suture is cut under the knot, close to the skin surface, so that, when it is pulled from the wound, the previously exposed and contaminated portion of the suture does not travel back through the wound. Although standard scissors can be used for most suture removal tasks, iris scissors or a #11 scalpel blade is recommended to cut the very fine sutures used on the face. Bandage or commercial suture-removal scissors have tips that are often too blunt to cut small, closely-spaced sutures easily. Before removal, all dried coagulum is gently removed from the suture line with cotton swabs and hydrogen peroxide. Cleaning away the coagulum makes locating small sutures and knots much easier. In addition, it pre-

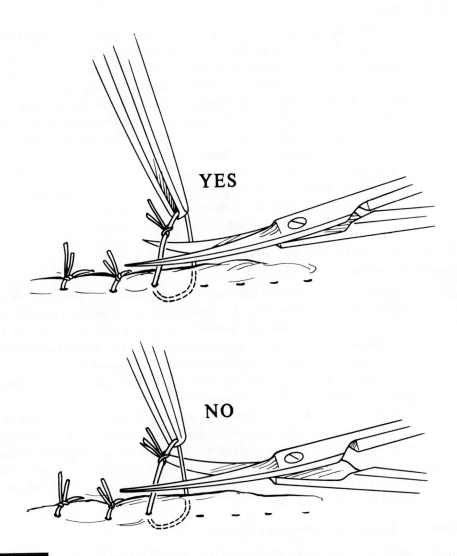

FIG. 20-1 Technique for correct removal of a suture. Note that the scissors cut between the knot and skin. The lower figure indicates the incorrect technique to remove sutures. (Modified from Zukin D, Simon R: *Emergency wound care: principles and practice*, Rockville, Md, 1987, Aspen Publishers.)

vents the unnecessary tugging and pulling that often accompany suture removal when sutures are excessively crusted.

ANALGESIA

Pain following wounding can range from the trivial to the severe. Simple lacerations are well tolerated by the patient after repair and dressing. Abrasions and partial-thickness (second-degree) burns can be unbearable. For most patients with uncomplicated lacerations, aspirin, acetaminophen, or other nonsteroidal antiinflammatory drugs relieve residual discomfort after repair. Occasionally, codeine or hydrocodone is necessary. Burn victims require more powerful analgesics such as oxycodone. In addition to drugs, pain relief can be greatly enhanced by elevation of the injured part, proper immobilization, and cool compresses to the affected area.

The pain of lacerations and burns tends to subside significantly within 24 to 48 hours. A key follow-up instruction to the patient is to be concerned when pain increases or recurs. The most likely cause of this change in the pain pattern is wound infection. Should pain increase, immediate physician notification is necessary.

INSTRUCTIONS TO THE PATIENT
Wound Protection

Patients need to be carefully instructed in nonmedical terms about how to care for their wound at home. The key principles of home care are protection, elevation, and cleanliness. Most patients instinctively protect wounds from further trauma, but a reminder that, although sutures are in place, undue pressure or other mechanical forces on the wound can cause disruption and possible infection. Counseling and admonition against premature use of the repaired hand or foot is especially necessary for patients who are anxious to return to work or sporting activities.

Elevation is particularly important in extremity wounds. The tendency of lower extremities and hands to develop edema from lymphatic stasis is well recognized. Elevation helps prevent these complications, lessens pain, and improves wound healing. Lower extremity wounds have a higher rate of wound infection, a complication that can be abetted by edema and stasis. Crutches and slings for extremity wounds are useful adjuncts for home wound care.

Dressing Change and Follow-Up Intervals

Dressing management and change intervals are discussed in Chapter 18.

Wound Cleansing and Bathing

Cleanliness is an important issue in wound aftercare. Sutured wounds of the scalp and face can be left open, provided that they are kept clean. In a controlled study of 200 head and neck incisions and traumatic lacerations, the investigators concluded that early washing (8 to 24 hours) after wound repair did not significantly alter wound healing or increase the potential for infection.[2] Wounds on other body sites can be gently cleansed 12 to 24 hours following suture repair without ill effect.[3]

Patients can begin to bathe 12 to 24 hours after wound repair. They can be allowed to bathe once a day, provided that the wound is not immersed and soaked in water. Dressings, unless instructed by the caregiver to be left intact, can be removed for cleansing. Showers are preferable to tub baths. Gentle soaping and rinsing are immediately followed by patting the wound dry with a soft towel. Application of an antibiotic ointment or reapplication of a dressing is recommended after each washing.

Signs of Wound Infection

Every patient has to be instructed in the signs of wound infection. Should any of these signs develop, the patient needs to return immediately for examination. The first sign of infection is usually excessive discomfort. The majority of minor wounds are only mildly uncomfortable. Early after repair, a small amount of bloody discharge can stain the dressing. Continued drainage, particularly if it is purulent appearing, is a sign of infection. Erythema from neovascularization and capillary dilatation accompanies most wounds. Redness that extends well beyond the wound margins (more than 5 mm) with accompanying swelling, induration, or tenderness does not occur in normal healing wounds. Lymphangitic streaks, local nodal enlargement, and fever are all signs of advanced infection.

Written Instructions

Finally, patients should be given specific written instructions reinforcing and detailing these general principles, as well as any other specifics for the given wound problem. Follow-up visits, dates, and times, have to be clearly written and understood by the patient and whenever possible, by accompanying family members. Fig. 20-2 provides an example of simple, yet effective, written wound care instructions.

UNDERSTANDING WOUND HEALING

Patients are most concerned about the size and appearance of the scar that will result from their laceration or wound. Because traumatic injuries occur randomly on the body surface, the final outcome, to a certain extent, is predetermined. It is the duty of the caregiver to advise the patient about the kind of scar he or she can expect. Candidly discussing various aspects of wound healing, such as the effects of wound mechanism, associated diseases, body region, and skin tension, allows the patient to better accept and cope with the healing process (see Chapter 3).

The appearance of a wound changes during the healing process, which often gives rise to patient concerns. It is important for patients to understand that, although stitches are removed within days of the injury and the wound appears to be sealed, tensile

Wound Care

You have been treated for a laceration. A laceration is a break in the skin that usually needs stitches or staples to close.

Treatment

On the first day, keep the wound clean and dry.

After the first day, you should look at the wound and clean it at least once a day. You can clean the wound with soap and water, and an ointment may be applied as directed by your doctor. The wound should be covered with a clean, dry bandage.

If you are given antibiotic medication, take the medication as prescribed, and take the medication until it is all gone.

Work limitations:
- ☐ Do not work until stitches or staples removed
- ☐ Light duty to protect the wound
- ☐ Full Duty
- ☐ Other_____

Return for stitches/staples removal on:_____

Notify Your Doctor Or Return To The Emergency Department If You Experience

Any signs of infection such as swelling, redness, drainage, increased pain, red streaks, or fever.

FIG. 20-2   Sample discharge instructions for patients with lacerations.

strength is very low. Reopening, or dehiscence, can occur if it is exposed to undue trauma. Wounds are often temperature- and touch-sensitive for weeks. Early scars appear red and raised, but eventual blanching and contraction eliminate those characteristics. People with dark skin have to be informed that scars may not regain lost pigmentation and might be lighter than the surrounding skin.

Finally, patients have to be counseled that scars mature and change in configuration for several months until they take on their final appearance. More often than not, an initially unsightly scar will likely become acceptable to the patient. However, a plastic surgeon can be consulted to assess for possible scar revision if concerns remain about the appearance of the scar.

REFERENCES

1. Crikelair CT: Skin suture marks, *Am J Surg* 96:631-632, 1958.
2. Goldberg HM, Rosenthal SAE, Nemetz JC: Effect of washing closed head and neck wounds on wound healing and infection, *Am J Surg* 141:358-359, 1981.
3. Noe JM, Keller M: Can stitches get wet? *Plast Reconstr Surg* 81:82-84,1988.

Index